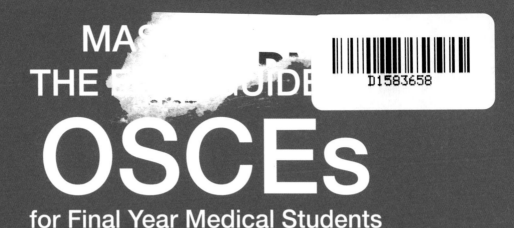

OSCEs

for Final Year Medical Students

NAZMUL AKUNJEE
MBBS MRCGP, London

MUHAMMED AKUNJEE
MBBS MRCGP (distinc) PgCert (Diabetes) PgCert (MedEd), London

Dr DOMINIC PIMENTA
MBBS, Core Medical Trainee at University College London Hospital

and

Miss DILSAN YILMAZ
MBBS MRCS, Academic Clinical Fellow in General Surgery based at The Royal London

Forewords by
NAZMUL and MUHAMMED AKUNJEE

and

EDWARD LAMUREN
Lead Consultant, A&E North Middlesex University Hospital;
Final Year Examiner, Royal Free and University College Medical Schools, London

Radcliffe Publishing London • New York

Radcliffe Publishing Ltd
St Mark's House,
Shepherdess Walk,
London N1 7BQ
United Kingdom

www.radcliffe-oxford.com
Electronic catalogue and worldwide online ordering facility.

The information provided in this textbook has been collated by the authors and has been checked against the most up to date and relevant hospital guidelines. Although great effort has been made to verify and check all aspects, the authors and publishers take no responsibility for any inaccuracies found within the book or for any medical advances which may affect any aspect of clinical practice. The authors also stress that the mock marks schemes in the book do not reflect on any university, medical school or other related official bodies involved in OSCE examination. They have been included to aid student OSCE revision and are subject to the authors' own discretion. The authors are in no way responsible for the candidate's performance in the examinations based upon the mark sheets or information contained in this work.

British Library Cataloguing in Publication Data

A catalogue record for this book is available from the British Library.

ISBN-10: 1 91022 708 0
ISBN-13: 978 191022 708 4

Typeset by codeMantra, India
Manufacturing managed by 21six

CONTENTS

PREFACE   vii
FOREWORD   ix
MARKING SCHEMES   xi

HISTORY TAKING   1

CHAPTER 1.1   General medical history   2
CHAPTER 1.2   Rheumatological history   5
CHAPTER 1.3   Chest pain   8
CHAPTER 1.4   Breathlessness   12
CHAPTER 1.5   Loss of consciousness   16
CHAPTER 1.6   Headaches   20
CHAPTER 1.7   General surgical history   24
CHAPTER 1.8   Urological history   27
CHAPTER 1.9   Abdominal pain   31
CHAPTER 1.10   Breast lump   35

EXAMINATIONS   39

CHAPTER 2.1   Cardiovascular   40
CHAPTER 2.2   Respiratory   48
CHAPTER 2.3   Abdomen   52
CHAPTER 2.4   Cranial nerve examination   61
CHAPTER 2.5   Upper limb neurological exam   68
CHAPTER 2.6   Lower limb neurological examination   74
CHAPTER 2.7   Cerebellar exam   81
CHAPTER 2.8   Speech   84
CHAPTER 2.9   Eye   87
CHAPTER 2.10   Ear   94
CHAPTER 2.11   Nose   98
CHAPTER 2.12   Arterial circulation   101
CHAPTER 2.13   Venous circulation   105
CHAPTER 2.14   Ulcers   109
CHAPTER 2.15   Neck lump   113
CHAPTER 2.16   Lymphatic system examination   116
CHAPTER 2.17   Thyroid   121
CHAPTER 2.18   Breast   124
CHAPTER 2.19   Rectal   129
CHAPTER 2.20   Inguinal scrotal   132
CHAPTER 2.21   Gals (gait, arms, legs, spine screen)   137

CONTENTS

CLINICAL SKILLS 141

CHAPTER 3.1   Hand washing   142
CHAPTER 3.2   Venepuncture   144
CHAPTER 3.3   Cannulation   146
CHAPTER 3.4   IV infusion   148
CHAPTER 3.5   Blood transfusion   150
CHAPTER 3.6   Intravenous injection   153
CHAPTER 3.7   Intramuscular injection   155
CHAPTER 3.8   Male catheterisation   158
CHAPTER 3.9   Nasogastric intubation   161
CHAPTER 3.10   Surgical gown and scrub   164
CHAPTER 3.11   Taking blood cultures   166
CHAPTER 3.12   Taking a blood pressure   169
CHAPTER 3.13   Blood glucose   171
CHAPTER 3.14   Urine dipstick   173
CHAPTER 3.15   Basic life support   176
CHAPTER 3.16   Oxygen therapy   179
CHAPTER 3.17   Setting up a nebuliser   182
CHAPTER 3.18   Arterial blood sampling   184
CHAPTER 3.19   Ankle brachial pressure index (using a doppler)   186
CHAPTER 3.20   Confirmation of death   189
CHAPTER 3.21   Recording an ECG   191

MANAGEMENT OF THE ACUTELY UNWELL PATIENT 193

CHAPTER 4.1   General schemata   194
CHAPTER 4.2   Palpitations   198
CHAPTER 4.3   Pulmonary embolism   202
CHAPTER 4.4   Sepsis   206
CHAPTER 4.5   Hypoglycaemia   210
CHAPTER 4.6   DKA   214
CHAPTER 4.7   Upper GI bleed   218

PRESCRIBING 223

CHAPTER 5.1   General tips   224
CHAPTER 5.2   GI bleed   227
CHAPTER 5.3   Acute asthma attack   232
CHAPTER 5.4   COPD exacerbation   234
CHAPTER 5.5   Acute coronary syndrome   236
CHAPTER 5.6   Acute left ventricular failure   238
CHAPTER 5.7   Hyperkalaemia   240

COMMUNICATION SKILLS 245

CHAPTER 6.1	HIV test counselling	246
CHAPTER 6.2	Peak flow	249
CHAPTER 6.3	CT head scan	251
CHAPTER 6.4	MRI scan	253
CHAPTER 6.5	OGD endoscopy	255
CHAPTER 6.6	Barium enema	257
CHAPTER 6.7	Transurethral resection of prostate	259
CHAPTER 6.8	Hernia repair	262
CHAPTER 6.9	Laparoscopic cholecystectomy	264
CHAPTER 6.10	Inhaler technique	267
CHAPTER 6.11	Spacer device	269
CHAPTER 6.12	GTN spray	271
CHAPTER 6.13	Instilling eye drops	273
CHAPTER 6.14	Blood pressure management	275
CHAPTER 6.15	Diabetic management	279
CHAPTER 6.16	Warfarin therapy	282
CHAPTER 6.17	Steroid therapy	285
CHAPTER 6.18	Epileptic starting a family	288
CHAPTER 6.19	Breaking bad news	291
CHAPTER 6.20	Angry patient	293
CHAPTER 6.21	Negotiation	295
CHAPTER 6.22	Interprofessional	297
CHAPTER 6.23	Cross cultural	299
CHAPTER 6.24	Radiology request	302
CHAPTER 6.25	Blood request	304
CHAPTER 6.26	Microbiology request form	307
CHAPTER 6.27	Death certification	309

DATA INTERPRETATION 311

CHAPTER 7.1	Chest radiograph	312
CHAPTER 7.2	Abdominal radiograph	318
CHAPTER 7.3	Interpreting the ECG	322
CHAPTER 7.4	Interpreting the ABG	329

EVIDENCE APPRAISAL 331

CHAPTER 8.1	How to approach an abstract	332
CHAPTER 8.2	Explaining an article to a patient	336

INDEX 339

PREFACE

Dear Reader,

Thank you for purchasing the expanded and fully revised edition of The Easy Guide to OSCEs for Final Year Medical Students. We have worked hard to embody the principle of the editing authors, Nazmul and Muhammed Akunjee, to create a single resource, with all the material a finals student could ever require to pass and excel, in their OSCE exam.

The OSCE is the time to test your ability to behave and act like a doctor, you will find it is a culmination of all your knowledge, written and practical, and a third component, your evolving professional personality that will be the seed that your career as a doctor will grow from.

For those of you just beginning your clinical training this book will be an entry point to examining and gaining practical experience. For those of you approaching finals, you already have all the knowledge you will ever need in your head. The secret to the exam, OSCE and written, is structure. By the end of the revision period you should be able to examine any part of the body, from top-to-toe, in a sensible, thorough manner without thinking about it. This book emphasises the structure that you need to learn as much as the individual steps, so that, as will be inevitable, when you find yourself presented with a situation you haven't prepared for, you will find that you have.

For those of you in between, keep going, and enjoy yourself! Medical school will be over far sooner than you'd think, or would like. Finally, when you get in to the OSCE, remember finals is the time to transition into the doctor you want to be. So, stand up straight, stethoscope behind your back, and begin.

Good luck for your exams,

Dr Dominic Pimenta MBBS, Core Medical Trainee, London
Miss Dilsan Yilmaz MBBS MRCS, Academic Clinical Fellow in General Surgery, London

FOREWORD

Despite being run for many years, the OSCE examinations still cause dread and panic in most medical students. The fear of being 'outed' as an incompetent diagnostician in front of your teachers or professors can even cause the most seasoned student to suffer a prolonged bout of palpitations. For this reason the concept of the 'Easy Guide to OSCE' series was conceived. Now running into its 8th year, the books have proved successful (locally and internationally) in guiding and ushering thousands of final year medical students into the world of being a junior doctor.

Although the core medical student curriculum has not changed greatly, the structure and make-up of OSCEs has undergone some advancement. To keep up with the times, we have recruited two budding young, newly qualified doctors to help refresh and update some of the material contained within this book.

The core of the book is essentially the same and we aim to still try and cover the vast bulk of the curriculum such that you should not need to purchase any other texts. In response to medical student feedback, we have kept the layout the same, so that in your practice groups you can still assess one another on how well you have performed. We have included more advice around how to present findings to the examiner, and introduced follow-up questions that some medical schools are employing in a PACEs / VIVA style assessment. We have added new sections and new style OSCE cases that are increasingly being used.

Having both sat and passed OSCE examinations as medical students, and now crossed over to the other side as OSCE examiners for 2 leading london medical schools, we feel more than ever that this book should be your OSCE companion to help you excel in your examinations!

Dr Muhammed & Dr Nazmul Akunjee
GP Partners, GP Appraisers
Former OSCE Examiners for UCL & Imperial Medical Schools
January 2015

The medical school curriculum has undergone much change in recent times, most notably with the introduction of an OSCE-style assessment. Although clinical examinations in the form of OSCEs have been present in the UK for the past 20 years, only in recent times have medical schools streamlined their courses fully incorporating the Objective Structured Clinical Examinations. Most medical schools now place a huge emphasis on the clinical OSCE stations as a way of assessing the clinical competency of future doctors.

This final year OSCE book has been devised to present the OSCEs in a way that gives the reader a simple and comprehensive system by which they should approach each station. The book is refreshing in its style with easily understood procedural explanation, a concise and highly relevant mark scheme which takes a similar format to those used by examiners and a broad range of covered topics which are routinely tested in the OSCEs. All clinical knowledge has been thoroughly researched and is in line with current evidence and guidelines. This is an excellent book that will reward all those who study and apply it in the all-important finals!

Mr Edward Lamuren
Lead Consultant, Accident & Emergency
North Middlesex University Hospital
Final Year Examiner (RF&UC Medical Schools)
January 2007

MARKING SCHEMES

For each OSCE station we have defined a set of criteria which can be used when assessing one's self under examination conditions. The figures of 0, 1 and 2 indicate how many marks have been allocated for performing the defined task. Some criteria have been allocated 2 marks and this indicates that more than one task must be accomplished in those criteria to attain the full marks. If only one task is completed then a score of 1 will be attained. A score of 0 is given if the task was omitted completely.

Some OSCE criteria have no marks allocated and this is to reflect that this is not a core competency skill, but inclusion of the task illustrates flair and higher achievement.

At the end of each OSCE station are five-point scores, one indicating the examiner's mark for overall ability and a second five-point scale (in stations where role players are used) for the role-player's overall assessment. 0 indicates extremely poor performance, with the candidate not fulfilling any of the OSCE criteria, poor communication skills and inconsideration for the role player's feelings. 3 indicates a fair performance, fulfilling most of the OSCE criteria and 5 an exceptional candidate who fulfilled the OSCE criteria, performing the tasks slickly and with confidence.

section 01

HISTORY
TAKING

01.1 GENERAL MEDICAL HISTORY

INSTRUCTIONS You are a foundation year House Officer in Accident & Emergency. Please elicit a full history relevant to this patient's complaints. You will have 10 minutes to complete this.

STAGE	KEY POINTS AND ACTIONS	SCORE		
	INTRODUCTION			
Introduction	Introduce yourself and establish rapport.	0	1	–
Name & Age	Elicit patient's name and age.	0	1	–
Occupation	Enquire about patient's present occupation.	0	1	–
	THE HISTORY			
Complaint	Elicit all of the patient's presenting complaints. Begin with an open question. What has brought you to hospital today?	0	1	2
History	For any symptom delineate the timing: When did it first start? What did you first notice? Is it getting better or worse? Have you ever had it before?			
Pain	For any history of pain ask the following: Where is the pain? When does it start? Does the pain move anywhere? What does the pain feel like? How severe is the pain? What makes it worse? What makes it better? Are there any other symptoms?	0	1	2
SOB	For any history of shortness of breath ask the following: When did your difficulty in breathing start? Is it there all the time? Does it come and go? What makes it worse? What makes it better? How many pillows do you sleep on? How far can you normally walk? How far can you walk now? Do you have a cough? Do you have any phlegm?	0	1	2
Concerns	Do you have any particular concerns or worries about the symptoms you are experiencing? Do you know what may be causing them?	0	1	–
Impact	How have these symptoms affected your life? And your family?	0	1	–
	ASSOCIATED HISTORY			
Medical History	Do you suffer from any medical illnesses?	0	1	–

STAGE	KEY POINTS AND ACTIONS	SCORE
	Do you have any of the following [Mnemonic—MJTHREADS]:	

Myocardial infarction
Jaundice
Tuberculosis
Hypertension/high cholesterol
Rheumatic fever
Epilepsy
Asthma/angina
Diabetes
Stroke

Have you ever been admitted to hospital?

Drug History Are you on any medications? Are you taking any over-the-counter preparations? Do you have any drug allergies? 0 1 –

Family History Has anyone in your family had similar troubles? Are there any inherited family disorders? Does anyone have diabetes or heart disease? 0 1 –

Social History [Mnemonic—HOSE PIPERS] 0 1 2

Home - Do you live in a house or flat? Does anyone else live with you? Do you have stairs at home? Is the condition of the flat good—boiler, paint, mould, etc.?
Occupation - What do you do for a living? Where is your work? Ask about exposures—inhaled gases, dust or metals, animal or travel exposures.
Smoking - Do you smoke? How many a day and for how long?
Ethanol - Do you drink alcohol? How many units a week do you drink? If > 21 units a day for a man or > 14 units for a woman ask about alcohol dependency—morning drinking, withdrawal symptoms, negative social or financial impact of drinking.

Pysch - Ask about mood and sleeping.
Independence - How are you coping at home? How do you mobilize? Ask about frames, sticks, scooters, etc. Can you look after yourself without help with dressing, washing, or feeding? Do you have carers? How many times a day? What do they do for you? Do you need more help?
Pets - Do you have any pets at home?
Expeditions/**E**xcursions - Have you been out of the country in the last six months? Have you ever visited Africa, Asia, or South America? Any freshwater swimming? Malaria areas? Insect or tick bites? Unwell contacts? Diarrhoea or fevers?
Recreational Drugs* - Do you use any recreational drugs?
Sexual History* - If relevant or appropriate, include menstrual history here for women if not already asked about. Sensitively ask about number of partners, protected or unprotected sex, and HIV risk factors—bisexual partners, known HIV contacts, partners from Asia or Sub-Saharan Africa, intravenous drug users, and sex workers.

*Preface these last two questions with some signposting. 'I'm going to ask you some questions some people find sensitive, but are important to the symptoms you have described' or 'Because the symptoms you are describing could suggest a sexually transmitted illness, I would like to ask more about that if that is okay'.

System Review A review of systems is a vital part of history taking and it is worthwhile practicing getting through all the systems in a coherent and logical manner. In very short stations it may not be possible to get through all of this but it is essential to ask about other symptoms related to the presenting complaint. If you do get a yes to any of the questions it is vital to further define the problem as you would a presenting symptom. 0 1 2

STAGE	KEY POINTS AND ACTIONS	SCORE

'I am now going to run through a list of quick questions to make sure I haven't missed anything....'

System	Symptoms
Constitutional	Weight loss, night sweats, malaise, itching, rashes, lumps, and bumps
Cardiovascular	Chest pain, orthopnoea, PND, palpitations, leg swelling
Respiratory	SOB, cough, sputum production, haemoptysis, pleuritic chest pain
Neurological	Headache, fits, faints, funny turns, hearing loss, sight disturbance, numbness, pins and needles, weakness, behavioural change
Gastrointestinal	Appetite, swallowing difficulty, vomiting, indigestion, abdominal pain, jaundice, change in bowel habit, malaena or fresh blood in the stool, tenesmus
Endocrine	Menstrual history in female, fertility problems, hair loss, heat/cold intolerance
Genitourinary	Urinary frequency, dysuria, haematuria, offensive or cloudy urine
Musculoskeletal	Joint/muscle/bone pain

COMMUNICATION SKILLS

Rapport	Establish and maintain rapport and demonstrate listening skills.	0 1 –
Responds	React positively to and acknowledge patient's emotions.	0 1 –
Fluency	General fluency and non-use of jargon.	0 1 –
Summarise	Check with patient and deliver an appropriate summary.	0 1 –

EXAMINER'S EVALUATION

Overall assessment of taking general medical history	0 1 2 3 4 5
Role player's score	0 1 2 3 4 5
Total mark out of 32	

01.2 RHEUMATOLOGICAL HISTORY

INSTRUCTIONS You are a foundation year House Officer in Rheumatology. Please elicit a full history relevant to this patient's complaints. You will have seven minutes to complete this.

STAGE	KEY POINTS AND ACTIONS	SCORE
	INTRODUCTION	
Introduction	Introduce yourself and establish rapport.	0 1 –
Name & Age	Elicit patient's name and age.	0 1 –
Occupation	Enquire about patient's present occupation.	0 1 –
	THE HISTORY	
Complaint	Elicit all of the patient's presenting complaints.	0 1 2
History	When did it first start? What did you first notice? Is it getting better or worse? Have you ever had it before? Have you had any recent trauma or infection?	
Pain	Where is the pain? When does it start? Did it start suddenly or gradually? Does the pain move anywhere? What does the pain feel like? How severe is the pain? What makes it worse? Is the pain worse after activity? What makes it better? Is the pain better on resting? Are there any other symptoms?	0 1 2
Stiffness	When do you notice stiffness in your joints? Did it start suddenly or gradually? Is it there all the time? Does it come and go? What makes it worse? What makes it better? Is it worse first thing in the morning or later on in the day? Do you find difficulty starting an action or maintaining an action?	0 1 2
Swelling	When did you notice swelling of the joints? Is it there all the time? Does it come and go? What makes it worse? What makes it better?	0 1 –
Distribution	Is only one joint (monoarticular), less than four joints (oligoarticular), or five or more joints (polyarticular) affected with the above symptoms? Are the problems on one side only (asymmetrical distribution) or on both sides (symmetrical)?	
Concerns	Do you have any particular concerns or worries about the symptoms you are experiencing? Do you know what may be causing them?	0 1 –
Impact	How have these symptoms affected your life? And your family?	0 1 –
Function	Are you able to dress yourself? Can you comb your hair? Are you able to feed yourself or hold a knife and spoon? Are you able to cook for yourself? Are you able to walk up the stairs? Are you able to work?	0 1 –

STAGE	KEY POINTS AND ACTIONS	SCORE

ASSOCIATED HISTORY

Medical History   Do you suffer from any medical illnesses?   0   1   2

Do you have any of the following [Mnemonic—GROSS]:
Gout
Rheumatoid arthritis
Osteoarthritis
SLE
Sarcoidosis

Do you have any of the following [Mnemonic—MJTHREADS]:
Myocardial infarction
Jaundice
Tuberculosis
Hypertension/high cholesterol
Rheumatic fever
Epilepsy
Asthma/angina
Diabetes
Stroke

Social History   **[Mnemonic—HOSE PIPERS]**   0   1   2
Home - Do you live in a house or flat? Does anyone else live with you? Do you have
stairs at home? Is the condition of the flat good—boiler, paint, mould, etc.?
Occupation - What do you do for a living? Where is your work? Ask about
exposures—inhaled gases, dust or metals, animal or travel exposures.
Smoking - Do you smoke? How many a day and for how long?
Ethanol - Do you drink alcohol? How many units a week do you drink? If > 21 units
a day for a man or > 14 units for a woman ask about alcohol dependency—morning
drinking, withdrawal symptoms, negative social or financial impact of drinking.

Pysch - Ask about mood and sleeping.
Independence - How are you coping at home? How do you mobilize? Ask about
frames, sticks, scooters, etc. Can you look after yourself without help with dressing,
washing, or feeding? Do you have carers? How many times a day? What do they do
for you? Do you need more help?
Pets - Do you have any pets at home?
Expeditions/Excursions - Have you been out of the country in the last six months?
Have you ever visited Africa, Asia, or South America? Any freshwater swimming?
Malaria areas? Insect or tick bites? Unwell contacts? Diarrhoea or fevers?
Recreational Drugs* - Do you use any recreational drugs?
Sexual History* - If relevant or appropriate, include menstrual history here for women
if not already asked about. Sensitively ask about number of partners, protected
or unprotected sex, and HIV risk factors—bisexual partners, known HIV contacts,
partners from Asia or Sub-Saharan Africa, intravenous drug users and sex workers.
In a rheumatological history ask specifically about pregnancies and miscarriages
and recent sexually transmitted infectious disease symptoms (important in reactive
arthritis).

*Preface these last two questions with some signposting. 'I'm going to ask you some
questions some people find sensitive, but are important to the symptoms you have
described' or 'Because the symptoms you are describing could suggest a sexually
transmitted illness, I would like to ask more about that if that is okay'.

STAGE	KEY POINTS AND ACTIONS	SCORE
System Review	Have you ever been admitted to hospital?	
Drug History	Are you on any medications? Are you taking diuretics (gout) or hydralazine (SLE-like symptoms)? Are you taking any over-the-counter preparations? Do you have any drug allergies?	0 1 –
Family History	Has anyone in your family had similar troubles? Are there any inherited family disorders? Do any of your family members suffer from psoriasis?	0 1 –
Extra-articular	Have you noticed your fingers change colour and go white in the cold (Raynaud's)? Have you had dry eyes (Sjögren's)? Or have your eyes gone red (keratoconjunctiva sicca, episcleritis, or scleritis—Sjögrens, RA, sarcoid)? Have you noticed any bloody diarrhoea (IBD)? Have you noticed any urethral discharge (Reiter's)? Have you noticed any rash, hair loss, or photosensitivity (SLE)?	0 1 2

COMMUNICATION SKILLS

STAGE	KEY POINTS AND ACTIONS	SCORE
Rapport	Establish and maintain rapport and demonstrate listening skills.	0 1 –
Responds	React positively to and acknowledge patient's emotions.	0 1 –
Fluency	General fluency and non-use of jargon.	0 1 –
Summarise	Check with patient and deliver an appropriate summary.	0 1 –

EXAMINER'S EVALUATION

Overall assessment of taking rheumatological history	0 1 2 3 4 5
Role player's score	0 1 2 3 4 5
Total mark out of 35	

01.3
CHEST PAIN

INSTRUCTIONS You are a foundation year House Officer in General Medicine. Mr Charles has presented with chest pain. Please take a brief history of his symptoms and establish a differential diagnosis.

STAGE	KEY POINTS AND ACTIONS	SCORE
	INTRODUCTION	
Introduction	Introduce yourself and establish rapport.	0 1 –
Name & Age	Elicit patient's name and age.	0 1 –
Occupation	Enquire about patient's present occupation.	0 1 –
	THE HISTORY	
Chest Pain	Ask patient all relevant questions regarding chest pain including site, onset, character, radiation, etc. [Mnemonic—SOCRATES]	
Site	Where exactly is the pain? Can you please point to it?	0 1 –
Onset	When did you first notice the pain? When did it first start?	0 1 –
Character	Can you describe how the pain feels? Is it sharp or dull? Does it feel like a pressure? Do you feel a burning sensation?	0 1 –
Radiation	Does the pain move anywhere? Does it go to your arms, jaw, or back?	0 1 –
Associated Symptoms	Have you noticed anything else with the pain such as difficulty in breathing? Palpitations or dizziness? Coughing? Are you bringing up any blood? Have you felt sick or actually vomited?	0 1 –
Timing	How long does the pain last? Have you ever had this pain before?	
Exacerbating and Relieving Factors	Does anything make the pain worse, such as exercising, taking a deep breath in, moving, coughing, eating a heavy meal, or the cold weather? Does anything make the pain better? For example, resting or taking GTN?	
Severity	On a scale of 1 to 10, one being the least pain and ten the worst pain you could ever imagine, how severe is the pain?	0 1 –

STAGE	KEY POINTS AND ACTIONS	SCORE
Risk Factors	Elicit relevant risk factors such as diabetes, smoking, previous hypertension, cholesterol, family history of cardiac problems (IHD), or recent travel, trauma or surgery (PE).	0 1 2
Concerns	Do you have any particular concerns or worries about the symptoms you are experiencing? Do you know what may be causing them?	0 1 –
Impact	How have these symptoms affected your life? And your family?	0 1 –

ASSOCIATED HISTORY

Medical History	Do you suffer from any medical illnesses?	0 1 –

Do you have any of the following [Mnemonic—MJTHREADS]:
Myocardial infarction
Jaundice
Tuberculosis
Hypertension/high cholesterol
Rheumatic fever
Epilepsy
Asthma/angina
Diabetes
Stroke

Have you ever been admitted to hospital? Any previous DVTs or PEs?

Drug History	Are you on any medications? Are you taking any over-the-counter preparations? Do you have any drug allergies?	0 1 –
Family History	Has anyone in your family had similar troubles? Are there any inherited family disorders? Does anyone have diabetes or heart disease?	0 1 –
Social History	[Mnemonic—HOSE PIPERS]	0 1 2

Home - Do you live in a house or flat? Does anyone else live with you? Do you have stairs at home? Is the condition of the flat good—boiler, paint, mould, etc.?
Occupation - What do you do for a living? Where is your work? Ask about exposures—inhaled gases, dust or metals, animal or travel exposures.
Smoking - Do you smoke? How many a day and for how long?
Ethanol - Do you drink alcohol? How many units a week do you drink? If > 21 units a day for a man or > 14 units for a woman ask about alcohol dependency—morning drinking, withdrawal symptoms, negative social or financial impact of drinking.

Pysch - Ask about mood and sleeping.
Independence - How are you coping at home? How do you mobilize? Ask about frames, sticks, scooters, etc. Can you look after yourself without help with dressing, washing, or feeding? Do you have carers? How many times a day? What do they do for you? Do you need more help?
Pets - Do you have any pets at home?
Expeditions/Excursions - Have you been out of the country in the last six months? Have you ever visited Africa, Asia, or South America? Any freshwater swimming? Malaria areas? Insect or tick bites? Unwell contacts? Diarrhoea or fevers? Any long-haul flights?
Recreational Drugs* - Do you use any recreational drugs?
Sexual History* - If relevant or appropriate, include menstrual history here for women if not already asked about.

*Preface these last two questions with some signposting. 'I'm going to ask you some questions some people find sensitive, but are important to the symptoms you have described' or 'Because the symptoms you are describing could suggest a sexually transmitted illness, I would like to ask more about that if that is okay'.

STAGE	KEY POINTS AND ACTIONS	SCORE
System Review	Run through the systems starting with the most relevant.	

COMMUNICATION SKILLS

STAGE	KEY POINTS AND ACTIONS	SCORE
Rapport	Establish and maintain rapport and demonstrate listening skills.	0 1 –
Responds	React positively to and acknowledge patient's emotions.	0 1 –
Fluency	General fluency and non-use of jargon.	0 1 –
Summarise	Check with patient and deliver an appropriate summary.	0 1 –

EXAMINER'S EVALUATION

Overall assessment of taking chest pain history		0 1 2 3 4 5
Role player's score		0 1 2 3 4 5
Total mark out of 32		

CHEST PAIN: DIFFERENTIAL DIAGNOSIS

Differential Diagnosis	Supporting Features	Risk Factors
Ischaemic Heart Disease: Includes: angina and ACS (unstable angina, NSTEMI, and STEMI)	Crushing in nature Pressure located over left chest Radiation to left arm or jaw May be alleviated by GTN spray **Stable angina:** pain induced by exercise, a large meal, or cold weather. Eventually abates on resting **ACS:** Pain comes on at rest and is associated with nausea/vomiting, sweating, and breathlessness	Strong family history of ischaemic heart disease Hypercholesterolaemia, hypertension Smoking Male gender Diabetes Obesity Raised stress levels Lack of regular exercise Cocaine use
Pericarditis: Inflammation of the pericardium Causes include: infection (Viral/TB), autoimmune processes, uraemia, metastatic disease, or as a complication of MI	Retrosternal chest pain May radiate to jaw, back, or left side of chest Pain worsened on deep inspiration and lying flat Improves when patient sitting up and leaning forward	Recent viral illness Rheumatological conditions (Churg-Strauss, SLE) Malignancy Recent MI (Dressler's syndrome)
Pulmonary Embolus: Blood clot embolised to the pulmonary vasculature Usually secondary to deep vein thrombosis	Sudden onset Sharp stabbing chest pain Pleuritic in nature (worsens on inspiration) Haemoptysis Palpitations (tachycardia) Breathlessness	Prolonged bed rest or immobility Oral contraceptive use Recent surgery (especially for lower limbs) Pregnancy/childbirth Cancer Chronic inflammatory conditions Thrombophilia (Factor V Leiden, anti-phospholipid syndrome)
Musculoskeletal Pain: Extremely common Origin of pain may be from: 1. muscle (myalgia) 2. bone (fractured rib) 3. cartilage (costochondritis)	Pain reproducible on certain movements and palpation History of trauma	Recent cough, cold, or muscle trauma Middle-aged women (Tietze's syndrome)
Aortic Dissection: A tear in the intimal wall of the aorta leading to blood tracking between layers of the vessel wall. Commonly occurring in the thoracic region	Sudden severe retrosternal chest pain Tearing in character Radiation to back / between shoulder blades Signs on examination: A difference of > 20mmHg between right and left brachial artery blood pressures Pericardial effusion (if aortic root involvement) Oliguria (if extending to renal arteries) Bilateral leg weakness (if involving the spinal artery of Adamkiewicz)	Uncontrolled high blood pressure Cocaine use Trauma Collagen disorders (Ehlers-Danlos/Marfan's) Bicuspid aortic valve

EXEMPLAR PRESENTATION

'This is Mr Charles, a 60-year-old landscape gardener with a background of angina, previous triple bypass this year, hypertension, type II diabetes, and hypercholesteraemia who has presented with central chest pain at rest. The pain started this morning, lasting for thirty minutes before he called an ambulance. The pain is dull and radiates to the left arm. The pain is partially relieved by GTN spray and unchanged with respiration or posture. He describes the pain as similar to his angina and is concerned that he is having another MI. He was admitted in May 04 when he suffered his first heart attack and had a three-vessel coronary artery bypass graft earlier this year. He is a smoker of 20 cigarettes a day and a social drinker. He suffers from hypertension, non-insulin dependent diabetes, stable angina, and hypercholesterolaemia; taking aspirin 75mg, metformin 500mg tds, gliclazide 40mg, bendroflumethiazide 2.5mg OD, ISMN M/R 30mg OD, and simvastatin 20mg at night. He denies any drug allergies. He has a strong family history of ischaemic heart disease, with his elder brother and father dying prematurely of heart attacks aged 50 and 45, respectively. He lives in a ground floor flat with his incapacitated wife, for whom he is the main carer. He has no children and is concerned about who will care for his wife if he is admitted to hospital.

The findings from the history are most consistent with an acute coronary syndrome and I would wish to exclude an acute myocardial infarction'. ■

01.4
BREATHLESSNESS

INSTRUCTIONS You are a foundation year House Officer in Accident & Emergency. Mr Brians, a former coal miner, has presented with difficulty in breathing. Please take a brief history of his symptoms and establish a differential diagnosis.

STAGE	KEY POINTS AND ACTIONS	SCORE		
	INTRODUCTION			
Introduction	Introduce yourself and establish rapport.	0	1	–
Name & Age	Elicit patient's name and age.	0	1	–
Occupation	Enquire about patient's present occupation.	0	1	–
	THE HISTORY			
Dyspnoea	Ask patient all relevant questions regarding shortness of breath including the following: [Mnemonic—ONE RESPS]			
Onset	When did you first notice your problem? When did it first start?	0	1	–
Nature	Is it present all the time? Or does it come and go?			
Exercise	How far can you walk before you feel breathless? How are you with stairs? How far could you walk before all of this started?	0	1	–
Relieving	What makes the breathlessness better? Resting? Inhalers?	0	1	–
Exacerbating	Is there anything that makes it worse, such as lying down (orthopnoea) or walking? Or is there anything that brings it on (allergen)?	0	1	–
Sleep	Is the breathlessness worse when you go to sleep? Does it ever wake you in the middle of the night (paroxysmal nocturnal dyspnoea)? How many times?	0	1	–
Pillows	How many pillows do you sleep on at night? Has this increased recently?	0	1	–
Symptoms	Have you noticed anything else such as cough, fevers, chest pain, wheezing, palpitations, dizziness? Have you noticed your ankles swell?	0	1	2

STAGE	KEY POINTS AND ACTIONS	SCORE
Concerns	Do you have any particular concerns or worries about the symptoms you are experiencing? Do you know what may be causing them?	0 1 –
Impact	How have these symptoms affected your life? And your family?	0 1 –

ASSOCIATED HISTORY

	Do you have any of the following [Mnemonic—MJTHREADS]: **M**yocardial infarction **J**aundice **T**uberculosis **H**ypertension/high cholesterol **R**heumatic fever **E**pilepsy **A**sthma/angina **D**iabetes **S**troke	0 1 –
	Have you ever had a PE or DVT?	
	Have you ever been admitted to hospital?	
Drug History	Are you on any medications? Are you taking any over-the-counter preparations? Do you have any allergies (drug or others)?	0 1 –
Family History	Has anyone in your family had similar troubles? Are there any inherited family disorders? Does anyone have emphysema or cystic fibrosis?	0 1 –
Social History	[Mnemonic—HOSE PIPERS] **H**ome - Do you live in a house or flat? Does anyone else live with you? Do you have stairs at home? Is the condition of the flat good—boiler, paint, mould, etc.? **O**ccupation - What do you do for a living? Where is your work? Ask about exposures—inhaled gases, dust or metals, animal or travel exposures. Ask specifically about asbestos exposure. **S**moking - Do you smoke? How many a day and for how long? **E**thanol - Do you drink alcohol? How many units a week do you drink? If > 21 units a day for a man or > 14 units for a woman ask about alcohol dependency—morning drinking, withdrawal symptoms, negative social or financial impact of drinking. **P**ysch - Ask about mood and sleeping. **I**ndependence - How are you coping at home? How do you mobilize? Ask about frames, sticks, scooters, etc. Can you look after yourself without help with dressing, washing, or feeding? Do you have carers? How many times a day? What do they do for you? Do you need more help? **P**ets - Do you have any pets at home? **E**xpeditions/**E**xcursions - Have you been out of the country in the last six months? Have you ever visited Africa, Asia, or South America? Any freshwater swimming? Malaria areas? Insect or tick bites? Unwell contacts? Diarrhoea or fevers? Any long haul flights? **R**ecreational Drugs* - Do you use any recreational drugs? **S**exual History* - If relevant or appropriate, include menstrual history here for women if not already asked about. *Preface these last two questions with some signposting. 'I'm going to ask you some questions some people find sensitive, but are important to the symptoms you have described' or 'Because the symptoms you are describing could suggest a sexually transmitted illness, I would like to ask more about that if that is okay'.	0 1 2
System Review	Run through the systems starting with the most relevant.	

STAGE	KEY POINTS AND ACTIONS	SCORE

Differential of Shortness of Breath [Mnemonic—AAAA PPPP]

Airway Obstruction	**P**neumonia
Angina Pectoris	**P**neumothorax
Anxiety	**P**ulmonary Oedema
Asthma	**P**ulmonary Embolus

COMMUNICATION SKILLS

Stage	Action	Score
Rapport	Establish and maintain rapport and demonstrate listening skills.	0 1 –
Responds	React positively to and acknowledge patient's emotions.	0 1 –
Fluency	General fluency and non-use of jargon.	0 1 –
Summarise	Check with patient and deliver an appropriate summary.	0 1 –

EXAMINER'S EVALUATION

	Score
Overall assessment of taking shortness of breath history	0 1 2 3 4 5
Role player's score	0 1 2 3 4 5
Total mark out of 32	

SOB: DIFFERENTIAL DIAGNOSIS

Differential Diagnosis	Supporting Features	Risk Factors
Asthma: Chronic respiratory disease characterised by hypersensitivity and reversible reduction in outflow (bronchospasm).	Breathlessness Chest tightness Wheezing Coughing (worse at night)	Family history of asthma Personal history of atopy (eczema or allergic rhinitis) An obvious allergen precipitating attacks such as pets, pollen, or foodstuffs
Chronic Obstructive Pulmonary Disease: - Chronic lung diseases including emphysema and chronic bronchitis. - The main cause of COPD is cigarette smoking (both active and passive).	Breathlessness Coughing with sputum production on most days for > 3 months Recurrent chest infections	Significant smoking history Family history of early COPD and liver disease (alpha-1-antitrypsin deficiency)
Bronchial Carcinoma: - The single most important causal factor for lung cancer is cigarette smoking (implicated in 90% of male lung cancers).	Cough Haemoptysis Dyspnoea Weight loss / Anorexia Lethargy Metastatic symptoms depend on site of infiltration and may include: - Horner's syndrome - Hoarseness of voice - Chest pain - Dysphagia	Smoking history Exposure to asbestos Family history Ionising radiation Coal miners
Pulmonary Oedema: - The accumulation of fluid in the lungs - Cardiac causes include heart failure (left ventricular failure), cardiac arrhythmias and myocardial infarction. - Non-cardiogenic causes include kidney failure, trauma (pulmonary contusion), and neurogenic (CVA/SAH).	Symptoms of pulmonary oedema from heart failure comprise: Breathlessness Orthopnoea Paroxysmal nocturnal dyspnoea Bipedal oedema Coughing Production of white/pink frothy phlegm Lethargy	Risk factors depend on cause of pulmonary oedema. As heart failure is a common cause enquire about cardiovascular risk factors and previous or recent MI.
Pneumonia: - Infection of the lung parenchyma - Broadly divided into community and hospital acquired depending on the source and causal organisms	Breathlessness developing over hours to days Fever Rigors Cough Pleuritic chest pain Haemoptysis Green/yellow sputum production (or rusty coloured in pneumococcal pneumonia)	Travel to endemic places Low immunity Infectious contacts

EXEMPLAR PRESENTATION

'This is Mr Brians, a 67-year-old former coal miner with a background of smoking who has presented with acute onset shortness of breath. The dyspnoea started a week ago, is present all the time, and is progressively getting worse. The dyspnoea is worse on lying flat and on exertion, and relieved by sitting up and resting. Previously, Mr Brians was able to walk 250 metres, but now is struggling to walk 4-6 metres. He is also having difficulty walking up stairs. He reports waking three or four times a night with coughing despite increasing the number of pillows from two to four over the past week. He denies any chest pain, weight loss, fevers, or haemoptysis. He also mentions that his lower legs are feeling more heavy and oedematous. He mentions that his uncle, who also was a coal miner, died from pneumoconiosis and is concerned that he has the same problem and may suffer the same fate. He is a light smoker of 5 cigarettes a day and drinks between 5 and 10 units of alcohol a week. He lives in a house with a single flight of stairs and is married with two children. He has not returned from holiday recently.

The findings from the history are consistent with a possible presentation of pulmonary oedema. However, I would wish to exclude coal miner's pneumoconiosis, bronchitis, emphysema, and infective causes'. ■

01.5 LOSS OF CONSCIOUSNESS

INSTRUCTIONS Mr Brooks has been admitted by Accident & Emergency with an episode of loss of consciousness. Take a relevant medical history of his complaint. Present your findings and differential diagnosis.

STAGE	KEY POINTS AND ACTIONS	SCORE
	INTRODUCTION	
Introduction	Introduce yourself and establish rapport.	0 1 –
Name & Age	Elicit patient's name and age.	0 1 –
Occupation	Enquire about patient's present occupation.	0 1 –
	THE HISTORY	
This Episode	Ask patient relevant questions regarding loss of consciousness including the following:	
	BEFORE THE EPISODE	
	Before you had this episode did you notice anything unusual? Did you know that you were going to pass out?	0 1 –
Circumstances	What were you doing at the time? Were you watching any bright flashing lights? Did you just wake up? Did you fall? Were you straining on the loo? Were you standing for a long time? Were you coughing or emotionally excited?	0 1 –
Symptoms Review	Any chest pains, dizziness, or palpitations? Any visual aura (scintillating scotoma), visual loss, phonophobia, or photophobia? Any nausea, vomiting, sweating, or agitation?	0 1 –
	DURING THE EPISODE	
	How long were you unconscious?	
Witness	Did anyone witness this episode? Did they report any limb or body shaking? Did you pass any urine or wet yourself? Did you bite your tongue?	0 1 –
	AFTER THE EPISODE	
Recovery	After you awoke how did you feel? Did you have a headache? Were you confused? How long did that last?	0 1 –
Amnesia	How much can you remember of what happened?	0 1 –

STAGE	KEY POINTS AND ACTIONS	SCORE
First Time	Have you ever had this problem before? When was the last time?	0 1 –
Concerns	Do you have any particular concerns or worries about the symptoms you are experiencing? Do you know what may be causing them?	0 1 –
Impact	How have these symptoms affected your life? And your family?	0 1 –

ASSOCIATED HISTORY

	Do you have any of the following [Mnemonic—MJTHREADS]: **M**yocardial infarction **J**aundice **T**uberculosis **H**ypertension/high cholesterol **R**heumatic fever **E**pilepsy **A**sthma/angina **D**iabetes **S**troke Have you ever been admitted to hospital?	0 1 –
Drug History	Are you on any medications (blood pressure, hypoglycaemics, antiepileptic)? Do you have any allergies?	0 1 –
Family History	Has anyone in your family had similar troubles? Are there any inherited family disorders? Does anyone have epilepsy or cardiac problems?	0 1 –
Social History	[Mnemonic—HOSE PIPERS]	0 1 2

Home - Do you live in a house or flat? Does anyone else live with you? Do you have stairs at home? Is the condition of the flat good—boiler, paint, mould, etc.?
Occupation - What do you do for a living? Where is your work? Ask about exposures—inhaled gases, dust or metals, animal or travel exposures. Ask specifically about asbestos exposure.
Smoking - Do you smoke? How many a day and for how long?
Ethanol - Do you drink alcohol? How many units a week do you drink? If > 21 units a day for a man or > 14 units for a woman ask about alcohol dependency—morning drinking, withdrawal symptoms, negative social or financial impact of drinking.

Pysch - Ask about mood and sleeping.
Independence - How are you coping at home? How do you mobilize? Ask about frames, sticks, scooters, etc. Can you look after yourself without help with dressing, washing, or feeding? Do you have carers? How many times a day? What do they do for you? Do you need more help?
Pets - Do you have any pets at home?
Expeditions/Excursions - Have you been out of the country in the last six months? Have you ever visited Africa, Asia, or South America? Any freshwater swimming? Malaria areas? Insect or tick bites? Unwell contacts? Diarrhoea or fevers? Any long haul flights?
Recreational Drugs* - Do you use any recreational drugs?
Sexual History* - If relevant or appropriate, include menstrual history here for women if not already asked about.

*Preface these last two questions with some signposting. 'I'm going to ask you some questions some people find sensitive, but are important to the symptoms you have described' or 'Because the symptoms you are describing could suggest a sexually transmitted illness, I would like to ask more about that if that is okay'.

STAGE	KEY POINTS AND ACTIONS	SCORE
System Review	Run through the systems starting with the most relevant.	0 1 2

COMMUNICATION SKILLS

Rapport	Establish and maintain rapport and demonstrate listening skills.	0 1 –
Responds	React positively to and acknowledge patient's emotions.	0 1 –
Fluency	General fluency and non-use of jargon.	0 1 –
Summarise	Check with patient and deliver an appropriate summary.	0 1 –

EXAMINER'S EVALUATION

Overall assessment of taking loss of consciousness history	0 1 2 3 4 5
Role player's score	0 1 2 3 4 5
Total mark out of 33	

LOSS OF CONSCIOUSNESS: DIFFERENTIAL DIAGNOSIS

Differential Diagnosis	Supporting Features	Risk Factors
Grand mal seizure: A transient surge of uncontrolled neuronal activity in the brain causing loss of consciousness and physical convulsions. Acute reversible underlying causes may be present and must be excluded before diagnosis of epilepsy is made.	Sudden onset loss of consciousness. Witnessed typical seizure like activity (tonic periods followed by repetitive jerks–clonic). Urinary incontinence. Lateral tongue biting. Lasts between 30 seconds and several minutes in most cases (rarely will not self-terminate–status epilepticus). Post-ictal drowsiness (typically 30-60 minutes)	Family history. Structurally abnormal brain. Space occupying lesion. Previous meningitis, traumatic brain injury, or other brain insult
Cardiac syncope: Transient loss of consciousness due to impaired brain perfusion	Typically sudden onset without warning–patients hurt themselves (as no time to put hands out to protect themselves). Visual loss–like a blind closing–reflects blood loss to the retina before event. Chest pain or palpitations may precede loss of consciousness. Recovery is usually quick if event is self-terminating–may present as out-of-hospital arrest.	Arrhythmias: VT (in young patients consider HOCM/ARVD). Massive myocardial infarct: (see CV risk factors under chest pain history)
Vasovagal: Overstimulation of vagal tone induces loss of sufficient blood pressure to perfuse the brain.	Definitive presyncopal symptoms – nausea, light-headedness, sweatiness. Usually patients manage to protect themselves, or collapse from a sitting position. Nearly instant recovery once supine.	Normally low blood pressures. Dehydration. Anxiety
Postural hypotension: Loss of compensated vascular tone when moving from sitting to standing	Typical change in position from sitting to standing. Ask about medications especially anti-hypertensives such as beta-blockers.	Low blood pressures. Diabetic autonomic neuropathy. Anti-hypertensive medication. Elderly

'This is Mr Brooks, a 29-year-old fishmonger with a background of alcohol dependence, who was brought in by ambulance, found unconscious in the street. He was witnessed to have had a full body fit lasting 5 minutes, during which time he was unconscious. He bit his tongue and had an episode of urinary incontinence. He mentions that he had a metallic taste in his mouth before he had the fit. He says that after he awoke, he had a headache and felt tired. He denies any chest pain, dizziness, falling, or headaches before the episode. He mentions that he has had two or three similar episodes before. He mentions that his mother was epileptic and died from a brain haemorrhage post fitting. He is concerned that he may suffer the same fate. He is a light smoker of 5 cigarettes a day and drinks 50 units of alcohol a week. He lives with his father in a new house with stairs.

The findings from the history are most consistent with an epileptic fit, which may be related to alcohol use. However, I would wish to exclude any metabolic or infective causes'. ∎

01.6
HEADACHES

INSTRUCTIONS You are a foundation year House Officer in General Practice. Ms McNair has attended with a history of headaches. Please explore the presenting complaint in detail including the areas of questioning relevant to it. Present your findings as well as a differential diagnosis to the examiner.

STAGE	KEY POINTS AND ACTIONS	SCORE
	INTRODUCTION	
Introduction	Introduce yourself and establish rapport.	0 1 –
Name & Age	Elicit patient's name and age.	0 1 –
Occupation	Enquire about patient's present occupation.	0 1 –
	THE HISTORY	
Headaches	Ask patient all relevant questions regarding headaches Including the following:	
	[Mnemonic—SOCRATES]	
Site	Where exactly is the pain? Can you please point to it?	0 1 –
Onset	When did you first notice the pain? When did it first start?	0 1 –
Character	Can you describe how the pain feels? Is it sharp or dull? Is it band-like, an ache, or a throbbing pain?	0 1 –
Radiation	Does the pain move anywhere?	0 1 –
Associated Symptoms	Have you noticed anything else such as feeling sick or vomiting? Do you have pain when you look at a strong light (photophobia)? Any changes in vision or visual disturbances, i.e. blurred vision? Any neck stiffness (meningeal irritation)? Any urinary incontinence? How is your concentration? Have you noticed any weakness, numbness, or pins and needles? Does it hurt when you chew food (jaw claudication) or when you comb your hair (scalp tenderness)?	0 1 2
Timing	How long does the pain last? Does the headache vary during the day? Are you able to know when the headaches will come on?	
Exacerbating and Relieving Factors	Does anything make the pain worse, such as stress, head movements, or coughing? Does anything make the pain better, like standing or lying in a certain position? Is the pain worse on exercise?	0 1 –

STAGE	KEY POINTS AND ACTIONS	SCORE		
Severity	On a scale of 1 to 10, one being the least pain and ten the worst pain you could ever imagine, how severe is the pain?	0	1	–
Head Injury	Have you had a head injury or fall recently? Have you ever had this problem before?	0	1	–
Concerns	Do you have any particular concerns or worries about the symptoms you are experiencing? Do you know what may be causing them?	0	1	–
Impact	How have these symptoms affected your life? And your family?	0	1	–

ASSOCIATED HISTORY

Medical History	Do you have any of the following [Mnemonic – MJTHREADS]: **M**yocardial infarction **J**aundice **T**uberculosis **H**ypertension/high cholesterol **R**heumatic fever **E**pilepsy **A**sthma/angina **D**iabetes **S**troke Have you ever been admitted to hospital before?	0	1	–
Drug History	Are you on any medications (nitrates)? Do you have any allergies?	0	1	–
Family History	Has anyone in your family had similar troubles? Are there any inherited family disorders? Does anyone suffer from migraines?	0	1	–
Social History	[Mnemonic – HOSE PIPERS] **H**ome - Do you live in a house or flat? Does anyone else live with you? Do you have stairs at home? Is the condition of the flat good – boiler, paint, mould, etc.? **O**ccupation - What do you do for a living? Where is your work? Ask about exposures – inhaled gases, dust or metals, animal or travel exposures. Ask specifically about asbestos exposure. **S**moking - Do you smoke? How many a day and for how long? **E**thanol - Do you drink alcohol? How many units a week do you drink? If > 21 units a day for a man or > 14 units for a woman ask about alcohol dependency – morning drinking, withdrawal symptoms, negative social or financial impact of drinking. **P**ysch - Ask about mood and sleeping, stress especially. **I**ndependence - How are you coping at home? How do you mobilize? Ask about frames, sticks, scooters, etc. Can you look after yourself without help with dressing, washing, or feeding? Do you have carers? How many times a day? What do they do for you? Do you need more help? **P**ets - Do you have any pets at home? **E**xpeditions/**E**xcursions - Have you been out of the country in the last six months? Have you ever visited Africa, Asia, or South America? Any freshwater swimming? Malaria areas? Insect or tick bites? Unwell contacts? Diarrhoea or fevers? Any long haul flights? **R**ecreational Drugs* - Do you use any recreational drugs? **S**exual History* - If relevant or appropriate, include menstrual history here for women if not already asked about. Think about catamenial migraine if headache and cycle coincide.	0	1	2

STAGE	KEY POINTS AND ACTIONS	SCORE

*Preface these last two questions with some signposting. 'I'm going to ask you some questions some people find sensitive, but are important to the symptoms you have described' or 'Because the symptoms you are describing could suggest a sexually transmitted illness, I would like to ask more about that if that is okay'.

Dietary
Do you eat a lot of cheese, chocolate, or yoghurts? Do you drink tea or coffee?

System Review
Run through the systems starting with the most relevant.

COMMUNICATION SKILLS

Rapport	Establish and maintain rapport and demonstrate listening skills.	0 1 –
Responds	React positively to and acknowledge patient's emotions.	0 1 –
Fluency	General fluency and non-use of jargon.	0 1 –
Summarise	Check with patient and deliver an appropriate summary.	0 1 –

EXAMINER'S EVALUATION

Overall assessment of taking headache history	0 1 2 3 4 5
Role player's score	0 1 2 3 4 5
Total mark out of 33	

HEADACHE: DIFFERENTIAL DIAGNOSIS

Differential Diagnosis	Supporting Features	Risk Factors
Subarachnoid Haemorrhage: Blood in the subarachnoid space May be traumatic or spontaneous	Sudden onset, occipital, maximal at onset May be associated with meningism - neck stiffness, photophobia, phonophobia	Family history - polycystic chronic kidney disease Collagen disorders Amyloidosis
Raised Intracranial Pressure:	Slow onset over weeks Typically worst in mornings Associated with vomiting without nausea Ask about blurred vision and small fields Loss of power and blood pressure changes are late signs	Variable - family history of space occupying lesions Idiopathic intracranial hypertension - overweight, young, and female
Migraine: The recurrence of debilitating headache	Typically unilateral, subacute onset over hours Photophobic, phonophobic Lasts hours and then subsides (can last for days) Sometimes associated with menstrual cycle in young women	Family history
Tension Headache: Commonest type of headache	Subacute onset over hours All-over headache No other features - may be stress-related	None
Cluster Headache: The recurrence of stereotyped severe pain usually unilateral	Very severe headaches that occur in 'clusters' of frequent episodes over several days or weeks and then subside for months Typically unilateral, behind one eye 'ice-pick' pain Injected eye, sinusitis, tearing pain Related syndromes - hemicrania, SUNCT syndrome	Family history Young men (cluster headache) Young women (hemicranias)
Sinusitis: Inflammation of the tissue lining the sinuses	Fullness or heaviness in face May have features of infection Nasal or postnasal drip	Abnormal sinuses - recurrent infections
Temporal Arteritis: A vasculitis requiring urgent attention due to risk of blindness preventable with steroids	Patients > 60 Palpable temporal artery Unilateral headache Amaurosis fugax - painless loss of vision secondary to ophthalmic artery involvement - late and irreversible	Elderly patients

'This is Ms McNair, a 24-year-old trainee solicitor previously fit and well who has had a six month history of headaches. The headaches are unilateral and have a severity of 7 out of 10. She also feels nauseous and tired when the headaches start. She mentions seeing flashing lights and zigzag lines half an hour prior to the headache starting and feels pain when she looks directly at light. She describes the headache as an intense throbbing pain mainly on the right side of her head. Consequently, she locks herself in her room for 4–6 hours until her symptoms resolve. She has had these symptoms every few days for the past six months and feels they are becoming more frequent and severe. She mentions that her elder sister suffers from migraines. She is concerned because she has missed one week of work this month due to the severity of the headaches and her employers want to know what the problem is. She has tried simple analgesia including paracetamol and neurofen with no relief. Her headaches are not related to her menstrual cycle. She mentions that she has been working as a trainee solicitor for the past eight months and that her work is extremely stressful.

The findings from the history are consistent with episodes of migraine. However, I would wish to exclude tension and cluster headaches'. ∎

01.7 GENERAL SURGICAL HISTORY

INSTRUCTIONS You are a foundation year House Officer in General Surgery. Please elicit a full history relevant to this patient's complaints. You will have ten minutes to complete this.

STAGE	KEY POINTS AND ACTIONS	SCORE
	INTRODUCTION	
Introduction	Introduce yourself and establish rapport.	0 1 –
Name & Age	Elicit patient's name and age.	0 1 –
Occupation	Enquire about patient's present occupation.	0 1 –
	THE HISTORY	
Complaint	Elicit all of the patient's presenting complaints.	0 1 2
History	When did it first start? What did you first notice? Is it getting better or worse? Have you ever had it before?	
Pain	Where is the pain? When does it start? Does the pain move anywhere? What does the pain feel like (constant, colicky, sharp, or dull)? How severe is the pain? What makes it worse? What makes it better? Are there any other symptoms?	0 1 2
Lump	When did you first notice a lump? Where exactly is it? Is it getting bigger or smaller? Are there any lumps elsewhere? Is it painful to touch?	0 1 –
Vomit	How much and how often do you vomit? Is the vomiting related to meals? Is it associated with pain or does vomiting cause some pain relief? Do you feel nauseous? What colour is the vomit? Is there any blood?	0 1 –

Different Colours of Vomit

Bile coloured	*(with bitter taste)* Small bowel intestinal obstruction
Faeculent	Large bowel or distal small bowel obstruction
Blood red	Oesophageal varices, gastric, or duodenal ulcers
Coffee ground	*(dark brown in appearance)* Bleeding from stomach

STAGE	KEY POINTS AND ACTIONS	SCORE
Stools	How often are you passing stools? Do you feel any pain on passing stools? Have you had any change in bowel motions? Suffered from any diarrhoea or constipation? Is there any blood in your stools? Is it fresh red blood or are the stools black? Are the stools difficult to flush? Is there any mucus in the stools? Do you feel you want to go to the toilet all the time?	

STAGE	KEY POINTS AND ACTIONS	SCORE

Different Colours of Stools

0 1 2

Dark tarry	(*Melaena*) Upper GI bleed (stomach, duodenum, oesophagus), iron, bismuth treatment	
Pale bulky	(*Steatorrhoea*) Fat malabsorption of small bowel (coeliac) or pancreatic disease (chronic pancreatitis)	
Blood red	Diverticulitis (large volume) Colorectal cancer (mixed with stool) UC & infective colitis (blood & mucus mixed in stool) Haemorrhoids (painless, fresh blood on stool & pan) Anal fissure (painful, fresh blood on paper & stool)	

Concerns — Do you have any particular concerns or worries about the symptoms you are experiencing? Do you know what may be causing them?

0 1 –

Impact — How have these symptoms affected your life? And your family?

0 1 –

ASSOCIATED HISTORY

Medical History

Do you have any of the following [Mnemonic—MJTHREADS]:

0 1 –

Myocardial infarction
Jaundice
Tuberculosis
Hypertension/high cholesterol
Rheumatic fever
Epilepsy
Asthma/angina
Diabetes
Stroke

Have you ever been admitted to hospital?

Surgical History — Have you ever had any surgical procedures? Did you have any reactions with the general anaesthetic?

0 1 –

Drug History — Are you on any medications? Are you taking any over-the-counter preparations? Do you have any drug allergies?

0 1 –

Family History — Has anyone in your family had similar troubles? Are there any inherited family disorders such as adenomatous polyposis or bowel cancers?

0 1 –

Social History

[Mnemonic—HOSE PIPERS]

0 1 2

Home - Do you live in a house or flat? Does anyone else live with you? Do you have stairs at home? Is the condition of the flat good—boiler, paint, mould, etc.?
Occupation - What do you do for a living? Where is your work? Ask about exposures—inhaled gases, dust or metals, animal or travel exposures. Ask specifically about asbestos exposure.
Smoking - Do you smoke? How many a day and for how long?
Ethanol - Do you drink alcohol? How many units a week do you drink? If > 21 units a day for a man or > 14 units for a woman ask about alcohol dependency—morning drinking, withdrawal symptoms, negative social or financial impact of drinking.

Pysch - Ask about mood and sleeping, stress especially.
Independence - How are you coping at home? How do you mobilize? Ask about frames, sticks, scooters, etc. Can you look after yourself without help with dressing, washing, or feeding? Do you have carers? How many times a day? What do they do for you? Do you need more help?
Pets - Do you have any pets at home?
Expeditions/Excursions - Have you been out of the country in the last six months? Have you ever visited Africa, Asia, or South America? Any freshwater swimming? Malaria areas? Insect or tick bites? Unwell contacts? Diarrhoea or fevers? Any long haul flights? Malaria prophylaxis and vaccines?
Recreational Drugs* - Do you use any recreational drugs?
Sexual History* - If relevant or appropriate, include menstrual history here for women if not already asked about.

STAGE	KEY POINTS AND ACTIONS	SCORE
	*Preface these last two questions with some signposting. 'I'm going to ask you some questions some people find sensitive, but are important to the symptoms you have described' or 'Because the symptoms you are describing could suggest a sexually transmitted illness, I would like to ask more about that if that is okay'.	
System Review	Run through the systems starting with the most relevant.	0 1 2

COMMUNICATION SKILLS

Rapport	Establish and maintain rapport and demonstrate listening skills.	0 1 –
Responds	React positively to and acknowledge patient's emotions.	0 1 –
Fluency	General fluency and non-use of jargon.	0 1 –
Summarise	Check with patient and deliver an appropriate summary.	0 1 –

EXAMINER'S EVALUATION

Overall assessment of taking general surgical history	0 1 2 3 4 5
Role player's score	0 1 2 3 4 5
Total mark out of 35	

01.8 UROLOGICAL HISTORY

INSTRUCTIONS You are a foundation year House Officer in Urology. Mr Chapman, a retired printer, has presented having passed frank blood in his urine. Assess his problems in relation to his symptoms and suggest a differential diagnosis to the examiner. You will be marked on your ability to elicit an appropriate urological history, to reach a diagnosis, and on your communication skills.

STAGE	KEY POINTS AND ACTIONS	SCORE
	INTRODUCTION	
Introduction	Introduce yourself and establish rapport.	0 1 –
Name & Age	Elicit patient's name and age.	0 1 –
Occupation	Enquire about patient's present occupation.	0 1 –
	THE HISTORY	
Haematuria	Ask relevant questions relating to haematuria including the following:	
	[Mnemonic – BONDS]	0 1 2
Blood	How much blood do you think you have lost? Did you notice any clots?	
Onset	When did you first notice blood in your urine? Is it there all the time or does it come and go?	
Number	How many times have you noticed blood in your urine?	
Duration	When in your stream do you notice the blood? Is it at the beginning of the stream, the middle, or toward the end?	0 1 –
Symptoms	Since the problem first started, do you feel things are improving or getting worse? Do you have any other symptoms like abdominal pain or sickness?	
Urology	Take a complete urological history to include infective symptoms, problems with stream, and pain.	
	[Mnemonic – PIS]	
Pain	Have you noticed any pain in your tummy? Any pain in your back (metastatic disease)? Take a full pain history, i.e. site, onset, character, radiation, associated, etc.	0 1 –

STAGE	KEY POINTS AND ACTIONS	SCORE
Infection	Are you passing urine more often (frequency)? Do you get any burning or pain when passing urine (dysuria)? Are you waking up at night to pass urine (nocturia)? Do you feel that when you want to go to the toilet you must go there and then (urgency)?	0 1 −
Stream	Do you notice when you pass urine you are unable to pass it straight away (hesitancy)? Have you noticed that your urine stream is not as strong as it used to be? Have you noticed when you finish passing urine that some still trickles out (dribbling)?	0 1 2
Concerns	Do you have any particular concerns or worries about the symptoms you are experiencing? Do you know what may be causing them?	0 1 −
Impact	How have these symptoms affected your life? And your family?	0 1 −
	ASSOCIATED HISTORY	0 1 −

Do you have any of the following [Mnemonic—MJTHREADS]:

Myocardial infarction
Jaundice
Tuberculosis
Hypertension/high cholesterol
Rheumatic fever
Epilepsy
Asthma/angina
Diabetes
Stroke

Have you ever been admitted to hospital?

Surgical History	Have you ever had any surgical procedures?	0 1 −
Drug History	Are you on any medications including anti-coagulants? Are you taking any over-the-counter preparations? Do you have any drug allergies?	0 1 −
Family History	Has anyone in your family had similar troubles? Are there any inherited family disorders (polycystic kidney disease, bladder cancer)?	0 1 −
Social History	[Mnemonic—HOSE PIPERS]	0 1 2

Home - Do you live in a house or flat? Does anyone else live with you? Do you have stairs at home? Is the condition of the flat good—boiler, paint, mould, etc.?
Occupation - What do you do for a living? Where is your work? Ask about exposures—inhaled gases, dust or metals, animal or travel exposures. Ask specifically about aniline dyes and rubber exposure (bladder cancer risk).
Smoking - Do you smoke? How many a day and for how long?
Ethanol - Do you drink alcohol? How many units a week do you drink? If > 21 units a day for a man or > 14 units for a woman ask about alcohol dependency—morning drinking, withdrawal symptoms, negative social or financial impact of drinking.

Pysch - Ask about mood and sleeping, stress especially.
Independence - How are you coping at home? How do you mobilize? Ask about frames, sticks, scooters, etc. Can you look after yourself without help with dressing, washing, or feeding? Do you have carers? How many times a day? What do they do for you? Do you need more help?
Pets - Do you have any pets at home?
Expeditions/Excursions - Have you been out of the country in the last six months? Have you ever visited Africa, Asia, or South America? Any freshwater swimming? Malaria areas? Insect or tick bites? Unwell contacts? Diarrhoea or fevers? Any long haul flights? Malaria prophylaxis and vaccines?
Recreational Drugs* - Do you use any recreational drugs?
Sexual History* - If relevant or appropriate, include menstrual history here for women if not already asked about.

STAGE	KEY POINTS AND ACTIONS	SCORE

*Preface these last two questions with some signposting. 'I'm going to ask you some questions some people find sensitive, but are important to the symptoms you have described' or 'Because the symptoms you are describing could suggest a sexually transmitted illness, I would like to ask more about that if that is okay'.

System Review — Run through the systems starting with the most relevant. `0  1  –`

COMMUNICATION SKILLS

Rapport — Establish and maintain rapport and demonstrate listening skills. `0  1  –`

Responds — React positively to and acknowledge patient's emotions. `0  1  –`

Fluency — General fluency and non-use of jargon. `0  1  –`

Summarise — Check with patient and deliver an appropriate summary. `0  1  –`

EXAMINER'S EVALUATION

Overall assessment of taking urology history and differential `0  1  2  3  4  5`

Role player's score `0  1  2  3  4  5`

Total mark out of 33

HAEMATURIA: DIFFERENTIAL DIAGNOSIS

DIFFERENTIAL DIAGNOSIS	SUPPORTING FEATURES	RISK FACTORS
Bladder Cancer Transitional cell carcinoma most common histological type in UK Rarer types: SCC (associated with Schistosoma Haematobium infection)	Painless gross haematuria (most common) Pain if associated with clot retention Metastatic disease: Bone pain, cachexia, lower limb oedema (from mass obstruction of vessels/lymphatics) Weight loss	Smoking Exposure to aniline dyes, aromatic amines Cyclophosphomide use Schistosomiasis infection
Urinary Tract Infection Infection of the lower or upper urinary tract most commonly bacterial, rarely mycobacterial	Dysuria Urgency Frequency Suprapubic discomfort Pyelonephritis/complicated UTI: Fever, flank pain, vomiting, rigors Haematuria Confusion (especially in the elderly)	Female gender Elderly Pregnancy Recent antibiotic use Diabetes (or other states of immunosuppression)
Urolithiasis Presence of stones in urinary tract Calcium containing stones (calcium oxalate, phosphate or urate) account for majority of stones seen	Pain Haematuria May have superimposed symptoms/sign of infection	Previous history of stones Dietary excess of spinach, tea and strawberries (causing hyperoxaluria) Drugs: Indinivir, sulfasalazine, magnesium silicate containing antacids
Prostate Cancer Adenocarcinoma most commonly seen subtype	Obstructive symptoms/overflow incontinence Haematuria Metastatic disease: Bone pain, cachexia, neurological defects (spinal cord compression)	Increasing age Family history Afro-Caribbean ancestry
Benign Prostatic Hypertrophy Smooth enlargement of the prostate gland associated with increasing age	Obstructive symptoms/overflow incontinence Haematuria	Increasing age Family history Men of Afro-Caribbean ancestry tend to have more severe disease

EXEMPLAR PRESENTATION

'This is Mr Chapman, a 60-year-old retired printer who has presented with a four-month history of worsening painless haematuria. The haematuria is more pronounced midway through voiding. He denies any burning, nocturia, frequency, or urgency. He also denies hesitancy, dribbling, or poor stream. He is a smoker of 30 cigarettes a day and drinks socially. He suffers from high blood pressure for which he is taking bendroflumethiazide. He also takes aspirin and denies any drug allergy. In addition to haematuria, he has noticed weight loss of a few kilograms and persistent night sweats. There has been no abdominal or back pain. There is no positive family history of urological or renal problems.

The findings on history are consistent with a presentation of possible bladder cancer. However, I wish to exclude other diagnoses such as a renal stone, infection, benign prostatic hypertrophy, glomerulonephritis, and prostatic carcinoma'. ■

01.9
ABDOMINAL PAIN

INSTRUCTIONS You are a foundation year House Officer in General Surgery. Mr Morden has presented with abdominal pain. Please take a brief history of his symptoms and establish a differential diagnosis.

STAGE	KEY POINTS AND ACTIONS	SCORE
	INTRODUCTION	
Introduction	Introduce yourself and establish rapport.	0 1 –
Name & Age	Elicit patient's name and age.	0 1 –
Occupation	Enquire about patient's present occupation.	0 1 –
	THE HISTORY	
Abdominal Pain	Ask patient all relevant questions regarding abdominal pain including the following:	
	[Mnemonic – SOCRATES]	
Site	Where exactly is the pain? Can you please point to it?	0 1 –
Onset	When did you first notice the pain? When did it first start?	0 1 –
Character	Can you describe how the pain feels? Is it sharp, dull, or an ache? Does it come and go? Do you feel a burning sensation?	0 1 –
Radiation	Does the pain move anywhere? For example, to your back, the tip of your shoulder, or towards your groin?	0 1 –
Associated Symptoms	Have you noticed any other problems such as constipation? Black stools? Change in urine habit? Nausea or vomiting? Pale stools?	0 1 –
Timing	How long does the pain last?	
Exacerbating and Relieving Factors	Does anything make the pain worse, such as eating a large meal? Spicy foods? Moving? Drinking alcohol?	
	Does anything make the pain better, such as lying in a certain position? Is the pain worse on exercise?	0 1 –
Severity	On a scale of 1 to 10, one being the least pain and ten the worst pain you could ever imagine, how severe is the pain?	0 1 –

STAGE	KEY POINTS AND ACTIONS	SCORE

Causes of Right and Left Iliac Fossa Pain   0 1 2

RIF pain [Mnemonic—APPENDICITIS]:
Appendicitis/Abscess (psoas)
Period pain/Pneumonia
Pelvic inflammatory disease
Ectopic pregnancy/Endometriosis
Neoplasia
Diverticulitis (Merkel's)
Intussusception
Crohn's disease/Cyst (ovarian)
Inflammatory bowel disease
Torsion (testis)
Irritable bowel syndrome
Stones (renal/ureteric)/Salpingitis

LIF pain [Mnemonic—SUPERCLOTS]:
Sigmoid diverticulitis
Ureteric colic
Pelvic inflammatory disease/Period pain
Ectopic pregnancy/Endometriosis
Rectus sheath haematoma
Colorectal carcinoma
Left lower lobe pneumonia
Ovarian cyst
Torsion (testicular)
Salpingitis/Stones (renal/ureteric)

Concerns	Do you have any particular concerns or worries about the symptoms you are experiencing? Do you know what may be causing them?	0 1 –
Impact	How have these symptoms affected your life? And your family?	0 1 –
Risk Factors	Elicit relevant risk factors such as previous ulcers, smoking, alcohol, and medicines such as aspirin or non-steroidal anti-inflammatories (e.g. ibuprofen).	0 1 2

ASSOCIATED HISTORY

Medical History	Do you have any of the following: [Mnemonic—MJTHREADS] Myocardial infarction Jaundice Tuberculosis Hypertension/high cholesterol Rheumatic fever Epilepsy Asthma/angina Diabetes Stroke Have you ever been admitted to hospital? Any previous endoscopies or ulcers?	0 1 –
Surgical History	Have you ever had any surgical procedures?	0 1 –
Drug History	Are you on any medications? Are you taking any over-the-counter preparations? Do you have any drug allergies?	0 1 –
Family History	Has anyone in your family had similar troubles? Are there any inherited family disorders? Does anyone have bowel problems (IBD, cancer)?	0 1 –

STAGE	KEY POINTS AND ACTIONS	SCORE

Social History

[Mnemonic—HOSE PIPERS]

Home - Do you live in a house or flat? Does anyone else live with you? Do you have stairs at home? Is the condition of the flat good—boiler, paint, mould, etc.?

Occupation - What do you do for a living? Where is your work? Ask about exposures—inhaled gases, dust or metals, animal or travel exposures. Ask specifically about aniline dyes and rubber exposure (bladder cancer risk).

Smoking - Do you smoke? How many a day and for how long?

Ethanol - Do you drink alcohol? How many units a week do you drink? If > 21 units a day for a man or > 14 units for a woman ask about alcohol dependency - morning drinking, withdrawal symptoms, negative social or financial impact of drinking.

0 1 2

Pysch - Ask about mood and sleeping, stress especially.

Independence - How are you coping at home? How do you mobilize? Ask about frames, sticks, scooters, etc. Can you look after yourself without help with dressing, washing, or feeding? Do you have carers? How many times a day? What do they do for you? Do you need more help?

Pets - Do you have any pets at home?

Expeditions/**E**xcursions - Have you been out of the country in the last six months? Have you ever visited Africa, Asia, or South America? Any freshwater swimming? Malaria areas? Insect or tick bites? Unwell contacts? Diarrhoea or fevers? Any long haul flights? Malaria prophylaxis and vaccines?

Recreational Drugs* - Do you use any recreational drugs?

Sexual History* - If relevant or appropriate, include menstrual history here for women if not already asked about.

*Preface these last two questions with some signposting. 'I'm going to ask you some questions some people find sensitive, but are important to the symptoms you have described' or 'Because the symptoms you are describing could suggest a sexually transmitted illness, I would like to ask more about that if that is okay'.

System Review

Run through the systems starting with the most relevant.

0 1 2

COMMUNICATION SKILLS

Rapport

Establish and maintain rapport and demonstrate listening skills.

0 1 –

Responds

React positively to and acknowledge patient's emotions.

0 1 –

Fluency

General fluency and non-use of jargon.

0 1 –

Summarise

Check with patient and deliver an appropriate summary.

0 1 –

EXAMINER'S EVALUATION

Overall assessment of taking abdominal pain history

0 1 2 3 4 5

Role player's score

0 1 2 3 4 5

Total mark out of 38

EXEMPLAR PRESENTATION

'This is Mr Morden, a 43-year-old meteorologist with a background of asthma who presents with constipation for the past three months in addition to a dull left sided abdominal pain which does not radiate. The pain is present all the time and worsens when eating. He mentions that he used to open his bowels once a day, but has not been for the past two weeks. Whenever he is able to pass stools he notices red blood mixed in with them. He often feels that he wants to go to the toilet but is unable to pass anything when he does go. He denies any urinary symptoms, nausea or vomiting. He says he has lost up to 4kg of weight but puts this down to his poor appetite for the past two months. He has had some shortness of breath especially when exercising but blames his asthma, for which he takes salbutamol and beclometosone inhalers. He is allergic to penicillin. He denies taking any aspirin, other NSAIDs or codeine containing painkillers. He smokes between 10 and 20 roll-ups a day and drinks 30 units of alcohol a week. He mentions that his uncle had rectal polyps and died of cancer, which is his main concern regarding his own symptoms. He lives in a house with two flights of stairs and is single with no children. He is planning to visit Central Asia on a business trip next week. He is concerned that he will have to cancel his trip for follow-up investigations which will result in loss of earnings.

The findings from the history are consistent with a possible presentation of bowel cancer. However, I would wish to exclude diverticular disease, inflammatory bowel disease, and haemorrhoids'. ■

ACUTE ABDOMINAL PAIN: DIFFERENTIAL DIAGNOSIS

DIFFERENTIAL DIAGNOSIS	SUPPORTING FEATURES	RISK FACTORS
Appendicitis Inflammation of the appendix	Classically umbilical pain followed by right iliac fossa pain Worse on coughing, jumping, and direct pressure Nausea and vomiting, anorexia, fever	Age over 6 years
Biliary Colic Pain associated with the temporary obstruction of cystic duct or common bile duct of gallstones	Right upper quadrant pain Associated with ingestion of meals with high fat content Radiation to back Subsides within hours Bloating Belching	Obesity Aged over 40 Female Pregnancy Haemolytic conditions such as thalassemia
Acute Cholecystitis Inflammation of gallbladder wall due to impaction of stone in cystic duct Acalculous cholecystitis occurs in conditions of extreme stress	Right upper quadrant pain similar to biliary colic Pain is persistent for longer periods than colic Nausea and vomiting Fever	As for biliary colic
Cholangitis Infection of the biliary tract E.coli is a common causative organism	Right upper quadrant pain Jaundice Fever Confusion	History of biliary colic Most common after age 50 Recent biliary tract procedure (e.g. stenting) History of hepatobiliary malignancy
Acute Pancreatitis Inflammation of the pancreas secondary to acute insult to the organ	Severe epigastric pain Pain constant and dull Radiation to back Nausea and vomiting Anorexia Temporary relief by curling up or bending forward	**GET SMASHED:** **G**allstone disease **E**thanol **T**rauma **S**teroids **M**umps **A**utoimmune disorders **S**corpion bite **H**ypercalcaemia post=**E**RCP **D**rugs (azathioprine)
Diverticulitis Inflammation or infection of diverticula (small pathological out-pouchings of large bowel) Left sided disease most common in UK population (opposite is true for the Asian population)	Lower left abdominal pain Fever Nausea and vomiting Change in bowel habit (especially constipation)	Known diverticular disease Elderly population

01.10
BREAST LUMP

INSTRUCTIONS Mrs J is a 57-year-old coming into clinic with a breast lump. Please take a thorough history.

STAGE	KEY POINTS AND ACTIONS	SCORE		
	INTRODUCTION			
Introduction	Introduce yourself and establish rapport.	0	1	–
Name & Age	Elicit patient's name and age.	0	1	–
Occupation	Enquire about patient's present occupation.	0	1	2
	THE HISTORY			
Lump	When and how was it noticed? Which breast? What size was it? What was the texture like? Any associated skin changes? Any associated trauma?	0	1	–
Change over Time	Has the lump changed over time (size, texture, pain, skin changes)? Have you noticed any other lumps?	0	1	2
Pain	Any pain or tenderness in the breasts or the lump? Unilateral or bilateral? Associated with menstruation? If pain is present take a full pain history.	0	1	–
Discharge	Is there any discharge? How much? From both nipples? What colour is the discharge (blood, yellow, milky?)	0	1	–
Menstrual History	When was your last period? Are they regular? Do you have any children? Are you breastfeeding? Could you be pregnant? Do the symptoms or the lump come and go with your period?	0	1	–
Risk Factors	Oral contraceptive pill and HRT? Family history of breast cancer or related cancers? Alcohol use and radiation exposure? Early menarche and late menopause?	0	1	–
	ASSOCIATED HISTORY			
	Do you have any of the following [Mnemonic—MJTHREADS]: **M**yocardial infarction **J**aundice **T**uberculosis **H**ypertension/high cholesterol **R**heumatic fever **E**pilepsy **A**sthma/angina **D**iabetes **S**troke	0	1	–

STAGE	KEY POINTS AND ACTIONS	SCORE
Surgical History	Have you ever had any surgery? Have you ever been admitted to hospital?	0 1 –
Drug History	Are you on any medications? Do you have any allergies?	0 1 –
Family History	Has anyone in your family had similar troubles? Are there any inherited family disorders? Is there any history of breast, ovarian, or bowel cancer in the family?	0 1 –
Social History	[Mnemonic—HOSE PIPERS] **H**ome - Do you live in a house or flat? Does anyone else live with you? Do you have stairs at home? Is the condition of the flat good—boiler, paint, mould, etc.? **O**ccupation - What do you do for a living? Where is your work? Ask about exposures—inhaled gases, dust or metals, animal or travel exposures. **S**moking - Do you smoke? How many a day and for how long? **E**thanol - Do you drink alcohol? How many units a week do you drink? If > 21 units a day for a man or > 14 units for a woman ask about alcohol dependency—morning drinking, withdrawal symptoms, negative social or financial impact of drinking. **P**ysch - Ask about mood and sleeping, stress especially. **I**ndependence - How are you coping at home? How do you mobilize? Ask about frames, sticks, scooters, etc. Can you look after yourself without help with dressing, washing, or feeding? Do you have carers? How many times a day? What do they do for you? Do you need more help? **P**ets - Do you have any pets at home? **E**xpeditions/**E**xcursions - Have you been out of the country in the last six months? Have you ever visited Africa, Asia, or South America? Any freshwater swimming? Malaria areas? Insect or tick bites? Unwell contacts? Diarrhoea or fevers? Any long haul flights? Malaria prophylaxis and vaccines? **R**ecreational Drugs* - Do you use any recreational drugs? **S**exual History* - If relevant or appropriate, include menstrual history here for women if not already asked about. *Preface these last two questions with some signposting. 'I'm going to ask you some questions some people find sensitive, but are important to the symptoms you have described' or 'Because the symptoms you are describing could suggest a sexually transmitted illness, I would like to ask more about that if that is okay'.	0 1 2
System Review	Run through the systems starting with the most relevant.	0 1 2

COMMUNICATION SKILLS

Rapport	Establish and maintain rapport and demonstrate listening skills.	0 1 –
Responds	React positively to and acknowledge patient's emotions.	0 1 –
Fluency	General fluency and non-use of jargon.	0 1 –
Summarise	Check with patient and deliver an appropriate summary.	0 1 –

EXAMINER'S EVALUATION

Overall assessment of taking abdominal pain history	0 1 2 3 4 5
Role player's score	0 1 2 3 4 5
Total mark out of 33	

EXEMPLAR PRESENTATION

'This is Mrs J, a 57-year-old Ancient History lecturer, otherwise fit and well who presents with a painless lump in the right breast which she noted a week ago whilst in the shower. The patient notes it to be about 2cm in diameter, with a craggy texture. She notes no other lumps, discharge, or associated skin changes. Systemically Mrs J feels well but has been experiencing some lower back pain for the past month which has been increasingly waking her from sleep.

Mrs J had her last menstrual over 10 years ago and received HRT therapy for 5 years thereafter. She has no significant past medical history and is otherwise fit and active for her age with no current medications or allergies. Her family history is positive for colon cancer—her brother and maternal aunt having died from it aged 57 and 63, respectively. She has never smoked but drinks up to 20 units of alcohol a week. She lives with her husband and never had any children. This patient has a worrying history and multiple risk factors for breast cancer. I would like to carry out an examination'. ■

BREAST LUMP: DIFFERENTIAL DIAGNOSIS

DIFFERENTIAL DIAGNOSIS	SUPPORTING FEATURES	RISK FACTORS
Breast Cancer A major cause of mortality and morbidity Adenocarcinoma most common subtype	Large size Irregular texture Growth over time Skin changes Axillary lumps Metastatic disease: bone pain, jaundice most common, symptoms of hypercalcaemia	Age Early menarche Late menopause Nulliparity BRCA genes Family history First pregnancy after the age of 30 HRT (especially combined) Obesity Not breast feeding Previous breast cancer The combined oral contraceptive pill
Breast Cyst Endothelial lined sac of fluid, may be multiple	Fluctuant texture May be associated to menstrual cycle	Age 30–40
Breast Abscess Most commonly caused by staphylococcus aureus	Fever Pain Skin erythema	Lactating women
Fibroadenoma Benign condition seen in young women	Well circumscribed 'breast mouse' Mobile Stable in size over time	Young women (20–30)

section 02

EXAMINATIONS

02.1
CARDIOVASCULAR

INSTRUCTIONS You will be asked to examine the cardiovascular system of this patient. Examine the CV system and present your findings as well as a differential diagnosis to the examiners.

STAGE	KEY POINTS AND ACTIONS	SCORE
	THE EXAMINATION	
Introduction	Introduce yourself. Elicit name, age, and occupation. Establish rapport.	0 1 –
Consent	Explain the examination to the patient and seek consent. 'The examination will involve looking at your hands, face, and legs and listening to your chest. Would that be okay'?	
Pain	Always ask about pain. 'Before we begin, do you have any pain anywhere'?	0 1 –
Position	Sit the patient at a 45 degree angle and expose the patient appropriately from the waist down.	0 1 –
	INSPECTION	
General	Stand and look at the patient from the edge of the bed. Observe for abnormal breathing, scars, added sounds, or a pacemaker.	0 1 –

General Observations in the Cardiovascular Examination

- **Bedside** – Heart monitors, fluid restriction signs, GTN sprays
- **Breathing at rest** – Comfortable, dyspnoeic, cough
- **Presence of scars** – Midline sternotomy (CABG, valve replacement), lateral thoracotomy (mitral valvotomy)
- **Malar flush** – Dusky pink discolouration of cheeks (mitral stenosis)
- **Added sounds** – Audible heart valves

Hands	Feel the hands for any temperature change.	0 1 –

Hand Signs in the Cardiovascular Examination

- **Temperature** – Warm and well perfused/poor perfusion
- **Peripheral cyanosis** – Blue nail beds
- **Clubbing** – Endocarditis, cyanotic congenital heart disease, atrial myxoma (see image)
- **Endocarditis** – Osler's nodes and Janeway lesions, splinter haemorrhages
- **Nicotine stains** – Peripheral vascular disease
- **Capillary refill** – Should be less than 2 seconds

STAGE	KEY POINTS AND ACTIONS	SCORE

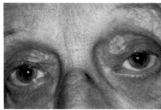

Fig. 2.1 Clubbing

Source: Tang T and Praveen B V. *MRCS Picture Questions Book 1*.
London: Radcliffe Publishing; 2006.

Pulse Feel the radial pulse with three fingers. Assess the rate, rhythm, and volume.

Rate Count for 15 seconds and multiply by 4. `0  1  –`
Normal – 60-100 beats per minute
Tachycardia – > 100 beats per minute
Bradycardia – < 60 beats per minute
Irregular heart rates should be timed at the apex with a stethoscope (distal-apical pulse mismatch).

Rhythm Establish the quality of the rhythm. `0  1  –`

- **Regular** – Sinus rhythm
- **Regularly irregular** – 2nd degree heart block, sinus arrhythmia (observe the respiratory pattern when timing the heart rate to identify a sinus arrhythmia)
- **Irregularly irregular** – AF or multiple ectopics (In order to distinguish these two you could ask the patient to touch their toes 10 times to increase their heart rate—AF will persist with increased heart rate, while ectopics will dissipate, becoming regular.)

Volume Establish the volume of the pulse.

- **Low volume** – Low cardiac output, heart failure, aortic stenosis *(see below)*
- **Bounding** – Thyrotoxicosis, CO_2 retention, aortic regurgitation, sepsis

Delay Compare the pulses in both arms assessing for radio-radial delay (coarctation of the aorta proximal to the left subclavian artery) and suggest assessing for radio-femoral delay (distal coarctation of the aorta).

Arms Indicate that you would like to measure the blood pressure in both arms (> 20mmHg `0  1  –`
difference is indicative of aortic dissection) and lying and standing blood pressures (early hypovolaemia, poor cardiac output, poor autonomic tone).

Face Look at the eyes for signs of anaemia. Inspect in and around the eyes for signs `0  1  2`
consistent with hyperlipidaemia (xanthelasma, corneal arcus), lens dislocation (Marfan's/homocystinuria). Inspect the tongue for central cyanosis, dental hygiene (bacterial endocarditis), macroglossia (amyloidosis), and a high arched palate (Marfan's syndrome).

Fig. 2.2 Xanthelasma

Source: Tang T and Praveen B V. *MRCS Picture Questions Book 1*.
London: Radcliffe Publishing; 2006.

Carotid Pulse Palpate the carotid pulse gently with your thumb to assess its character. Never `0  1  –`
compress or palpate both carotids simultaneously.

Character The carotid pulse is palpable in the neck and provides more accurate information of `0  1  –`
volume and character than the radial pulse.

STAGE	KEY POINTS AND ACTIONS	SCORE

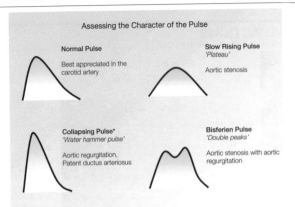

Assessing the Character of the Pulse

Normal Pulse
Best appreciated in the carotid artery

Slow Rising Pulse
'Plateau'
Aortic stenosis

Collapsing Pulse*
'Water hammer pulse'
Aortic regurgitation, Patent ductus arteriosus

Bisferien Pulse
'Double peaks'
Aortic stenosis with aortic regurgitation

* To feel the collapsing pulse, raise the patient's arm while feeling the pulse with your fingers.
- Pulsus alternans is alternating strong and weak beats (left ventricular failure).
- Pulsus paradoxus is detected when the pulse is weaker or absent on inspiration (Tamponade).

JVP   0 1 2

Assess the jugular venous pressure and waveform by ensuring that the patient is lying at 45 degrees and asking them to look to one side. Locate the internal jugular vein between the sternal and clavicular heads of the sternocleidomastoid muscle and observe for JVP pulsations. Measure the height of the JVP from the sternal angle. Normal JVP is no more than 4cm above the sternal angle.

Distinguishing features between the jugular and carotid impulses
Jugular impulse
Most rapid movement inward, two peaks per heartbeat (sinus rhythm), impalpable, obliterated with pressure at the base of the neck, changes with inspiration and degree of inclination, transient increase with abdominal pressure

Carotid impulse
Most rapid movement outward, one peak per heartbeat, palpable, unaffected with pressure at base of neck, unaffected with respiration and inclination, independent of abdominal pressure

A pulsating raised jugular venous pressure commonly suggests right heart failure. A paradoxical rise in JVP during inspiration (Kussmaul's sign) indicates constrictive pericarditis (also seen in restrictive cardiomyopathy and right heart failure). However, marked fixed elevation in JVP with no pulsations suggests superior vena caval obstruction, often caused by bronchial carcinoma or a large mediastinal mass.

Causes of raised jugular venous pressure
[Mnemonic—**PQRST**]

- **P**ericardial effusion/Pulmonary embolism/Pericardial constriction/Pulmonary hypertension (asthma/COPD)
- **Q**uantity of fluid increased (iatrogenic fluid overload)
- **R**ight heart failure or congestive heart failure
- **S**uperior vena caval obstruction
- **T**ricuspid regurgitation/Tricuspid stenosis/Tamponade (Cardiac)

Hepatojugular Reflex   0 1 2

Warn the patient first and ask about pain in the abdomen. Apply firm pressure over the abdomen for about 15 seconds and look for a rise and subsequent fall of about 2cm in the JVP. A persistent rise in JVP over 15 seconds of compression is a positive hepatojugular sign (right ventricular failure).

STAGE	KEY POINTS AND ACTIONS	SCORE

CHEST

Inspection

Look again closely at the chest shape, presence of scars, and implanted devices.   0 1 2

- **Scars** – Midline thoracotomy – CABG, aortic valve replacement – check legs for saphenous venous harvest scars, lateral thoracotomy – mitral valve replacement, lobectomy
- **Chest shape** – Pectus carinatum, pectus excavatum
- **Implanted devices** – Pacemakers (large, typically round devices in left upper chest), implantable heart monitors (small devices, left upper chest)

PALPATION

Apex Beat

Palpate the apex beat by feeling the furthest pulsatile point of the heart. It is normally   0 1 – located in the 5th intercostal space mid-clavicular line. Note the character of the apex beat and whether it is displaced laterally (left ventricular dilatation).

Assessing the character of the apex beat
- **Tapping** – Mitral stenosis
- **Heaving** – Aortic stenosis
- **Thrusting** – Aortic regurgitation, mitral regurgitation
- **Diffuse, weak** – Left ventricular failure, dilated cardiomyopathy
- **Double impulse** – HOCM

Heaves & Thrills

Feel for the presence of thrills (palpable murmurs – AS, VSD) by using the flat of the   0 1 2 hand to palpate over the precordium. Use the flat of the hand to palpate over the left sternal edge, feeling for a parasternal heave (right ventricular hypertrophy).

AUSCULTATION

Listen

Auscultate over the four areas of the heart with a stethoscope listening for heart   0 1 2 sounds, additional sounds (extra heart sounds, clicks, or snaps), murmurs, or pericardial rubs. Time the murmurs with carotid pulse using your thumb to establish if it is a systolic or diastolic murmur. [You can remember the order of the auscultate of the heart using the following mnemonic—**A P**lace **T**o **M**eet.]

Neck
Aortic stenosis murmurs often radiate here from the aortic area

Axilla
Mitral regurgitation murmurs radiate here

Aortic Area
Aortic stenosis best heard here

Pulmonary Area
Pulmonary stenosis is best heard here

Tricuspid Area
Aortic and tricuspid regurgitation best heard here

Mitral Area (apex)
Mitral regurgitation and mitral stenosis is best heard here

Aortic

Located over the 2nd intercostal space, right sternal edge. Listen for aortic stenosis   0 1 – and aortic sclerosis in this area. Check for radiation of the murmur to the carotids.

Pulmonary

Located over the 2nd intercostal space, left sternal edge. Listen for pulmonary   0 1 – stenosis and the flow murmur of an atrial septal defect here.

STAGE	KEY POINTS AND ACTIONS	SCORE
Tricuspid	Located over the 5th intercostal space, left sternal edge. Listen for aortic regurgitation with the patient leaning forward and asking them to take a deep breath in and out, holding it in full expiration. Listen for tricuspid regurgitation with the patient leaning forward, holding their breath in full inspiration.	0 1 –
Mitral	Located over the apex, 5th intercostal space, mid-clavicular line. Listen for mitral stenosis here using the bell to hear the low pitched murmur. Ask the patient to hold their breath in expiration, leaning over to the left hand side. Next listen for mitral regurgitation by using the diaphragm of the stethoscope at the apex. Check for radiation of the murmur to the axilla.	0 1 –
Murmurs	Listen for cardiac murmurs noting the timing, intensity, site, character, pitch, radiation, and the effect of respiration and position.	0 1 2
Timing	Establish if the murmur is systolic, diastolic, or continuous in nature. • **Systolic** – Ejection (AS, PS, ASD), pansystolic (MR, TR, VSD-'harsh') • **Diastolic** – Early diastolic (AR, PR), mid-diastolic (MS, TS) • **Continuous** – Patent ductus arteriosus (PDA)	
Intensity	**Grade the intensity of the murmur between 1 and 6 (Levine grading)** • **Grade 1-3** Thrill absent: 1 Faint and hard to hear with stethoscope, 2 Louder and heard easily with stethoscope, 3 Very loud with stethoscope. No thrill present. • **Grade 4-6** Thrill present: 4 Heard with stethoscope on chest with thrill, 5 Heard over wide area with stethoscope and thrill, 6 Very loud, audible without stethoscope.	
Site	Determine the location on the precordium where the murmur is best heard. Note if it is best heard in the mitral, pulmonary, aortic, or tricuspid area.	
Character	Assess whether it is a crescendo-decrescendo, decrescendo, crescendo, or plateau type of murmur.	
Pitch	Assess the pitch of the murmur. High-pitch murmurs are best heard with the diaphragm (AS) while low-pitch murmurs are best heard with the bell (MS).	
Radiation	Check if the murmur radiates to the carotids (AS), axilla (MR), left sternal edge (AR), or back (PDA).	
Respiration	[Mnemonic for the effect of respiration on murmurs—RILE: **R**ight sided murmurs are heard with greatest intensity in **I**nspiration while **L**eft sided murmurs are heard with greatest intensity in **E**xpiration.]	
Position	Note if the murmur is best heard in the supine position (most murmurs), leaning forward with breath held in exhalation (AR) or in inspiration (TS), or in the left lateral position (MS).	
Manoeuvres	The Valsalva manoeuvre increases the intensity of hypertrophic cardiomyopathy while softening aortic stenosis. Squatting increases the intensity of AS but softens HOCM.	
Lung Bases	Keep the patient leaning forward and auscultate the lung bases listening for crackles of pulmonary oedema and the absent breath sounds of a pleural effusion (left ventricular failure).	0 1 –

ADDITIONAL POINTS

Oedema	Examine for sacral oedema by applying firm pressure against the lower back and for pedal oedema by pressing down over the ankle. Observe pitting oedema by looking for an indentation of your finger after applying pressure. Ensure that you ask the patient if they feel any pain whilst pressing.	0 1 2
	Palpate the abdomen for a pulsatile (tricuspid regurgitation) or enlarged liver (hepatic congestion) and ascites (severe right heart failure).	

STAGE	KEY POINTS AND ACTIONS	SCORE

Causes of oedema
- **Pitting oedema** – Heart failure, nephrotic syndrome, decompensated cirrhosis, malnutrition, severe anaemia
- **Non-pitting oedema** – Lymphatic obstruction, deep vein thrombosis

STAGE	KEY POINTS AND ACTIONS	SCORE
Pulses	Palpate the peripheral pulses (femoral, popliteal, posterior tibial, dorsalis pedis).	0 1 –
Finishing Off	Thank the patient and offer to help them get dressed.	0 1 –
Request	Request to measure the BP and oxygen saturations, take an ECG tracing and chest x-ray of the patient (if appropriate). State you would also like to dipstick the urine and carry out fundoscopy (looking for signs of hypertension and/or endocarditis). Mention that you would review the observations chart.	0 1 –
Present	Present a structured, complete and thorough presentation and offer your differential diagnosis with investigation and management (if appropriate).	0 1 –

EXAMINER'S EVALUATION

Overall assessment of examination of the cardiovascular system	0 1 2 3 4 5

Total mark out of 41

NOTES ON THE CARDIOVASCULAR EXAMINATION FOR THE OSCE

Aortic stenosis – main indications for replacement

[European Society of Cardiology Guidelines: Valvular Heart Disease 2012]

1. Any symptomatic patient with severe AS
2. Asymptomatic severe AS undergoing CABG
3. Asymptomatic severe AS with LVEF <50% due to no other cause
4. Asymptomatic severe AS with abnormal exercise testing related to AS

**consider severe gradient >40-50mmHg or valve area <1.0cm. Beware low-flow aortic stenosis.
http://www.escardio.org/guidelines-surveys/esc-guidelines/GuidelinesDocuments/Guidelines_Valvular_Heart_Dis_FT.pdf

Anticoagulation and prosthetic valves

[European Society of Cardiology Guidelines: Valvular Heart Disease 2012]

Bioprostheses – first three months only (although controversial)

Mechanical prostheses – lifelong warfarin. Target INR between 2.5-4.0 depending on thrombogenicity of the valve and other risk factors.

EXEMPLAR PRESENTATION

'Today I examined the cardiovascular system of Mrs X, a 52-year-old florist. There was an audible valvular click at the bedside but the patient was comfortable at rest with no signs of cardiorespiratory distress. Peripherally the patient had a regular pulse with a normal volume and a medical alert bracelet. On inspection of the chest there was a midline sternotomy scar with no saphenous vein harvesting scars on the legs. On palpation the apex was non-displaced and of a normal character. The first heart sound was normal. Auscultation revealed a loud, ejection systolic murmur, loudest in the 2nd intercostal space at the right sternal edge in expiration, with radiation to both carotids. The second heart sound was loud with a metallic click. There were no diastolic murmurs. There was no peripheral or sacral oedema.

These findings are most consistent with a diagnosis of aortic prosthetic valve replacement, in this age group most likely secondary to previous rheumatic heart disease or a bicuspid valve. I would take a full history and monitor the function of the valve clinically for signs of failure including regurgitation, obtain a full blood count for anaemia and clotting, and request initial transthoracic echocardiography should there be any sign of prosthetic valve endocarditis'. ■

COMMON OSCE MURMURS

Pathology	Pulse rate	Pulse character	Apex	Systolic/Diastolic	S1	S2
Aortic stenosis	Reg	**Slow-rising	Thrusting **Displaced	Ejection Systolic	N	**Quiet
Aortic sclerosis	Reg	Normal	Normal	Ejection systolic	N	N
Aortic regurg	Reg	Collapsing (Corrigans/Watsons)	Heaving & displaced	Early diastolic	N/Soft	N
Mitral stenosis	AF often	Normal	**Tapping	Mid-to-late diastolic	?	N
Mitral regurg	Reg/AF	Normal/ pulsus alternans (HF)	**Thrusting and displaced	Pansystolic	Quiet	N
Tricuspid regurg	Reg/AF	Normal	Normal /Displaced **Left parasternal heave	Pansystolic	Quiet	N/ Loud S2
VSD	Normal	Normal/**collapsing	Normal	Pansystolic 'HARSH'	N	N
PDA	Normal	Collapsing	Normal	Continuous machinery	N	N

** Indicate severe disease

Modified Duke Criteria Endocarditis
2 MAJOR, 1 MAJOR + 3 MINOR, or 5 minor
(a pair, a full-house, or a straight)

MAJOR
1. Positive blood culture with likely organism
2. Positive echocardiogram

MINOR [mnemonic – PIPER]
1. **P**yrexia (>38°C)
2. **I**mmunological phenomena: evidence of glomerulonephritis, Osler's nodes
3. **P**ositive culture or positive serology (but not a typical organism)
4. **E**mbolic phenomena – PE, arterial, stroke, Janeway lesions
5. **R**isky patient – IVDU, known cardiac abnormality

First line investigation is a transthoracic echo (transoesophageal is more sensitive but only indicated if negative TTE).

[European Society of Cardiology: Infective Endocarditis Essential Messages 2009]

Position	Radiation	Other associations	Causes	Diagram
2nd ICS R sternal edge in expiration	Carotids	**Reversed splitting S2 Gets louder with Valsava **Progressively later peak of murmur in systole	Rheumatic heart disease, bicuspid valve	S1 / Soft S2 / EC - Ejection click
2nd ICS R sternal edge Expiration	Nil	Old age Can progress to AS over time	Age	Same as Aortic stenosis
4th ICS L sternal edge Expiration Leaning forward	Nil	Quinckes, Landolfis, Mullers, DeMussets, Corrigans, Traubes, Duroziez, **Left ventricular failure, **S3 **Austin-Flint Murmur	Rheumatic fever, bacterial endocarditis, Ankylosing spondylitis, Marfans, Syphilis	S1 / S2
Apex Expiration Left lateral position	No	Malar flush **Enlarged left atrium- Ortner's syndrome	Rheumatic heart disease	S1 Loud / S2 / Opening Snap – OS
Apex Expiration	Axilla	Left ventricular dysfunction 3-4 days post-MI secondary to papillary muscle ruptureRheumatic heart	Rheumatic heart disease, Mitral valve prolapse, endocarditis	Soft S1 / S2 / Third heart Sound – S3
4th ICS L sternal edge Inspiration (Carvallho's sign)	Mid-chest	Cannon CV waves in the JVP	Cor pulmonale- think idiopathic pulmonary hypertension, COPD, chronic VTEs and scleroderma	
4th ICS L sternal edge Expiration or inspiration (depending on shunt)	Liver	Maladie de Roger: the loudness of the murmur bears no relation to severity of defect Eisenmenger's: reversal to R>L Pulmonary hypertension	Congenital Post-MI (septum rupture)	
Mid-scapula region on back	Back	Bears no relation to the cardiac cycle May progress to heart failure (high output)	Congenital	

02.2
RESPIRATORY

INSTRUCTIONS Examine the respiratory system and present your findings as well as a differential diagnosis to the examiners.

STAGE	KEY POINTS AND ACTIONS	SCORE
	THE EXAMINATION	
Introduction **Consent**	Introduce yourself. Elicit name, age, and occupation. Establish rapport.	0 1 –
	Explain the examination to the patient and seek consent. 'The examination will involve looking at your hands, face, and legs and listening to your chest. Would that be okay'?	
Pain	Always ask about pain. 'Before we begin, do you have any pain anywhere'?	0 1 –
Position	Sit the patient at 45 degrees and expose the patient appropriately.	0 1 –
	INSPECTION	
General	Stand and observe the patient from the edge of the bed.	0 1 2

General observations in the Respiratory Examination

- **Bedside** – 'Paraphenalia of respiratory disease'; specifically oxygen masks, nebulisers, peak flow meters, inhalers (*see* box) and sputum pots
- **Body habitus** – Cachectic, Cushingoid (reflected long-term steroid use)
- **Breathing at rest** – Comfortable, dyspneoa
- **Added sounds** – Cough, wheeze, stridor
- **Presence of scars** – Thoracotomy scar, operative scars
- **Chest shape** – Barrel chest, pectus excavatum, pectus carinatum
- **Chest movements** – Asymmetrical chest expansion, use of accessory muscles
- **Intercostal recession** – Asthma, COPD (With pursed lips so-called 'auto-PEEPing')
- **Respiratory rate** – Count for 30 seconds and multiply by 2; normal 16-20 breaths per minute, tachypneoa > 20 breaths per minute.

Hands	Note the following in the hands.	0 1 2

Hand signs in the Respiratory Examination

- **Temperature** – Warm and well perfused/poor perfusion
- **Tremor** – Resting tremor (beta agonist – Salbutamol)
- **Peripheral cyanosis** – Blue nail beds
- **Nicotine stains** – Evidence of smoking
- **Clubbing** [ABCDEF] – **A**sbestosis/Abscess, **B**ronchiectasis/Bronchial Carcinoma, **C**ystic fibrosis, **D**ecreased O_2 (hypoxia), **E**mpyema, **F**ibrosing alveolitis
- **CO_2 retention** (Asterixis) – Examine for an irregular jerking of the hands after the wrists have been cocked back in wrist extension.

STAGE	KEY POINTS AND ACTIONS	SCORE
Pulse	Feel the radial pulses and assess the rate and rhythm. Assess for the presence of a bounding pulse (CO_2 retention).	
Arms	Indicate that you would like to measure the patient's blood pressure.	0 1 –
Face & Neck	Look at the eyes for signs of anaemia. Inspect the tongue for central cyanosis. Examine the jugular venous pressure looking for a raised and pulsatile JVP (cor pulmonale) or raised and fixed (SVC obstruction).	0 1 2

Fig. 2.3 **SVC syndrome**

Source: Tang T and Praveen B V. *MRCS Picture Questions Book 1.* London: Radcliffe Publishing; 2006.

PALPATION

Lymph Nodes	Sit the patient forward and palpate the lymph nodes in the cervical region and supraclavicular fossa. Observe for any enlarged lymph nodes (TB, cancer of the bronchus).	0 1 –
Trachea	Palpate the tracheal position by placing the index and ring fingers either side of the trachea and the middle finger tracing the centre. Warn the patient that it may feel uncomfortable. Determine if it is central (trachea is normally slightly deviated to the right) or deviated to one side.	0 1 –
Apex Beat	Palpate the apex beat by feeling the furthest pulsating point of the heart. It is normally located in the 5th intercostal space mid-clavicular line. Determine if the apex beat is displaced (large pleural effusion, tension pneumothorax) suggestive of lower mediastinal shift.	0 1 –
Expansion	Assess chest expansion by placing your hands on the patient's chest with the thumbs just touching in the midline and fingers spread along the ribcage. Ask the patient to breath normally and then to take deep breaths. Measure the distance between your thumbs (normal chest expansion >5cm). Note if chest expansion is bilaterally or unilaterally reduced. Palpate the upper and lower chest on the front and back.	0 1 –

PERCUSSION

Chest	Place the middle finger of one hand on the patient's chest wall in the intercostal space and percuss the centre of the middle phalanx with the middle finger or middle and index fingers of the other. Percuss the upper, middle, and lower zones, including the axilla, lateral areas, and apex, comparing the percussion note on both sides.	0 1 2

Character of percussion note

- **Stony dull** – Pleural effusion
- **Dull** – Consolidation, pulmonary fibrosis, lung collapse
- **Resonant** – Normal lung
- **Hyper-resonant** – Pneumothorax, hyperinflation (COPD)

Vocal Fremitus	Use the ulnar border of your hand to assess for vocal fremitus by asking the patient to say '1,1,1,1'. Elicit the vocal fremitus and note whether it is increased (consolidation, fibrosis), decreased (pneumothorax, COPD), or absent (collapse, effusion).	0 1 –

AUSCULTATION

Chest	With the patient relaxed, request them to breathe deeply through their mouth, demonstrating how to do so if necessary. Use a stethoscope to listen over the different lung areas mentioned above for breath sounds (bronchial breathing, vesicular breathing, absent) or added sounds (wheeze, crackles). Assess for change in the crackles with coughing or position.	0 1 2

STAGE	KEY POINTS AND ACTIONS	SCORE

Added chest sounds on auscultation
- **Wheeze** (rhonchi) – Asthma, COPD
- **Crackles** (crepitations) –
  - **Fine**: Pulmonary oedema, pulmonary fibrosis
  - **Coarse**: Bronchiectasis, pneumonia, exacerbation of COPD
  - **Early**: Pneumonia, bronchiectasis
  - **End-inspiratory**: Pulmonary fibrosis
- **Pleural rub** – Pneumonia, pulmonary embolism

Vocal Resonance
Assess vocal resonance by asking the patient to say '1,1,1,1' while listening over the lung areas.

Repeat
Sit the patient forward and repeat chest expansion, percussion, and auscultation on the back.   0 1 –

ADDITIONAL POINTS

Oedema
Examine for sacral oedema by applying firm pressure against the back and for ankle oedema by pressing down over the ankle. Observe pitting oedema by looking for an indentation of your finger after applying pressure. Ensure that you ask the patient if they feel any pain whilst pressing.
Palpate the abdomen for a pulsatile (tricuspid regurgitation) or enlarged liver (hepatic congestion) and ascites (severe right heart failure).   0 1 –

Request
Request to measure the BP and oxygen saturations, take an ECG tracing and chest x-ray of the patient (if appropriate). Mention that you would review the observations chart. Send any sputum for microbiology (Gram and Acid-fast bacilli staining [Auramine stain more commonly used than the traditional ZN stain]), culture, and cytology.   0 1 –

Present
Present a structured, complete, and thorough presentation and offer your differential diagnosis with investigation and management (if appropriate).   0 1 –

EXAMINER'S EVALUATION

Overall assessment of examination of the respiratory system   0 1 2 3 4 5

Total mark out of 28

	Pathology	Patient	Peripheral signs	Trachea	Chest expansion
COMMON OSCE CONDITIONS	Pneumonia	Unwell Tachypnoeic**	Flushed, septic**	Central	Reduced affected side
	PE	Unwell**, Tachypnoeic	Nil +/– DVT signs	Central	Normal
	COPD	Well or unwell**	Tar staining, cyanotic**, asterixis**	Enlarged cricosternal distance	Hyperexpanded, symmetrical
	Bronchiectasis	Well typically	Clubbed, nebulisers (antibiotics)	Central	Normal, maybe hyperexpanded
	Pulmonary fibrosis	Well or unwell**	Clubbed, cyanotic**	Central	Reduced bilaterally
	Pleural effusion	Well or unwell**	Nil- clubbed if empyema	Deviated away**	Decreased on affected side
	Massive collapse	Depending on cause	Nil- clubbed if carcinoma	Deviated towards	Decreased on affected side
	Pneumothorax	Well or Unwell**	Nil	Deviated away in tension	Decreased on affected side
	Pneumonectomy	Well	Depending on cause- if clubbed think of TB, bronchiectasis or carcinoma	Deviated towards	Decreased on affected side

** Indicate severe disease

EXEMPLAR PRESENTATION

'Today I examined the respiratory system of Mrs F, a 60-year-old retired deep sea diver. The patient was comfortable at rest, with no accessory muscle use, and had a respiratory rate of 14. There was a nebuliser by the bedside and a sputum pot; the sputum was mucoid and green. Peripherally the patient was clubbed, with no tar staining or cyanosis. The chest was normally expanded. The apex was non-displaced and of a normal character. Anteriorly chest expansion was equal, with a resonant percussion note throughout. Tactile vocal fremitus was equal and normal. Breath sounds were vesicular, a normal inspiratory/expiratory phase ratio with coarse crackles in the mid-zones which altered with coughing. Apices were clear. Posteriorly expansion was symmetrical, percussion note was resonant. Breath sounds were vesicular, with good air entry to the bases. There were coarse, early-inspiratory crackles of the same character from the bases to the midzones bilaterally. There was no wheeze. There was no peripheral or sacral oedema. In summary this is a well-looking 60-year-old woman productive of green sputum with a home nebuliser, with coarse, early-inspiratory crackles to the mid-zones with no signs of heart failure, COPD, or acute infection.

These findings are most consistent with a diagnosis of bronchiectasis in this age group possibly secondary to previous viral or bacterial infection. I would take a full history including risk factors for bronchiectasis, arrange a peak flow, chest x-ray, and medicines review that would inform my further management'. ∎

Sputum

- **Green:** Pneumonia (acute), abscess (chronic) COPD, bronchiectasis
- **Ask if it has changed**
- **Yellow:** Suppurative diseases as above
- **Grey/White:** Chronic smoker's sputum
- **Black:** Asbestosis
- **Rusty-gold:** Said to be typical of pneumococcal pneumonia
- **Blood stained:** Haemoptysis – think PE, TB, Goodpasture's
- **Pink, frothy:** Pulmonary oedema

Tactile fremitus	Percussion	Auscultation	Other signs
Increased affected side	Dull	Bronchial breathing, early, coarse crackles, reduced air entry	Rusty-sputum, herpetic lip ulcers (pneumococcus) +/– Pleural rub, confusion
Normal	Normal	Normal	+/– Pleural rub
Reduced (aerated lung)	Normal (hyperinflated lungs)	Prolonged expiratory phase, wheeze, +/– crackles (in infective exacerbation)	Home O2**, auto-PEEPing** Raised JVP**, peripheral oedema**, tricuspid regurgitation**
Normal	Normal	Coarse, early inspiratory crackles, usually bibasally	CF: diabetes paraphenalia, young patient RA: rheumatoid hands, nodules Green sputum
Increased	Dull in severe disease	Fine, end-inspiratory crackles, apical or bibasal depending on cause	TB: Apical fibrosis
Absent	Stony dull	Absent (bronchial breathing above fluid level), listen for pleural rub	Think effusion, haemothorax, empyema or chylothorax
Absent	Dull	Decreased	Think foreign body or bronchial obstruction (monophonic wheeze)
Absent	Hyperresonant	Decreased	Tension is a medical emergency and requires immediate Thoracostomy
Absent	Dull (filled with fluid)	Absent breath sounds	Look for lateral thoracotomy scars

02.3
ABDOMEN

INSTRUCTIONS Examine the abdominal system of this patient and present your findings as well as a differential diagnosis to the examiners.

STAGE	KEY POINTS AND ACTIONS	SCORE
	THE EXAMINATION	
Introduction	Introduce yourself. Elicit name, age, and occupation. Establish rapport.	0 1 –
Consent	Explain the examination to the patient and seek consent. 'The examination will involve looking at your hands, face, and chest and listening to and examining your stomach area. Would that be okay'?	
Position	Lie the patient flat and expose the patient appropriately from 'nipple to knee'. Maintain the patient's dignity as much as possible.	0 1 –
Pain	Ask the patient if they are comfortable and if they are in pain.	0 1 –
	INSPECTION	
General	**Bedside** – Look for fluid or diet restriction warnings, dialysis units and urinary, ascitic, or biliary catheter bags – inspect the contents.	0 1 –
	Stand and observe the patient from the edge of the bed. Look for scars, distension, masses, stoma sites (ileostomy, colostomy), hernias, discolouration, or the presence of any indwelling catheters. Note any movements including visible gastric peristalsis or pulsations.	

STAGE	KEY POINTS AND ACTIONS	SCORE

Describe the abdominal contour as flat, scaphoid (sunken abdomen), or protuberant.

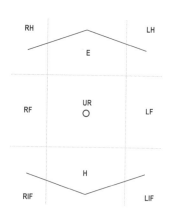

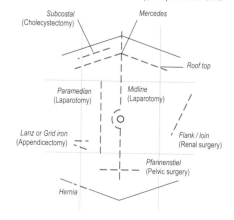

RH	Right Hypochondrium	RF	Right flank or lumbar area
RIF	Right iliac fossa	E	Epigastrium
UR	Umbilical region	H	Hypogastric or suprapubic area
LH	Left hypochondrium	LF	Left flank or lumbar area
LIF	Left iliac fossa		

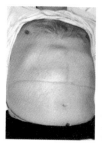

Fig. 2.4 'Mercedes Benz' scar

Source: Tang T and Praveen B V. *MRCS Picture Questions Book 2.*
London: Radcliffe Publishing; 2006.

Hands

Feel the hands and inspect the nails. Look in the hands for:

0 1 2

Hand signs in the Abdomen Examination

- **Clubbing** – Liver cirrhosis, IBD, coeliac disease, cystic fibrosis
- **Leukonychia** (whitening of the nails) – Cirrhosis, hypoalbuminaemia
- **Koilonychia** (spoon-shaped nails) – Iron deficient anaemia
- **Palmar erythema** – Chronic liver disease
- **Dupuytren's contracture** – Liver cirrhosis
- **Asterixis** – Look for a flapping tremor by asking the patient to cock back their wrist (hyperextension) with the arms outstretched (decompensated hepatic encephalopathy).
- **Scars** – Current or old fistula sites

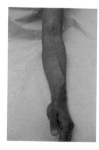

Fig. 2.5 Radiocephalic AV fistula

Source: Tang T and Praveen B V. *MRCS Picture Questions Book 2.*
London: Radcliffe Publishing; 2006.

STAGE	KEY POINTS AND ACTIONS	SCORE

Face   Look at the eyes for signs of jaundice and anaemia.

Look around the lips for brown freckles (Peutz-Jeghers syndrome).

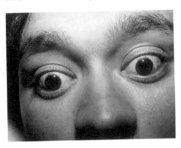

Fig. 2.6 Icteric sclera

Source: Shiv Shanker Pareek. *The Pictorial Atlas of Common Genito-Urinary Medicine*. London: Radcliffe Publishing; 2012.

Inspect the mouth for:

Signs in the Tongue in the Abdomen Examination

- **Central cyanosis** – Blue tongue
- **Macroglossia** – Hypothyroidism, acromegaly, or amyloidosis
- **Atrophic glossitis** – Iron, folate, B12 deficiency
- **Dry tongue** – Dehydration
- **Apthous ulcers** – Crohns, coeliac disease, Behcets
- **Breath** – Ketosis, ethanol, foetor hepaticus

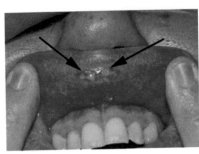

Fig. 2.7 Apthous ulcers

Source: Shiv Shanker Pareek. *The Pictorial Atlas of Common Genito-Urinary Medicine*. London: Radcliffe Publishing; 2012.

Chest/Body   Inspect the rest of the body for skin changes including Campbell de Morgan spots (normally benign, although a sudden eruption can be a sign of new malignancy), or striae and signs of chronic liver disease including spider naevi, gynaecomastia, loss of body hair (chest and axilla in men), and caput medusa (dilated collateral veins around umbilicus).

PALPATION

Lymph Nodes   Feel for cervical, axillary, and femoral lymphadenopathy. Feel especially for Virchow's node in the left supraclavicular fossa (gastric carcinoma).

0 1 –

ABDOMEN

Ask the patient if there is any tenderness in the abdomen before proceeding.

Warm your hands and examine the patient at the same level.

Without touching the patient, ask them first to distend their abdomen as fully as they can, and then to suck it in again. Ask if this is painful (early peritonism). Ask them to cough and look for obvious herniation or pain. Ask them to flex their head forward and look at their feet; this is to identify divarication of the rectus muscle.

Look at the patient's face while palpating for signs of pain.

STAGE	KEY POINTS AND ACTIONS	SCORE

Light Palpation

Palpate all quadrants of the abdomen starting away from the site of the pain.

Note any tenderness, rebound tenderness (greater pain felt on releasing pressure), guarding (reflex contraction of abdominal muscles), or rigidity. You may find distracting the patient helpful to get them to relax the abdominal muscles.

Signs on Palpation in the Abdomen Examination

- **Murphy's sign** – Apply gentle but firm pressure over the right hypochondrium and ask the patient to breathe in deeply. In acute cholecystitis the patient experiences intense pain with arrest of inspiration as the enlarged and inflamed gallbladder descends and contacts the palpating hand. Conclude the test by palpating the left hypochondrium noting absence of pain. Murphy's sign is absent in chronic cholecystitis.
- **Rovsing's sign** – Apply gentle but firm pressure in the left iliac fossa. The patient will describe that they experience more pain in the right iliac fossa than the left when doing so. Test is suggestive of acute appendicitis (distal-local sign).

Deep Palpation

Palpate all quadrants more deeply. Feel for masses and deep tenderness. If a mass is detected note its size, shape, edge, consistency, percussion note, and the presence of bowel sounds or thrills, and its movement with respiration.

Signs on Palpation in the Abdomen Examination

- **Abdominal distension** [Mnemonic—9 Fs] – **F**at, **F**aeces, **F**luid, **F**latus, **F**etus, **F**ull-sized tumours, **F**ull bladder, **F**ibroids, **F**alse pregnancy.
- **Right iliac fossa mass** – Appendix mass or abscess, caecal cancer, Crohn's disease, transplanted kidney, tuberculosis mass, actinomycosis.

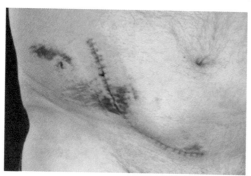

Fig. 2.8

Source: Tang T and Praveen B V. *MRCS Picture Questions Book 2*. London: Radcliffe Publishing; 2006.

Liver

Palpate the liver from the right iliac fossa. Ask the patient to take deep breaths. During inspiration, press firmly inward and upward using the flat of your hand to palpate the liver. Allow the liver edge to slip under your fingertips as the liver descends. Progressively palpate toward the costal margin. Feel for an enlarged liver, describing its edge (smooth, irregular), size (in centimetres below costal margin), consistency (soft, firm, hard), nodularity, and tenderness.

0 1 –

Spleen

Palpate the spleen from the right iliac fossa toward the left hypochondrium using the same technique as for the liver edge. The spleen should be found between the 9th and 11th ribs extending to the anterior axillary line. Remember the spleen has to be enlarged by 2-3 times before it is palpable. Feel for a notch, size, consistency, and tenderness.

0 1 –

Kidneys

Ballot the kidneys on inspiration. Position one hand beneath the patient's lower rib cage and the other hand on the surface of the abdomen. Ask the patient to breathe in deeply. Attempt to push kidney with the lower hand into the fingertips of the resting hand. Note for tenderness or enlargement.

0 1 2

STAGE	KEY POINTS AND ACTIONS	SCORE

Differentiating between the Left Kidney and enlarged Spleen

- **Splenomegaly** – Notched edge, moves early in inspiration, dull to percussion in Traube's space, cannot get above the spleen (ribs on stop), enlarges toward the RIF.
- **Left kidney** – Smooth shape, moves late in inspiration, resonant to percussion, possible to get above the kidney, directed downwards.

Aorta   Feel for an aortic aneurysm by placing two fingers along the midline above the umbilicus and feel for an expansile pulsation (distinguish from a transmitted pulse).   0   1   –

PERCUSSION

Liver   Percuss the upper and lower liver borders detecting any enlargement. Note a change of percussion from resonant to dull. Determine the upper border from the 4th intercostal space and the lower border from the costal margin. The liver should be 10cm in height.   0   1   –

Spleen   Percuss the spleen, employing a similar technique as for the liver.   0   1   –

Ascites

- **Assess for shifting dullness.** Percuss from the umbilicus toward the flanks while noting the point of dullness. Roll the patient toward you keeping your finger over the same point. Wait 30 seconds. Now percuss the marked point to see if the point of dullness has shifted. Return the patient to the supine position and check if dullness is in the same place as initial percussion.
- **Fluid thrill.** To assess for the presence of a fluid thrill, ask the patient to place his hand along the midline of his abdomen. Place the detecting hand on the patient's flank while flicking the opposite flank area with the index finger. Presence of a fluid thrill suggests severe ascites.

Bladder   Percuss the suprapubic area for dullness (bladder distension).   0   1   –

AUSCULTATION

General   Listen over the abdomen with a stethoscope for peristaltic bowel sounds. Listen for 30 seconds and establish the number of sounds heard (at least 2-3 in 30 seconds). Determine if they are hyperactive ('tinkling' – obstruction), hypoactive, or absent (general peritonitis, paralytic ileus).   0   1   –

Aorta   Auscultate over the aorta for aortic bruits (arteriosclerosis, aneurysm).

Renal Artery   Listen over the renal or femoral arteries, approximately 2-3cm superior and lateral to the umbilicus, for bruits (renal artery stenosis).

Liver   Listen over the liver for a hepatic bruit (hepatocellular carcinoma) or a hepatic rub (hepatitis, rapid liver enlargement).

ADDITIONAL POINTS

Hernias   Feel for a cough impulse over the hernial orifices as the patient coughs (see Hernia Examination).   0   1   –

Nodes   Feel for inguinal lymph nodes.

Pulses   Check for leg varicosities (new onset abdominal tumour), palpate the distal peripheral pulses. Examine the feet carefully for signs of small emboli (trash foot – indicative of abdominal aortic aneurysm).   0   1   –

Finishing Off   Thank the patient and offer to help them get dressed.   0   1   –

STAGE	KEY POINTS AND ACTIONS	SCORE
Request	Request to perform a full inguinal and scrotal examination and PR. Also request to dipstick the urine and mention that you would review the observations chart.	0 1 –
Present	Present a structured, complete, and thorough presentation and offer your differential diagnosis with investigation and management (if appropriate).	0 1 –

EXAMINER'S EVALUATION

Overall assessment of examination of the gastrointestinal system	0 1 2 3 4 5

Total mark out of 28

EXEMPLAR PRESENTATION

'Today I examined the abdominal system of Mr X, a 45-year-old pet-shop owner. The patient was comfortable at rest and pain free. There was a low potassium diet sign at the bedside. Peripherally the patient was warm, and well perfused. A 2cm scar was noted on the inner aspect of the right medial forearm. The abdomen was flat, with an obvious horizontal scar in the right iliac fossa. There was a palpable right iliac fossa mass, approximately 10cm in length, firm, non-fluctuant and non-tender, with a smooth edge. It did not move with respiration, percussion note was dull and no bowel sounds were heard over it. There were bilaterally palpably enlarged, nodular kidneys. There was no obvious hepatosplenomegaly. Bowel sounds were present, of normal character, with no ascites. There were no other scars. In summary this is a 45-year-old man with a right forearm scar, bilateral nodular large kidneys, and a right iliac fossa scar and mass.

These findings are most consistent with a diagnosis of renal transplant, with an underlying diagnosis of autosomal dominant polycystic kidney disease and previous dialysis, with reversal of the fistula in the right forearm. I would take a full history, including risk factors for renal disease and medication history, dip the urine, and order basic blood tests including full blood count, urea, and electrolytes that would inform my further management'. ∎

NOTES FOR THE ABDOMINAL EXAMINATION IN THE OSCE

Hepatomegaly

Hepatomegaly is enlargement of the liver. The normal liver is palpable in thin individuals 1cm below the right costal margin. It is smooth, uniform, non-tender, and descends to meet the palpating fingers on inspiration. An enlarged liver expands down and across toward the left iliac fossa. (Beware of Riedel's lobe, this is a normal anatomical variant with extension of the right lobe of the liver inferiorly.)

Causes of hepatomegaly

Large, smooth, and tender liver – Hepatitis, chronic heart failure, sarcoidosis, early alcoholic cirrhosis, tricuspid regurgitation with a pulsatile liver

Large, hard, and craggy liver – Primary hepatoma or secondary tumours

Note: A small liver is typical in late cirrhosis and nodular cirrhosis producing a small shrunken liver and not a large craggy one.

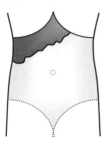

Splenomegaly

Splenomegaly is an enlarged spleen. It enlarges from the left costal margin to the right iliac fossa leading with the notched edge. An enlarged spleen may not be palpable until it is 3 times its normal size. A palpable spleen is always pathological while a spleen that can only be felt in expiration is grossly enlarged.

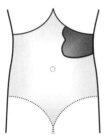

Causes of splenomegaly

Pathology	Spleen size	Associated features – history	Associated signs
Chronic myeloid leukaemia	Massive	Failure of haematopoiesis- fatigue, pale (low Hb), easy bruising, epistaxis (low platelets), recurrent infections (immunoparesis)	Lymphadenopathy (cervical, axillary and femoral) Bruising Hepatomegaly
Myelofibrosis	Massive	As above	Bruising
Malaria	Massive	Exposure to malaria zone +/–prophylaxis, time delay can be present up to a year, cyclical fevers	CNS involvement, rigors
Leishmaniasis	Massive	Kala-azar (visceral leishmaniasis) – exposure to leishmania zone, fevers	
Gauchers	Massive	Positive family history, at-risk background, failure of other organ systems (pancytopenia see above)	CNS signs Yellow/brown skin Bruising, pallor Hepatomegaly
Lymphoma	Moderate to massive	Weight loss, night sweats, B-symptoms, pain with alcohol, itching	Lymphadenopathy
TB	Moderate to massive	Dry cough, weight loss, night sweats, at-risk population	CNS signs Lymphadenopathy, apical fibrosis
Infectious mononucleosis	Mild to moderate	Fever, malaise (weeks duration), sore throat, rash, kissing contact, generally young adult population	Maculopapular rash Pharyngitis Hepatomegaly
Other haematological malignancies e.g. CLL	Mild to moderate	As CML, younger age group in general	As CML

Causes of hepatosplenomegaly

Infective – Viral hepatitis, infectious mononucleosis, CMV

Haematological – Leukaemia, myeloproliferative disease, lymphoma

Other – Amyloidosis, acromegaly, SLE

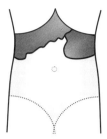

Enlarged kidneys

The kidneys are not usually palpable except in a thin individual where normal sized kidneys can be felt. The right kidney is found below the left kidney. If a kidney shows cystic qualities it is possibly due to polycystic kidney disease; if it is hard it could be due to the presence of a renal cell carcinoma. If a kidney is tender consider infection (pyelonephritis) or obstruction (hydronephrosis).

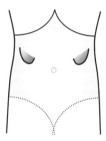

Causes of enlarged kidneys

Pathology	Unilateral/bilateral	Associated features – history	Associated signs
Polycystic kidney disease	Bilateral (often asymmetric with unilateral enlargement)	Autosomal dominant family history 30% have Berry aneurysms – history of subarachnoid haemorrhage	Bilateral, cystic enlarged kidneys Look for renal fistula and transplant kidney sites in older adults (>40)
Hydronephrosis	Unilateral/bilateral	Unilateral: Children – recurrent UTIs (vesicoureteric reflux); Adults: Urinary tract tumours (weight loss, exposure to aniline dyes, smoking) Bilateral: Children – abnormal stream (urethral valves); Adults: weight loss, fatigue (bladder cancer or other malignancy), urinary frequency and hesitance (prostate cancer/hypertrophy)	Variable with cause
Renal malignancy	Unilateral	Children: nephroblastoma (Wilms), Adults: Renal cell carcinoma, transitional cell carcinoma Weight loss, fevers (RCC especially)	Metastases to lungs Lymphadenopathy Hypercalcaemia signs (dehydrated, neuropsychiatric changes)
Perinephric abscess	Unilateral	Often secondary to obstruction Fevers, sepsis, unwell, constipation	Tender flank Fever

Ascites

Ascites is the presence of excess fluid in the peritoneal cavity. Mild ascites is often impalpable and only detectable on skilled ultrasonography. Moderate ascites leads to abdominal distension that can be palpated and detected with flank bulging and shifting dullness on physical examination, while severe ascites can be confirmed by the presence of a fluid thrill. Ascites can be broadly divided into two categories depending on its protein content and/or serum albumin ascites gradient (SAAG) which is the serum albumin concentration – ascites albumin concentration.

Common causes of ascites

Transudate (ascitic albumin <30g/L or SAAG > 11g/L)	Exudate (ascitic albumin >30g/L or SAAG <11g/L)
Liver cirrhosis, hepatitis	Malignancy (ovarian, breast, occult primary)
Constrictive pericarditis	Infective causes: Tuberculosis, pneumococcal
Renal failure (nephrotic syndrome)	Pancreatitis
Cardiac failure	Serositis (e.g. SLE)
Hepatic metastases	

**Budd-Chiari – high SAAG, high protein (due to portal hypertension)*

Liver notes:

Differential for acute liver failure
Paracetamol-induced, ETOH-induced
Infective: Hepatitis A, B, rarely E in pregnancy especially
Bacterial: Leptospirosis, severe sepsis
Vascular: Budd-Chiari, infarct
Drug-induced: methotrexate, idiosyncratic
Autoimmune: Autoimmune hepatitis, Primary biliary cirrhosis
Metabolic: Wilson's

Childs-Pugh Classification
Is for calculating prognosis in liver cirrhosis, predominantly for survival in shunt surgery. It is made up of 3 blood markers and 2 clinical findings;
Albumin
Bilirubin
Clotting – PT/INR
Distension – Ascites present/absent
Encephalopathy

A newer score, the **Model for End Stage Liver Disease (MELD)** score, consists of 3 blood markers and aetiology of cirrhosis and is used for transplant decisions.
Bilirubin
Bleeding – PT/INR
Creatinine
Cause – etiology of cirrhosis

Management of decompensated liver failure
-ABCDE approach
-Careful fluid balance – may require restriction and catheterisation in extremis
-The role of steroids is controversial
-Therapeutic paracentesis
-Careful monitoring for spontaneous bacterial peritonitis (mortality 15-20%) or variceal bleeding and hepatorenal syndrome
-Correction of clotting and electrolyte abnormalities
-Nutrition
-Ultimately, transplant if possible

Scoring system for transplant;
Kings College Criteria – Two scores exist for paracetamol and non-paracetamol induced liver failure.

02.4 CRANIAL NERVE EXAMINATION

INSTRUCTIONS Examine this patient's cranial nerves from I to XII and present your findings as well as a differential diagnosis to the examiners.

STAGE	KEY POINTS AND ACTIONS	SCORE
	THE EXAMINATION	
Introduction	Introduce yourself. Elicit name, age, and occupation. Establish rapport.	0 1 –
Consent	Explain the examination to the patient and seek consent. 'The examination will involve examining the nerves and muscles in your face, and testing your vision and hearing. Would that be okay'?	
Position	Sit the patient at 90 degrees facing directly opposite you at eye level.	0 1 –
Pain	Ask about any pain and check that the patient is comfortable.	0 1 –
	INSPECTION	
	Look for facial asymmetry, craniotomy scars, hydrocephalus. Look specifically for nasolabial fold asymmetry, ptosis, unequal pupils, and temporalis muscle wasting.	0 1 –
	Olfactory (I) Nerve	
Smell	Ask the patient if they have noticed a change in their sense of taste or smell. Offer to test these sensations using peppermint or coffee beans with their eyes shut and check whether the patient can breathe through each nostril.	0 1 –
	Optic (II) Nerve	
	[Mnemonic—AFRO-C] • Visual **A**cuity • Visual **F**ields • **R**eflexes • **O**pthalmoscopy • **C**olour Vision	
Visual Acuity	Ask the patient if they have any difficulty with their vision. Test acuity with the patient's glasses on. Test each eye separately, preferably using a proper eye occluder, avoid using the patient's hands. Ask them to read a Snellen chart at 6 metres or at 3 metres.	0 1 –

STAGE	KEY POINTS AND ACTIONS	SCORE

If the patient cannot read down to 6/6 see if this corrects with the addition of a pinhole (uncorrected refractive error; e.g. the patient needs glasses). If the largest letters on the chart can still not be read at 6 metres move the patient forward by 1 metre and repeat. Continue to do so until the letters can be read. If they are still not able to read the highest line at 1 metre away, ask the patient first to count fingers, and then perception of hand movements, and then perception of light. Legally blind is no perception of light (*see* Chapter 2.09 Eye Exam).

Near Vision

Ask the patient to read a page in a book to test near vision.

Visual Fields

Test visual field by confrontation. Sit directly opposite the patient and at the same level. Ask the patient to cover their right eye while you cover your left eye. Ask the patient to look straight into your eye. Test the outer aspects of their visual field by moving a slowly wagging finger (or white hat pin) from the periphery to the centre. Test nasal fields with the same technique. Check both eyes.

0 1 2

Blind Spot

Use the red hat pin to establish the blind spot and the presence of a central scotoma (multiple sclerosis, B12 deficiency).

Inattention

Test visual inattention by waggling two fingers simultaneously on either side of the patient's head and ask him to report whether he saw one or both move. With a parietal lobe lesion, only the ipsilateral finger to the lesion is observed.

Reflexes

Assess the 2nd and 3rd nerves together by testing the pupillary reflexes. Ask the patient to fixate on an object in the distance. Inspect the pupil size (constriction/dilatation) and shape (irregular).

0 1 2

Direct & consensual: Shine a light directly at the eye looking for a pupillary response, observing the pupillary constriction. Illuminate one eye, observing for pupillary constriction in the adjacent eye. Repeat for both eyes.

Swinging light test: Swing a light from one eye to the next, observing for sustained pupillary constriction. Interrupted constriction suggests a relative afferent pupillary defect (Marcus Gunn pupil – retina or optic nerve damage).

Common Types of Visual Defects

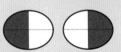

Mononuclear Field Loss
Lesions at the level of the retina cause unilateral visual loss. Causes include central retinal artery occlusion (giant cell arteritis), demyelination (multiple sclerosis), trauma and papilloedema.

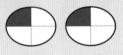

Bitemporal Hemianopia
Lesions at the chiasm classically produce a bitemporal hemianopia. They are commonly caused by pituitary adenoma, pressing on the chiasm from below, as well as craniopharyngioma, pressing from above.

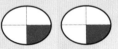

Upper Left Homonymous Quadrantanopia
Lesions in the lower fibres of the temporal radiation cause congruous upper quadrantic homonymous anopia.

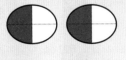

Lower Right Homonymous Quadrantanopia
Lesions in the upper fibres of the parietal radiation cause inferior quadrantic homonymous anopia without macular sparing.

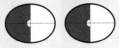

Left Homonymous Hemianopia
Lesions in the optic tract and radiation cause a contralateral homonymous hemianopia without macular sparing. Causes include a stroke (middle cerebral artery infarction), abscess or a tumour.

Left Homonymous Hemianopia (with macular sparing)
Lesions in the visual cortex produce a contralateral homonymous hemianopia with macular sparing. This is caused by a posterior cerebral artery occlusion.

STAGE	KEY POINTS AND ACTIONS	SCORE
Accommodation	Ask the patient to fixate on an object in the distance and then to look at a finger held close to the patient's face. Observe for any changes in pupillary size.	
Opthalmoscopy	State that you would like to inspect the retina using a fundoscope.	
Colour Vision	Assess colour vision by asking the patient to view a series of Ishihara plates.	

Oculomotor (III), Trochlear (IV), Abducens (VI) Nerves

STAGE	KEY POINTS AND ACTIONS	SCORE
Inspect	Ptosis (unilateral: 3rd nerve palsy, Horner's, bilateral: myotonic dystrophy, myasthenia gravis, congenital), pupil size, strabismus (squint), proptosis.	0 1 –
Slow Pursuit	Ask the patient to keep their head fixed when following your finger with their eyes. Make a sign of an 'H' with your finger. Move your finger horizontally and vertically, an arm's length distance from their face, and to a maximum of 30 degrees from the midline in either extreme. Ask the patient if they notice any double vision or pain at any time. Look for signs of nystagmus. Look specifically for lid lag with a finger drawn down quickly in the midline (hyperthyroidism).	0 1 2
Double Vision	Elicit whether the images are separated vertically or horizontally and in which direction the separation is maximal. Ask the patient to close one eye and note which image disappears. (The outer image is the false one; i.e. the eye with pathology.)	
Internuclear Opthalmoplegia	A lesion in the medial longitudinal fasciculus creates an inability to coordinate ipsilateral adduction with contralateral abduction. The patient appears to have an inability to adduct the affected eye, with contralateral nystagmus. This is most commonly seen in multiple sclerosis.	

Trigeminal (V) Nerve

STAGE	KEY POINTS AND ACTIONS	SCORE
Sensation	Ask the patient for any numbness or altered sensation (pain) in the face. Use cotton wool to test light touch in the opthalmic, maxillary, and mandibular regions. Compare the right and left areas, asking if both sensations were equal. Test sharp touch using a pin prick.	0 1 2
Corneal Reflex	State that you would test this with a wisp of cotton wool on the cornea (not sclera). Do not do this without warning the patient. The afferent arm is the ophthalmic branch of the trigeminal nerve. Efferent arm is the facial (VII) nerve.	0 1 –
Motor	Inspect the muscles of mastication for wasting and test strength by asking the patient to carry out the following commands: Clench their teeth together – Masseters/Temporalis Open mouth against resistance – Pterygoids Move the open jaw side to side – Masseters	0 1 –
Jaw Jerk	Place your index finger above the tip of the mandible with the mouth slightly open. Gently strike your finger with a tendon hammer (brisk jaw jerk – UMN).	0 1 –

Facial (VII) Nerve

STAGE	KEY POINTS AND ACTIONS	SCORE
Inspect	Facial asymmetry and asymmetrical wrinkling of the forehead (lower facial motor neurone lesion; e.g. Bell's Palsy). Remember 'upper spares upper' – in upper motor neurone lesions the upper facial muscles are relatively spared. Upper involvement therefore suggests a lower motor neurone lesion.	0 1 –

STAGE	KEY POINTS AND ACTIONS	SCORE

Types of Facial Nerve Weakness

Lower motor neurone lesion	Upper motor neurone lesion
Affects all muscles on the same side as the lesion. There is loss of frontal wrinkling, impaired blinking and eye closure with lower facial weakness. Also there is a loss of taste in anterior ⅔ of tongue. The spectrum of deficit varies with aetiology.	'Upper spares upper.' There is normal forehead and eye closure. However, there is weakness in the lower part of the face on the opposite side with sparing of the forehead as the upper part of the face is bilaterally innervated.
Causes Bell's Palsy Herpes Zoster (Ramsey-Hunt syndrome type II) Cerebellopontine angle lesion (e.g. acoustic neuromas) Lyme Disease (bilateral) Sarcoid (bilateral)	**Causes** Stroke Multiple Sclerosis Cerebral tumour

Facial Muscles

Test the muscles of facial expression by asking the patient to carry out the following commands:

Raise the eyebrows – Frontalis

Screw the eyes tight (try to open) – Orbicularis oculi

Show the teeth – Orbicularis oris

Blow out the cheeks (try to push air out)

Taste – Ask about taste in the anterior ⅔ of the tongue. Could test with ascorbic acid tablets, sugar, or salt if required.

0 1 2

Vestibular Cochlear (VIII) nerve

Hearing

Ask the patient if they have any problems with hearing. Stand behind the patient and repeat a set of letters and numbers in each ear and ask the patient to recall them. Mask the non-examined ear by rubbing your finger and thumb together in front of it at the same time. Repeat three times if the patient makes a mistake.

0 1 –

Request

State that you would like to perform the Weber's and Rinne's tests using a 512 Hz tuning fork and that you would examine the ears with an otoscope.

0 1 –

Weber's

This tests for lateralisation. Strike the tuning fork sturdily and press the end of the instrument on the middle of the patient's forehead. Ask the patient where they hear the sound the loudest (in the centre or lateralised to one side). Normally, the sound is heard equally in both ears.

Rinne's

This test compares air conduction with bone conduction. Strike the tuning fork firmly and place the end on the mastoid. Tell the patient to indicate when they no longer feel the vibrations. Remove the butt from the mastoid process and place the tuning fork near the ear without touching it. Establish whether the tuning fork can be heard. Normally air conduction is more sensitive than bone conduction and the patient should be able to still hear the tone at the ear when they could no longer hear it at the mastoid. Repeat the test on the other side.

	Rinne's (R)	Rinne's (L)	Weber's
Conductive hearing loss – Right ear	Bone conduction > Air conduction	Air conduction > Bone conduction	Loudest in right ear
Conductive hearing loss – Left ear	Air conduction > Bone conduction	Bone conduction > Air conduction	Loudest in left ear
Sensorineural hearing loss – Right ear	Air conduction > Bone conduction (quiet/absent)	Air conduction > Bone conduction	Loudest in left ear
Sensorineural hearing loss – Left ear	Air conduction > Bone conduction	Air conduction > Bone conduction (quiet/absent)	Loudest in right ear

Easy way to remember this;
1. Bone conduction should NEVER be louder than air conduction; wherever that is the case that ear is abnormal.
2. Weber's lateralises to the same ear in conductive hearing loss, and the opposite in sensorineural.

STAGE	KEY POINTS AND ACTIONS	SCORE
	Glossopharyngeal (IX) and Vagus (X) Nerves	
Gag Reflex	Indicate that you test the gag reflex by touching the posterior wall of the pharyngeal arches with an orange stick (afferent is 9th nerve, efferent is 10th nerve).	0 1 –
Uvula Deviation	Ask the patient to say 'ahh'. Using a pen torch and tongue depressor, look for the soft palate rising. The palate immediately adjacent to the uvula should rise equally. A glossopharyngeal nerve defect will therefore deviate the uvul**A A**way from the side of the lesion.	
	Hypoglossal (XII) Nerve	
Inspect	Ask the patient to open their mouth. With the aid of a torch, look at the tongue for wasting and fasciculation (LMN sign – commonly seen in motor neurone disease). Ask the patient to protrude their tongue. Observe for deviation of the tongue. The tongue will deviate to the side of the lesion. Assess the movement of the tongue as the patient waggles it from side to side.	0 1 2
	Accessory (XI) Nerve	
Inspect	Inspect for wasting of both the trapezius and sternocleidomastoid muscles.	
Resistance	Ask the patient to shrug their shoulders (trapezius) against resistance and then to turn their head against your hand (sternocleidomastoid). Remember to feel the left sternocleidomastoid when the head turns right and vice versa.	0 1 2
	ADDITIONAL POINTS	
Finishing Off	Thank the patient and offer to help them get dressed.	0 1 –
Request	Request to complete a full neurological assessment, including upper and lower limb neurology, swallow, and speech assessment.	0 1 –
Present	Present a structured, complete, and thorough presentation and offer your differential diagnosis with investigation and management (if appropriate). (*See* Chapter 2.31 for a useful structure.)	0 1 –
	EXAMINER'S EVALUATION	
	Overall assessment of examination of the cranial nerves	0 1 2 3 4 5
	Total mark out of 36	

EXEMPLAR PRESENTATION

'Today I examined the cranial nerves of Mrs F, a 40-year-old police officer. She was comfortable at rest, with no paraphernalia of neurological deficit at the bedside. She had noticed no alteration in her sense of smell, her visual acuity was 6/6 in both eyes and her visual fields were intact peripherally, but with a central scotoma present in the right eye. Pupils were equal, direct, and consensual reflexes were intact bilaterally. Accommodation reflex was normal. There was impaired adduction of both eyes, with contralateral nystagmus on lateral gaze. Eye movements were slightly painful in the right eye. Fundoscopy was not performed. Sensation and power was intact in the trigeminal nerve. There was weakness in the left facial nerve, sparing the upper face. The right side was intact. Cranial nerves eight, nine, ten, eleven, and twelve were intact. In summary, this is a 40-year-old woman with a right central scotoma and painful eye movements, an internuclear opthalmoplegia, and a left-sided upper seventh cranial nerve lesion.

These findings are most consistent with a unifying diagnosis of multiple sclerosis. I would like to take a full history, including medication review and full systems review. I would like to perform a full neurological assessment, including upper and lower limb, speech, and swallow, as well as assessing basic Activities of Daily Living. To establish a diagnosis in this case it might be appropriate to perform MRI imaging of the brain and spinal cord. I would use this information to inform my further management'. ■

NOTES ON THE CRANIAL NERVE EXAMINATION FOR THE OSCE

Bell's Palsy

Bell's palsy is a temporary palsy of the facial nerve (VII) usually caused by a viral infection, and causes unilateral paralysis of the facial muscles. It usually begins to resolve from three weeks of onset. The symptoms are quite acute and include paralysis or weakness on one side of the face (including the forehead), sagging of the eyebrow, and difficulty in closing the eye. Other less common symptoms include numbness of the face, dry mouth, difficulty in speaking, dribbling when drinking, ear pain, and impairment of taste in the anterior ⅔ of the tongue.

Common Features of Bell's Palsy
[Mnemonic – **BELL'S P**alsy]

- **B**link reflex is abnormal (mediated by the seventh)
- **E**arache
- **L**acrimation (lack of or excess)
- **L**oss of taste in anterior ⅔ of tongue
- **S**udden onset in nature
- **P**alsy of VII nerve muscles

*It is important to remember that all symptoms are unilateral to the side affected.

Horner's Syndrome

Horner's syndrome is caused by an interruption or injury to the sympathetic fibres that run to the eye. It is characterised by pupillary miosis (constriction), ptosis (drooping eyelid), and facial ipsilateral anhydrosis (dryness of the face) often with contralateral flushing. Other features include apparent enopthalmos, which can be assessed by standing behind the patient, and changes in tear viscosity. There is a huge array of causes of Horner's syndrome including interruption to the sympathetic nerve fibres from a stroke in the brain stem, injury to the carotid artery, Pancoast tumour (tumour in the apex of the lung), and cluster headaches.

Localising the lesion in Horner's

	Brainstem	Pre-ganglionic	Post-ganglionic
Features	Flushing present	Flushing present	Flushing absent Ocular/headache pain present
Differential	PICA Stroke (Wallenberg or lateral medullary syndrome) MS Malignancy Syringobulbia/syringomyelia Basal meningitis	Cervical rib Aortic aneurysm Pancoast tumour	Internal carotid artery dissection Cluster headaches

Common Features of Horner's Syndrome

[Mnemonic — **SAMPLE**]

- **S**ympathetic fibres injury
- **A**nhydrosis (ipsilateral facial dryness with contralateral flushing in pre-ganglionic and brainstem injury)
- **M**iosis (pupil constriction)
- **P**tosis (drooping eyelid)
- **L**oss of ciliospinal reflex
- **E**nopthalmos

Bulbar Palsy

Bulbar palsy results from impairment of the function of the IXth, Xth, and XIIth cranial nerves usually because of motor neurone disease, Guillain-Barré (Miller-Fisher variant) syringobulbia, or brainstem stroke. Paralysis of the lower cranial nerves affecting the tongue, muscles for swallowing, and facial muscles gives rise to symptoms including difficulty in speaking (dysarthria), choking or nasal regurgitation of foods (dysphagia), hoarseness of voice, nasal speech, and susceptibility to aspiration pneumonia (due to impaired swallow). It usually presents with features of a lower motor neurone lesion; i.e wasting and fasciculation of the tongue.

Pseudobulbar Palsy

This is more common than bulbar palsy and presents with an upper motor neurone lesion (UMN). It usually results from the degeneration of neurological pathways to the V, VII, X, XI, and XII cranial nerve nuclei. Common causes include hemispheric stroke (CVA), multiple sclerosis, and motor neurone disease (can cause both upper and lower motor signs). Symptoms include problems swallowing, husky voice ('Donald Duck' speech), immobile protruding tongue, emotional lability, brisk jaw reflexes, and UMN signs in limbs.

Cranial Nerve Syndromes

These come up in exams more than OSCEs but are useful whenever you see a collection of cranial nerve palsies.

Cranial nerves involved	Pathology	Associated features
III, IV, VI (V1)	Cavernous sinus thrombosis	Ipsilateral signs, acne
V, VII, VIII	Cerebello-pontine angle (CPA) syndrome	Acoustic neuroma (NF II), meningioma, astrocytoma
IX, X, XII	Pseudobulbar and bulbar palsies	As above
IX, X, XI	Jugular foramen syndrome	Glomus jugulare paraganglioma
Bilateral VII	May be a part of CPA syndrome or alone	Bilateral acoustic neuromas, Lyme disease, Sarcoidosis

02.5 UPPER LIMB NEUROLOGICAL EXAM

INSTRUCTIONS You will be asked to perform a neurological exam of this patient's upper limbs. Examine both the sensory and motor systems and present your findings to the examiners as well as a differential diagnosis.

STAGE	KEY POINTS AND ACTIONS	SCORE
	THE EXAMINATION	
Introduction	Introduce yourself. Elicit name, age, and occupation. Establish rapport.	0 1 –
Consent	Explain the examination to the patient and seek consent. 'The examination will involve looking at your arms, asking you to copy some movements and testing the sensation in the arms. Would that be okay'?	
Position	Sit the patient upright and expose the patient's arms adequately.	0 1 –
Pain	Before beginning the examination ask the patient if they are in pain and are comfortable.	0 1 –
Handedness	Check if the patient is left- or right-handed.	
	INSPECTION	
General	Inspect for skin and muscle signs including the presence of a tremor.	0 1 –

Observations in the Nervous System Examination

- Skin
- **Neurofibromas** (Neurofibromatosis type I) – Multiple soft nodules and tumours
- **Café au lait spots** – Oval-shaped light brown patches (Neurofibromatosis I, tuberous sclerosis)
- **Muscle wasting** – In any muscle group
- **Fasciculation** – Twitching in resting muscles
- **Tremor** – Resting, postural or action
- **Chorea** – Irregular, jerking movements
- **Athetosis** – Involuntary writhing movements
- Scars

STAGE	KEY POINTS AND ACTIONS	SCORE

Hand Signs

- **Peri-ungual fibromas** – Tuberous sclerosis
- **BM puncture marks** – Diabetes mellitus
- **Hypopigmented patches** – Vitiligo/ leprosy
- **Thickened nerves** – Leprosy, acromegaly, amyloidosis

MOTOR

Ask the patient to fully extend their arms in front of them with plantar surfaces pointing upward and eyes closed. Observe for slow pronation – unilateral pronator drift implies a pyrimadal distribution of weakness (old stroke or hemispheric insult) or if bilateral implies weakness in both arms. Look for upward motion and test rebound by gently tapping the arms down and releasing them; observe for an overcompensated upward movement. Upward drift and rebound phenomenon are signs of cerebellar disease.
[Mnemonic—**ToP RaCk**]

0 1 2

TONE

Ask the patient to relax their body and muscles; it is useful to tell them to pretend to be asleep. Passively flex and extend the wrists and elbows as well as supinating and pronating the forearm. Note the presence of increased or reduced tone.

0 1 –

Different Characters of Tone

- **Hypotonia** – LMN and cerebellar lesions
- **Spastic rigidity** – UMN (clasp knife phenomenon) (increased resistance variable with velocity of movement and direction)
- **Leadpipe** – Extrapyramidal (Parkinson's) (increased resistance independent of velocity or direction)
- **Cog-wheeling** is the combination of tremor and leadpipe rigidity.

POWER

Muscle Power

Each joint should be tested in isolation. Compare both sides in antagonistic pairs and grade them (see below). Test like-for-like; i.e. test biceps with your flexed arm, test fist power with your fists, test finger abduction with your outstretched index and little finger. Demonstrate each movement to facilitate the examination.

Shoulder Abduction (Deltoid – C5)
'Raise your elbows like wings. Don't let me push them down'.

0 1 –

Shoulder Adduction
'Now push my hands down'.

Elbow Flexion (Biceps – C6) – stabilize the joint above.
'Bring your arms up like a boxer. Pull me toward you'.

0 1 –

Elbow Extension (Triceps – C7)
'Push me away'.

0 1 –

Long Wrist Extensors (Radial nerve)
'Put your fists out like you're riding a bike. Don't let me push them down'.

0 1 –

Long Wrist Flexors
'Now push my fists down'.

Finger Extension (Extensor digitorum – C7)
'Extend your fingers and stop me from pushing down'.

0 1 –

STAGE	KEY POINTS AND ACTIONS	SCORE
	Finger Flexion (Grip – C8) 'Clasp my fingers and squeeze them as hard as possible'.	0 1 –
	Finger Abduction (Dorsal interossei muscles – T1/Ulnar nerve) 'Spread your fingers like you're playing the piano. Keep them spread and don't let me close them'.	0 1 –
	Thumb Abduction (Abductor pollicis brevis – T1/Median nerve) 'Turn your palms up. Now raise your thumb to the ceiling; don't let me push it down'.	0 1 –
Power Grading	Grade the power of each muscle according to its strength as detailed below. **Medical Research Council (MRC) Scale for Muscle Power** • 0 – No visible muscle contraction • 1 – Flicker of muscle contraction only • 2 – Movement of muscle at joint only when gravity is eliminated • 3 – Movement of muscle at joint against gravity but not against resistance • 4 – Movement against resistance but incomplete • 5 – Normal power	
	REFLEXES	
Elicit Reflexes	Have the patient lying comfortably with their hands resting loosely over their abdomen. Use a tendon hammer to elicit the reflexes and compare both sides. For an absent reflex use the reinforcement technique (Jendrassik) by asking the patient to clench their teeth.	0 1 2
Biceps	Place the thumb over the biceps tendon and strike it with the patella hammer (Biceps reflex – C5, C6).	
Brachioradialis (Supinator)	Locate the supinator tendon on the radial margin of the extensor surface forearm just above the wrist, observe a slight supination of the forearm (Brachioradialis reflex – C5, C6).	
Triceps	Have the elbow flexed to 90 degrees and strike the triceps tendon located just above the elbow (Triceps reflex – C7).	
Hoffmann's Reflex	Flick the nail base of the middle finger between your thumb and index finger and observe for involuntary flexion of their thumb. Positive – seen in upper motor neurone disease and some normal individuals.	0 1 2
	Grading Reflexes • 0 Completely absent • +/– Present only with reinforcement • 1 or + A hypoactive slight jerk • 2 or ++ A normal average response • 3 or +++ A hyperactive reflex not associated with clonus • 4 or ++++ An extremely hyperactive reflex associated with clonus	
	CO-ORDINATION	
Finger-Nose	Perform the finger-nose test by asking the patient to touch his nose and then your finger at an arm's length from the patient as fast as possible, looking for an intention tremor and past pointing (dysmetria).	0 1 –
Dysdiachokinesia	Ask the patient to clap their hands and then to clap again but alternating one hand between the palmar and dorsal surfaces. Repeat the test with the other hand testing for dysdiachokinesia (cerebellar disorder).	0 1 –

STAGE	KEY POINTS AND ACTIONS	SCORE

Upper & Lower Motor Neurone Signs

- **Lower Motor Neurone Signs** – Wasting, fasciculation, hypotonia, muscle weakness, depressed or absent reflexes
- **Upper Motor Neurone Signs** – Spasticity, brisk reflexes, muscle weakness, clonus (>5 beats), extensor plantar response, positive Hoffmann's reflex, depressed abdominal response

[handwritten: → flick nail down]
[handwritten: absent ...]
[handwritten: ⓂⒷ thumb + index]

SENSATION

Light Touch
(Dorsal Column)

Before you begin examining the patient, ask if they have any numbness, pins and needles (paraesthesia), or pain. If present ask the patient to demarcate the areas. **0 1 2**

Ask the patient to close their eyes, so that they are unable to obtain any visual clues, and ask them to respond verbally to each touch. Apply a wisp of cotton wool to the sternum (as a reference point) and ask if they are able to sense it. Ideally use a 10g monofilament–press it into the skin until it bends–this is a consistent method of delivering pressure at 10g, and therefore reproducible between examiners. Then apply the cotton wool to the dermatomes within the arms. Have the patient's palms facing upward. Compare both sides symmetrically. Always start distally, working proximally.

Check for glove and stocking distribution (peripheral neuropathy – commonest causes diabetes, ETOH). If there is any sensory loss attempt to identify dermatomal versus peripheral nerve distribution.

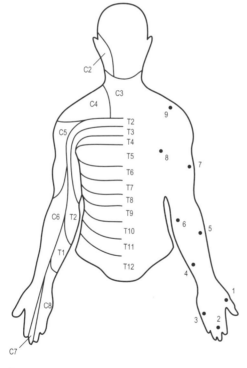

Sensory Dermatome Distribution
Anterior surface of the upper body. The points suggest the areas to test for disturbances.

1.	Thumb & 1st finger	C6
2.	Middle finger	C7
3.	Fourth & fifth digits	C8
4.	Med distal forearm	T1
5.	Lateral forearm	C6
6.	Med prox. forearm	T2
7.	Lateral arm	C5
8.	Armpit	T3
9.	Shoulder	C4

Peripheral Nerves

- **Median nerve** – Over the thenar eminence
- **Radial nerve** – Over the anatomical snuff box (dorsum of the hand at the base of the thumb between the tendons of extensor pollicis longus and extensor pollicis brevis with abductor pollicis longus)
- **Ulnar nerve** – Over the hypothenar eminence

STAGE	KEY POINTS AND ACTIONS	SCORE
Pain (Sharp Touch or Pin Prick) *(Spinothalamic Tract)*	Request to test pain sensation using a neurological pin; the standard in most hospitals is a disposable neurotip. Dispose of it in the sharps bin when you are finished. Ask the patient to close their eyes and apply a pin to the sternum then to the dermatomes, comparing both sides as demonstrated above. Ask the patient to state if the sensation changes, becoming more blunt (hypoaesthesia) or more painful (hyperaesthesia). If there is any abnormality delineate the loss by testing distally and working proximally. Map out any area of abnormal sensation and determine the type of distribution. Test specifically for dermatomal, peripheral nerve, or glove-and-stocking distributions. Compare both sides.	0 1 2
Proprioception *(Dorsal Column)*	Hold the distal interphalangeal joint of the index finger *by its sides* with your thumb and forefinger of one hand and move the distal phalanx up and down with the other hand while describing its direction; i.e. up or down. Next ask the patient to close their eyes whilst moving the distal phalanx and request them to identify its direction. Repeat the test up to three times while comparing both sides. If unsuccessful or the responses are inaccurate, test the proximal interphalangeal joint (IPJ), moving to the metacarpophalangeal (MCO) joints, wrist joints, elbow, and then shoulder if each is impaired.	0 1 2
Vibration Sense *(Dorsal Column)*	Ask the patient to close their eyes. Apply a vibrating 128Hz *(mnemonic – 12eight-vibrate)* tuning fork over the sternum. Then place it over a bony prominence of the upper limbs (interphalangeal joint of thumb). Ask the patient to identify when the fork begins to vibrate and when the vibration stops. Compare both sides. If unsuccessful, test the MCP joint of the thumb, moving to the wrist and elbow if each is impaired.	0 1 2
Temperature *(Spinothalamic Tract)*	Ask the patient if the vibrating tuning fork feels cold.	0 1 –

ADDITIONAL POINTS

STAGE	KEY POINTS AND ACTIONS	SCORE
Two-Point Discrimination	Test ideally using a specific 2-point discriminator, but if not, then two monofilaments or neurotips at a set distance apart. Place both pins or one on the patient's skin and ask if one point or two is felt. Normally two discrete points can be felt at a distance of 3-5mm apart.	0 1 –
Neglect	Using light or sharp touch, test both sides in comparable positions at the same time. Ask on which side sensation was felt. A normal response is both. Parietal lobe lesions can be subtly detected if there is relative neglect; attention is only paid to the non-affected side when both are touched.	0 1 –
Finishing Off	Thank the patient and offer to help them get dressed. Offer to examine the lower limbs.	0 1 –
Request	Request to measure the BM, examine the lower limbs, gait, cranial nerves and speech, and Mini Mental State Examination.	0 1 –
Present	Present a structured, complete, and thorough presentation and offer your differential diagnosis with investigation and management (if appropriate). *(See Chapter 2.31 for a useful structure.)*	0 1 –

EXAMINER'S EVALUATION

Overall assessment of examination of the neurological system of the upper limb	0 1 2 3 4 5
Total mark out of 40	

EXEMPLAR PRESENTATION

'Today I examined the neurological system in the upper limbs of Mr X, a 74-year-old, right-handed, retired sound engineer. He was comfortable at rest, with a wheeled walker at the bedside. On inspection there was nasolabial asymmetry, with weakness on the right and the upper limb was held in flexion at the shoulder and elbow with the right hand held with fingers flexed. The lower limb was held in extension at the hip, knee, and ankle. This pattern is consistent with a pyramidal distribution of weakness. On inspection of the upper limb there was no slight asymmetry of muscle bulk in the right arm versus the left, and no visible rashes, fasciculations, or scars. Tone was markedly increased in the right arm compared to the left, with clasp knife spasticity present. Power in the left arm was 5/5 throughout. Power in the right arm was 4/5 in shoulder abduction and 3/5 in adduction, 4/5 in elbow flexion and 3/5 in elbow extension, and 4/5 in wrist extension and flexion. Power grip was much reduced, 3/5. Reflexes were normal in the left arm, and hypertonic on the right. Co-ordination was much impaired due to weakness in the right arm, and normal on the left. On examining sensation light touch, vibration sense, and proprioception were reduced in the right arm compared to the left, as were sharp touch and temperature sensation. In summary, this is a 74-year-old man with a pyramidal distribution of weakness on the right, with decreased power and increased tone in the right upper limb and normal sensation.

These findings are most consistent with a diagnosis of middle cerebral artery territory stroke – some time previously due to the development of hypertonicity. I would like to take a full history, including medication review and full systems review. I would like to complete a full neurological assessment, including upper and lower limb, speech and swallow, as well as assessing basic Activities of Daily Living. Management in this case is primarily supportive and rehabilitative in a multidisciplinary approach including GPs, physiotherapists, occupational therapists, dieticians, and speech and language therapists. Secondary prevention includes antiplatelet therapy, smoking cessation, and investigation and treatment of carotid artery stenosis and atrial fibrillation'. ■

Notes on the upper limb examination for the OSCE

The common exam scenarios you may come across and the individual signs to point you toward them:

Condition	Inspection	Tone	Power	Co-ordination	Reflexes	Sensation	Special tests
Multiple sclerosis	Variable depending on syndrome	Increased/ normal	Reduced/ normal	Impaired – cerebellar signs (*see below*)	Hypertonic/ normal	Spinal syndrome – impaired, band-like level/normal	Lhermitte's Sign – lean the patient's head back – sensation of shooting pain down spine, painful eye movements in optic neuritis
MCA stroke	Late – arms tonic and weak in a pyramidal distribution**	**Early** – hypotonia **Late** – increased	Decreased affected side	Impaired due to weakness	Late – hypertonic	Normal	Face and leg weakness Hoffmann's reflex Impaired speech in left MCA stroke
ACA stroke	Arms > Legs/Face	As above	As above	As above	As above	Normal	As above
Parkinson's	Resting tremor Hypokinetic facies	Leadpipe rigidity Cogwheeling (rigidity + tremor)	Normal/ Reduced in severe	Resting tremor, hypokinetic movements	Normal	Normal	Hypokinetic faces Glabellar tap reflex Festinant gait Slow turn Micrographia
Peripheral neuropathy	BM marks, hypopigmented spots	Normal	Normal	Propioceptive loss (Ask patient to close eyes)	Impaired in severe disease	Impaired – glove and stocking, distal > proximal	Depending on cause

*(UL flexors stronger > extensors, LL extensors stronger > flexors)

02.6 LOWER LIMB NEUROLOGICAL EXAMINATION

INSTRUCTIONS You will be asked to examine the neurological system of the patient's lower limbs. Present your findings as well as a differential diagnosis to the examiners.

STAGE	KEY POINTS AND ACTIONS	SCORE
	THE EXAMINATION	
Introduction	Introduce yourself. Elicit name, age, and occupation. Establish rapport.	0 1 –
Consent	Explain the examination to the patient and seek consent. 'The examination will involve looking at your legs, asking you to copy some movements, and checking the sensation in the lower limbs. Would that be okay'?	
Position	Sit the patient at 45 degrees and expose the patient appropriately from waist down. Preserve their dignity as much as possible.	0 1 –
Pain	Before beginning the examination ask the patient if they are in pain and are comfortable.	0 1 –
	INSPECTION	

Observations in the Nervous System Examination

- Skin
- **Neurofibromas (Neurofibromatosis I)** – Multiple soft nodules and tumours
- **Café au lait spots** – Oval-shaped light brown patches (Neurofibromatosis I, tuberous sclerosis)
- **Muscle wasting** – In any muscle group
- **Fasciculations** – Twitching in resting muscles
- **Tremor** – Resting or intentional
- **Chorea** – Irregular, jerking movements
- **Scars**
- **Hypopigmented patches** – Vitiligo / leprosy
- **Thickened nerves** – Leprosy, acromegaly, amyloid

STAGE	KEY POINTS AND ACTIONS	SCORE

MOTOR

[Mnemonic — **T**o**P** Ra**C**k]

TONE

Test Tone — Ask the patient to relax their body and muscles – it is useful to tell them to pretend to be asleep. Roll each leg on the couch and quickly flex the knee by lifting it off the bed. It is important to vary the rate and amplitude of your movements. Note the presence of increased tone or reduced tone. | 0 1 –

Clonus — Elicit ankle clonus by sharply dorsiflexing the foot with one hand while supporting the flexed knee with the other. More than 3-5 beats of clonus is abnormal (upper motor neurone). Warn the patient first, and check specifically for ankle pain beforehand.

POWER

Muscle Power — Each joint should be tested in isolation. Compare both sides in antagonistic pairs and grade them (see below). It is difficult to test like-for-like in the lower limbs. Remember that gait is a better test of power, especially of ankle dorsiflexion and plantarflexion.

Hip Flexion (Iliopsoas – L1/2)
'Raise your leg straight off the bed'. Place hand on thigh. 'Keep it there, don't let me push you down'. | 0 1 –

Hip Extension (Gluteus maximus – S1)
Place hand under thigh. 'Now push me down'. | 0 1 –

Knee Extensors (Quadriceps- L3/4)
'Bend your knee'. Place one hand on the ankle and the other on the knee. 'Push my hand away'. | 0 1 –

Knee Flexion (Hamstrings – L5, S1)
'Now pull my hand toward you'. | 0 1 –

Ankle Dorsiflexion (Tibialis anterior – L4)
Hold patient's medial and lateral malleoli with one hand. Place ulnar part of the other hand against the dorsal aspect of the foot. 'Push your foot up against my hand'. | 0 1 –

Ankle Plantarflexion (Gastrocnemius & Soleus – S1)
Place ulnar part of the hand against the plantar aspect of the foot. 'Push down against my hand'. | 0 1 –

Big Toe Extension (Extensor hallucis longus – L5)
Place finger against the dorsal aspect of the big toe. 'Push your toe up against my finger'. | 0 1 –

Power Grading — Grade the power of each muscle according to its strength against resistance, against gravity, and whether fasciculations are visible.

REFLEXES

Elicit Reflexes — Have the patient lying comfortably on the couch. Use a tendon hammer to elicit the reflexes and compare both sides. For an absent reflex use the reinforcement technique (Jendrassik) by asking the patient to clench their teeth or to interlock their fingers and tighten them. | 0 1 2

Knee — Have the patient's knees flexed to 60 degrees and resting on top of the examiner's arm. Strike the patella tendon to obtain a knee jerk (knee reflex – L3, L4).

STAGE	KEY POINTS AND ACTIONS	SCORE
Ankle	Have the patient's leg abducted and externally rotated at the hip while flexed at the knee and ankle. Alternatively, ask the patient to kneel on a chair while standing facing away from you, with ankles dangling freely. Strike the Achilles tendon to obtain an ankle jerk (ankle reflex – S1, S2).	
Plantar Response (Babinski)	Elicit a plantar response by scraping the lateral plantar surface of the patient's foot with an orange stick. A normal response is flexion of the big toe (downgoing plantar response). Extension of the big toe (upgoing plantar response) is always abnormal in adults and is an upper motor neurone sign.	0 1 –
Nerve Root Supply for Tendon Reflexes	**[Mnemonic – 1234567]** • **One, two**, buckle my shoe – S1, 2 – ankle reflex • **Three, four**, kick the door – L3, 4 – knee reflex • **Five, six**, pick up sticks – C5, 6 – biceps and brachioradialis • **Seven, eight**, shut the gate – C7 – triceps reflex	
	CO-ORDINATION	
Heel/Shin	Ask the patient to run their left heel over their right shin (from knee down to ankle) and then up to touch your hand. Repeat the test on the other leg. Observe for jerky motion, difficulty hitting targets, tremor, or initiating movement.	0 1 –
Gait	Ask the patient to walk to the end of the room, turn around, and return. Observe the gait, commenting on the type of gait and presence of arm swing. Ask the patient to walk heel-to-toe (cerebellar function), on heels, and tip-toes (true tests of power of dorsi and plantarflexion).	0 1 –
Romberg's Test	Have the patient standing upright, feet together, with eyes open. Stand nearby with your arms encircling them, reassuring them they won't fall. Observe for unsteadiness. Then ask the patient to close their eyes. Observe if the patient is less stable (positive Romberg's test – propioceptive loss).	
	Upper & Lower Motor Neurone Signs • **Lower Motor Neurone Signs** – Wasting, fasciculation, hypotonia, muscle weakness, depressed or absent reflexes • **Upper Motor Neurone Signs** – Spasticity, brisk reflexes, muscle weakness, clonus (>5 beats), extensor plantar response, positive Hoffmann's reflex, depressed abdominal response	
	SENSATION	
Light Touch *(Dorsal Column)*	Before you begin examining the patient, ask if they have any numbness, pins and needles (paraesthesia), or pain. If present ask the patient to demarcate the areas.	0 1 –
	Ask the patient to close their eyes, so that they are unable to obtain any visual clues, and ask them to respond verbally to each touch. Apply a wisp of cotton wool to the sternum (as a reference point) and ask if they are able to sense it. Ideally use a 10g monofilament–press it into the skin until it bends–this is a consistent method of delivering pressure at 10g, and therefore reproducible between examiners. Then apply the cotton wool to the dermatomes within the legs. Compare both sides symmetrically. Always start distally, working proximally. Check for glove and stocking distribution (peripheral neuropathy – commonest causes diabetes, ETOH).	

STAGE	KEY POINTS AND ACTIONS	SCORE

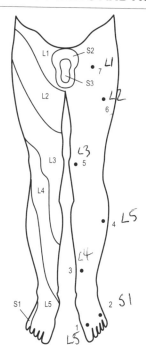

Sensory Dermatome Distribution
Anterior surface of the lower body. The points suggest the areas to test for disturbances.

1.	Big toe - 4th digit	L5
2.	Little toe	S1
3.	Med distal lower leg	L4
4.	Lat proximal lower leg	L5
5.	Med distal thigh	L3
6.	Lat proximal thigh	L2
7.	Inner thigh (groin)	L1

Pain (Sharp Touch or Pin Prick) *(Spinothalamic Tract)*

Request to test pain sensation using a neurological pin; the standard in most hospitals is a disposable neurotip. Dispose of it in the sharps bin when you are finished. Ask the patient to close their eyes and apply a pin to the sternum then to the dermatomes, comparing both sides as demonstrated above. Ask the patient to state if the sensation changes, becoming more blunt (hypoaesthesia) or more painful (hyperaesthesia). If there is any abnormality delineate the loss by testing distally and working proximally. Map out any area of abnormal sensation and determine the type of distribution. Test specifically for dermatomal, peripheral nerve, or glove and stocking distributions. Compare both sides.

0   1   2

Proprioception *(Dorsal Column)*

Hold the distal interphalangeal joint of the big toe by its sides with your thumb and forefinger of one hand and move the distal phalanx up and down with the other hand while describing its direction; i.e. up or down. Next ask the patient to close their eyes whilst moving the distal phalanx and request them to identify its direction. Repeat the test up to three times while comparing both sides. If unsuccessful or the responses are inaccurate, move to the metatarsophalangeal joint (MTPJ), and then the knee joint if each is impaired.

0   1   2

Vibration Sense *(Dorsal Column)*

Ask the patient to close their eyes. Apply a vibrating 128Hz [mnemonic—12eight-vibrate] tuning fork over the sternum. Then place it over a distal bony prominence, i.e. the metatarsophalangeal joint of the big toe. Ask the patient to identify when the fork begins to vibrate and when the tuning fork stops. Compare both sides. If unsuccessful, test the medial malleolus, tibial shaft, knee, hip, and then sternum.

0   1   2

Temperature *(Spinothalamic Tract)*

Ask the patient if the vibrating tuning fork feels cold.

0   1   –

ADDITIONAL POINTS

Two-Point Discrimination

Test ideally using a specific two-point discriminator, but if not, then two monofilaments or neurotips at a set distance apart. Place both pins or one on the patient's skin and ask if one point or two is felt. Normally two discrete points can be felt at a distance of 3-5mm apart.

0   1   –

STAGE	KEY POINTS AND ACTIONS	SCORE
Neglect	Using light or sharp touch, test both sides in comparable positions at the same time. Ask on which side sensation was felt. A normal response is both. Parietal lobe lesions can be subtly detected if there is relative neglect – attention is only paid to the non-affected side when both are touched.	0 1 –
Finishing Off	Thank the patient and offer to help them get dressed.	0 1 –
Request	Request to measure the BM, examine the upper limbs, gait, cranial nerves and speech, and Mini Mental State Examination.	0 1 –
Present	Present a structured, complete, and thorough presentation and offer your differential diagnosis with investigation and management (if appropriate). (See Chapter 2.31 for a useful structure.)	0 1 –

EXAMINER'S EVALUATION

Overall assessment of examination of the neurological system of the lower limb	0 1 2 3 4 5
Total mark out of 34	

EXEMPLAR PRESENTATION

'Today I examined the neurological system of the lower limb of Mr D, a 32-year-old graphic designer. Around the bedside were two crutches. The patient appeared comfortable at rest, with obvious facial asymmetry, muscle wasting, scar, rashes, or fasciculations. Tone in the lower limbs was markedly increased bilaterally, with >5 beats of clonus left and right. Power was reduced in all muscle groups bilaterally to 4/5. Reflexes were brisk at the knee and ankle, and plantars were upgoing bilaterally. Sensation was intact, in light touch, vibration, and proprioception bilaterally, and temperature and sharp touch. There was a scissor gait, requiring crutch support and difficulty with turning. Romberg's test could not be performed due to lack of power. In summary this is a 32-year-old gentleman with a bilateral upper motor neurone deficit in the lower limbs, scissoring gait requiring crutch support, and intact sensory examination. Given the crutch use the upper limbs appear relatively intact, therefore these findings are most consistent with a diagnosis of a spastic diplegia – the most common cause in this age group would be cerebral palsy.

My differential diagnosis would include thoracic to lumbar spinal cord injury, anterior spinal artery infarct, and sagittal meningioma, although all of these except the last would have some sensory level. I would like to take a full medical history, including medications and Activities of Daily Living, complete a full neurological examination including the upper limbs, speech, swallow, and MMSE. Management in this case is supportive, and multidisciplinary in nature, involving GP, physiotherapy, and occupational therapy'. ∎

NOTES ON THE NEUROLOGICAL EXAMINATION OF THE LOWER LIMB

Sensory deficits

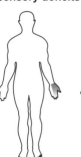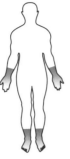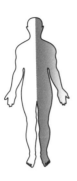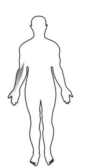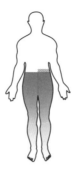

Mononeuropathy	Polyneuropathy	Hemisensory loss	Spinal root lesion	Dissociated sensory loss
Carpal tunnel syndrome	Diabetes	Stroke, brain tumour	Herniated disc, OA	Brown-Séquard lesion

Mononeuropathy

Mononeuropathy involves damage to or destruction of an isolated nerve. It is most often caused by damage to a local area resulting from injury or trauma, although systemic disorders such as diabetes, sarcoidosis, and rheumatoid arthritis can also cause it. If more than two peripheral nerves are affected it is known as mononeuritis multiplex, typically associated with vasculitis. Symptoms include pain, numbness, and diminution of all sensory modalities to the area the nerve supplies. There may also be muscle weakness in the corresponding muscle groups; i.e. median nerve (C6-T1), ulnar nerve (C7-T1), and radial nerve (C5-T1).

Polyneuropathy

Polyneuropathy is the simultaneous damage or destruction of many peripheral nerves affected throughout the body. It may develop acutely or gradually depending on the cause. It is usually a diffuse symmetrical disease of the peripheral nerves affecting the distal parts of the limbs classically in the 'glove and stocking' distribution. Often in polyneuropathies the legs are affected before the hands due to the length-dependant process of most causes (see below). The sensory loss may progressively extend proximally from the extremities. Polyneuropathies can involve motor, sensory, and autonomic function. Symptoms depend on the nerves affect and include pain, paraesthesia, or numbness in the glove and stocking distribution as well as weakness of distal muscles, unsteadiness of feet (due to proprioceptive loss), and lower motor neurone signs. There may be autonomic features such as postural hypotension, constipation, diarrhoea, impaired pupillary responses, impotence, urinary retention, and diminished sweating.

Causes of Polyneuropathy

[Mnemonic—**ABCDEFGH**]

- **A**lcohol
- **B** vitamin deficiency (B1 [Thiamine], B6 [Niacin], B12 [Hydroxycobalamin])
- **C**ancer/**C**onnective tissue disease (paraneoplastic; e.g. SLE) CKO
- **D**iabetes mellitus/**D**rugs (nitrofurantoin, isoniazid, phenytoin, metronidazole)
- **E**ndocrine (hypothyroidism)
- **F**riedreich's Ataxia
- **G**uillain-Barré syndrome (proprioception and areflexia > spinothalamic loss)
- **H**ereditary motor sensory neuropathy (e.g. Charcot-Marie-Tooth)

Hemisensory loss

Hemisensory loss is the loss of sensation including pain, temperature, vibration sense, and joint position sense affecting one side of the body. The most common cause is stroke, which normally presents with an array of symptoms including hemiplegia to one side of the body. Symptoms are usually on the contralateral side to the lesion.

Spinal root lesions (Radiculopathy)

Spinal cord lesions at any level tend to produce sensory and motor loss over areas of the body below the level of the lesion. In contrast, spinal root lesions at one level are restricted to a single dermatome and myotome. Pain, paraesthesia, and numbness are often the chief complaint, with symptoms limited to a particular dermatome which the spinal root supplies. Other symptoms include weakness to the muscles supplied by the spinal root with lower motor neurone signs such as hyporeflexia, hypotonia, and atrophy. Causes include herniated intervertebral discs, degenerative disc disease, and osteoarthritis.

Bilateral and Dissociated Sensory Loss of the Legs

A bilateral sensory loss distribution confined to the legs is synonymous with a spinal cord lesion below the level of T1. There may be loss of all the sensory modalities as well as muscle paralysis in the legs. Often the level of the sensory loss is indicative of the vertebral level of the spinal lesion. Brown-Séquard syndrome, on the other hand, is a unilateral spinal cord lesion that causes dissociated sensory loss. Spinal trauma accounts for the vast majority of cases, with spinal neoplasms, infections, and multiple sclerosis rounding out the differential. It presents with ipsilateral loss of light touch, vibration sense, and motor function (spastic paralysis) at the level of the lesion and contralateral loss of pain and temperature sense beginning just below the level of the lesion (due to the spinothalamic tract decussating a few segments above entering the spinal cord). These symptoms can be explained by taking into account the distribution of the corticospinal, dorsal column, and spinothalamic tract and the level at which they cross the midline in the spinal cord. Other features include a localised zone of hyperpathia with lower motor neurone signs often at the same level and ipsilateral to the lesion. Some other types of spinal cord lesions can cause dissociated sensory loss such as syringomyelia. This results in the loss of pain and temperature sensation but preservation of joint position and vibration sense below the level of the lesion. Dorsal column lesions cause loss of joint position and vibration sense but retain temperature and pain sensation (e.g. tabes dorsalis – tertiary syphilis).

Motor
[handwritten annotation: Genetic cysts in spinal cord]

Clinical syndrome	Site of the lesion	Differential	Presenting features	Associations
Monoplegia – paralysis of a single limb	Peripheral spinal nerves – cortical, root or plexus lesion	Brachial plexus: Erb's paralysis – C5/6, Klumpke's – C8/T1 Pelvic paralysis – L4-S2 nerve or lumbosacral plexus	Erb's: 'Waiters tip' posture Klumpke's: Claw hand Pelvis injury – 'sciatica' distribution of weakness Common peroneal nerve: foot drop ALL LMN signs: wasting, fasciculations, areflexia	Erb's: Shoulder dystocia Klumpke's: trauma Sciatic nerve injury: hip replacement Common peroneal nerve: plaster casts, ITU stay
Hemiplegia: complete paralysis affecting one half of the body	Corticospinal tract *Thalamus* *Brainstem*	Middle cerebral artery stroke > Anterior cerebral artery Thalamic/Brainstem stroke Other: subdural haematoma, brain abscess, multiple sclerosis, space-occupying lesion	Contralateral upper motor neurone weakness, pyramidal distribution of weakness (upper limb flexed, lower limb extended) ALL UMN signs: brisk reflexes, hypertonia	
Paraplegia: complete paralysis of both legs	Spinal cord (compression > infarct) Cerebral hemispheres	Spastic: spinal cord compression (<T1) Parasagittal meningioma Anterior spinal artery infarct, cerebral palsy, MS, motor neurone disease, spinal cord tumours, syringomyelia, subacute combined degeneration of the spinal cord Flaccid: cauda equina, below L1/L2 (LMN)	Spastic: UMN signs Cauda equina: LMN signs, wasting, fasciculation and areflexia, painless urinary retention, constipation, and perineal numbness Spinal cord lesion: usually associated with a sensory level	SACD: optic atrophy, glossitis, peripheral neuropathy MS: cerebellar signs, optic neuritis MND: fasciculations, cranial nerve involvement Syringomyelia: dissociated spinothalamic loss
Quadriplegia (paralysis of all four limbs)	High spinal cord compression (<C3/C4) Brainstem lesion ('locked in' syndrome)	Trauma Cervical spondylosis Brainstem infarct	UMN signs: spastic paralysis in all limbs, absent sensation throughout	
Myopathies and dystrophies	Muscle/ Neuromuscular junction	Congenital: Duchennes/ Beckers/ fascioscapulohumeral Autoimmune: polymyositis, polymyalgia rheumatica Other: hypothyroidism, statin induced	Typically proximal > distal muscle weakness (exception inclusion body myositis distal > proximal)	DM: X-linked recessive, early in childhood, difficulty in standing Beckers: similar to DM but milder course FSHMD – AD, early teens, winged scapulae and facial weakness, shoulder and pelvic girdle PMR: associated with giant cell arteritis
Mixed UMN and LMN signs	Predominantly spinal pathologies	[Mnemonic—**F**red's **T**abby **C**at **S**eeks **M**ice] **F**riedrich's Ataxia **T**aboparesis (syphilis) **C**onus medullaris (cervical spondylosis) **S**ubacute Combined Degeneration of the Spinal Cord **M**otor neurone disease (ALS)	Mixed LMN and UMN signs, usually in the legs Friedrich's Ataxia: young patient, with cerebellar signs Taboparesis: older patient, dorsal column loss MND: no sensory component	FA: visual impairment, cardiac involvement, dorsal column loss SACD: as above MND: as above

02.7
CEREBELLAR EXAM

INSTRUCTIONS You will be asked to examine the cerebellar system of this patient. Please present your findings as well as a differential diagnosis to the examiners.

STAGE	KEY POINTS AND ACTIONS	SCORE
	THE EXAMINATION	
Introduction	Introduce yourself. Elicit name, age, and occupation. Establish rapport.	0 1 –
Consent	Explain the examination to the patient and seek consent. 'The examination will involve listening to your speech, looking at the movements of your arms and walking, and testing your reflexes. Would that be okay'?	
Position	Sit the patient upright initially.	0 1 –
Pain	Check the patient is comfortable and not in any pain.	0 1 –
	INSPECTION	
	[Mnemonic for examination—**DANISH-P**astry]	
Dysdiachokinesia	Ask the patient to hold their left hand out with the palm facing the ceiling then to place the right hand on top palm-to-palm. Now ask them to turn the right hand over to face back-to-palm. Ask them to alternate back-and-forth between the two as fast as possible, then to repeat this with the opposite hand. In cerebellar disease the ability to perform repetitive rapidly alternating movements is impaired.	0 1 2
	This can also be tested in the lower limb by asking the patient to tap their foot up and down against your hand as fast as possible.	
Ataxia	**Truncal ataxia** Observe the patient sitting. Ask them to cross their arms across their chest and look for any imbalance.	0 1 –
	Gait ataxia Observe the patient walking. Look for a wide-based gait. Ask them to walk heel-to-toe.	0 1 –
	Limb ataxia Ask the patient to place both hands in front them, palms facing down, with eyes closed. Observe for cerebellar drift (one arm rising involuntarily). Gently tap down on both arms at once. Normally the arms should return to their original position. In cerebellar disease they may shoot past this (known as rebound phenomenon).	0 1 –

STAGE	KEY POINTS AND ACTIONS	SCORE
Romberg's Test	Have the patient standing upright, feet together, with eyes open. Stand nearby with your arms encircling them, reassuring them they won't fall. Observe for unsteadiness. Then ask the patient to close their eyes. Observe if the patient is less stable (positive Romberg's test – proprioceptive loss, negative – cerebellar disease).	
Nystagmus	Place one hand on the patient's head. Observe for resting nystagmus. Ask the patient to follow your finger at a distance approximately equal to one arm's length. Ask if they see one finger or two and observe for nystagmus; this may be in any direction in cerebellar disease, usually maximal at the extremes of eye movement. Stay within 30 degrees of the midline in either direction – beyond this is more likely to induce end-gaze physiological nystagmus. If there is an ophthalmoscope handy, examine the eyes (looking for Keyser-Fleischer rings seen in Wilson's disease).	0 1 –
Intention Tremor	**Finger-nose test** Test finger to nose coordination by asking the patient to move their index finger between your finger and their nose as fast as possible. Position your index finger at a distance from the patient that requires them to fully extend their arm. Reposition your finger after each touch. Test both arms. Observe for past pointing (dysmetria) and an intention tremor. **Heel/shin test** Ask the patient to run their left heel over their right shin (from knee down to ankle) and then up to touch your hand. Repeat the test on the other leg. Observe for tremor or past pointing.	0 1 2
Slurred speech	Ask the patient to repeat the phrases 'Baby Hippopotamus' and 'British Constitution'. Assess for slurring vowel sounds and 'staccato' speech where each syllable is given equal weight and said separately; i.e. 'Ba-Bee-Hip-Po-Po-Ta-Mus'.	0 1 2
Hypotonia	Assess tone in the upper and lower limbs. **Reflexes** Assess biceps, triceps, brachioradialis, knee, and ankle jerks. Cerebellar lesions cause 'pendular' reflexes, where the muscle will contract and return, and then contract and return several times. This is best seen with the lower leg dangling freely on the knee jerk.	0 1 2
Past Pointing	This is tested with the finger-nose test as above (making the **P**astry part of the mnemonic somewhat redundant).	0 1 –
Finishing Off	Thank the patient.	0 1 –
Request	Request to complete a full neurological exam, including cranial nerves, upper and lower limbs, swallow, and speech examination.	0 1 –
Present	Present a structured, complete, and thorough presentation and offer your differential diagnosis with investigation and management (if appropriate). (*See* Chapter 2.31 for a useful structure.)	0 1 –

EXAMINER'S EVALUATION

Overall assessment of examination of the cerebellar system	0 1 2 3 4 5

Total mark out of 24

'Today I examined the cerebellar system of Mr C, a 54-year-old antiques trader with a history of epilepsy. At the bedside there were no neurological aids, and Mr C looked comfortable sitting in the chair. There was bilateral dysdiadochokinesia, with a markedly ataxic, wide-based gait and slurred speech with staccato intonation. Nystagmus was present in horizontal extreme lateral gaze left and right, with the fast phase variable with the direction of movement. Ophthalmoscopy was normal. There was bilateral intention tremor with no past pointing and reflexes were pendular in the biceps and knee, left and right. In summary, this is a 54-year-old gentleman with known epilepsy with a bilateral cerebellar syndrome.

These findings are most consistent with a diagnosis of anti-epileptic induced global cerebellar degeneration. My differential in this age group would include alcoholism, multiple sclerosis, and paraneoplastic syndrome. I would want to take a full history, including medication, social and family histories, and risk factors for neoplasm, especially smoking. I would complete a full neurological exam of the cranial nerves, upper and lower limbs, swallow, speech assessment, and MMSE. My immediate plan would be some basic blood tests including FBC, U&E, and LFT and then MRI imaging of the head, the results of which would inform my further management. Management in cerebellar dysfunction is primarily supportive; reversible cerebellar dysfunction occurs in post-varicella cerebellitis and sometimes in paraneoplastic disease'. ∎

NOTES ON THE CEREBELLAR EXAM

Differential diagnosis of cerebellar lesions

	Cause	Associated features
Unilateral (ipsilateral)	Stroke	PICA syndrome (lateral medullary syndrome – Wallenberg's) – ipsilateral Horner's, vertigo, dysphagia, contralateral spinothalamic sensory loss
	Tumour	Check for cerebellopontine angle syndrome (CN V, VII, VIII)
Bilateral	Alcoholism	Thiamine deficiency – Wernicke's (ataxia, confusion, and opthalmoplegia)
	Multiple sclerosis	Optic neuritis/atrophy, spinal cord involvement
	Paraneoplastic syndrome	Anti-Jo Antibodies – cachexia, smoker, lung mass
	Drug-induced	Anti-epileptics, chemotherapy
	Metabolic	Wilson's disease: Keyser-Fleischer rings, neuropsychiatric disturbance Coeliac: dermatitis herpetiformis, loose, malabsorptive stools
	Congenital	Friedrich's Ataxia, Arnold-Chiari, Dandy-Walker

P
A
S
T
R
I
E
S

02.8
SPEECH

INSTRUCTIONS Examine the speech of this patient and present your findings as well as a differential diagnosis to the examiners.

STAGE	KEY POINTS AND ACTIONS	SCORE
	THE EXAMINATION	
Introduction	Introduce yourself. Elicit name, age, and occupation as far as possible. Establish rapport. Comment on any obvious speech deficits with your opening question.	0 1 –
Consent	Explain the examination to the patient and seek consent. 'The examination will involve asking you to answer a few questions, repeat a few sentences, and having a look at your face and throat. Would that be okay'?	
Position	Sit the patient upright.	0 1 –
Questions	'Are you hard of hearing'? 'Is English your first language'?	0 1 –
	INSPECTION	
	Inspect the face for nasolabial folds asymmetry, tongue fasciculations, facial deformities, and hearing aids.	
	Inspect the patient for pyramidal distribution of weakness, tremor, or walking aids.	
Opening	Ask an open question which requires the patient to talk in a few full sentences. Ask follow-up questions if this is too short. 'How did you get to here today? (Follow up) – How was the journey'? or 'What did you do for breakfast this morning? (Follow up) – Is that what you normally do'?	0 1 2
	Assess and comment on each of the following: Appropriate use of nouns and overall response. Rhythm of speech: staccato, slurred, or stuttered speech. Volume: appropriate level and pitch.	
	Then go on to assess each of three speech areas independently.	
Dysphasia	**Wernicke's Receptive Dysphasia** Ask the patient to complete a three-stage command; e.g. 'Please put your left index finger to your nose and then to your right ear'. If they fail this, then try a two-stage command. Then a one-stage command.	0 1 2

STAGE	KEY POINTS AND ACTIONS	SCORE
	Broca's Dysphasia Ask the patient to write a sentence – this is a good marker of expressive dysphasia – although the whole exam will find this deficit, this is a good demonstration. Be cautious with patients who have motor deficit or are illiterate. 'Could I ask you to write a sentence'? Assess for noun use, structure, and overall sense.	0 1 2
	Nominal Aphasia Ask the patient to name several objects; e.g. a watch and a pen. Ask the patient to name five nouns from a category; e.g. five animals. This can be a sign of a global deficit.	0 1 2
	Conductive Aphasia Ask the patient to repeat a nonsensical phrase immediately back to you. 'Repeat after me, No Ifs, Ands or Buts'. This tests the ability to transfer information between the receptive and expressive speech areas.	0 1 2
Dysarthria	Ask the patient to repeat the following vowel sounds: 'La, la, la' or 'ta, ta, ta' – tongue (cranial nerve XII) 'Ma, ma, ma' or 'ba, ba, ba' – lips (cranial nerve VII) 'Ka, ka, ka' or 'ga, ga, ga' – palate (cranial nerve IX/X) Then the following phrases: 'Baby Hippopotamus, British Constitution, 52 Western Avenue'. Assess for slurred or staccato speech (cerebellar dysfunction).	0 1 2
Dysphonia	Ask the patient to cough (bovine cough – laryngeal nerve palsy) Reassess volume of speech – Quiet volume (Parkinson's); loud (hearing impairment) Nasal speech – Bulbar palsy 'Donald Duck' voice – Pseudobulbar palsy Hoarse voice – Myasthenia gravis, laryngeal nerve palsy	0 1 2
	ADDITIONAL POINTS	
Finishing Off	Thank the patient and offer to help them get dressed.	0 1 –
Request	Request to complete a full neurological examination including cranial nerves, upper and lower limb, swallow assessment, and MMSE.	0 1 –
Present	Present a structured, complete and thorough presentation and offer your differential diagnosis with investigation and management (if appropriate). (*See* Chapter 2.31 for a useful structure.)	0 1 –
	EXAMINER'S EVALUATION	
	Overall assessment of examination of speech	0 1 2 3 4 5
	Total mark out of 25	

EXEMPLAR PRESENTATION

'Today I examined the speech of Mrs X, a 44-year-old retired pilot. On inspection there was a walker next to the bed, no nasolabial fold asymmetry but tongue fasciculations were present at rest. On opening questioning there was quiet, nasal speech, slightly slurred, with a normal rhythm and appropriate sentence structure, and some difficulty in vowel sounds 'Ta' and 'Ka'. On systematic testing there was no dysphasia, bilateral cranial nerves XII and X weakness, and some slurring of speech. The voice was quiet with a nasal quality.

These findings, taken with the observation of tongue fasciculations, are most consistent with a diagnosis of a bulbar palsy, secondary to amyotrophic lateral sclerosis or other motor neurone disease. I would like to take a full history, specifically inquiring about medications and Activities of Daily Living. I would like to perform a complete neurological examination, including cranial nerves, upper and lower limbs, swallow assessment, and MMSE. Management in this case is primarily supportive in a multidisciplinary approach including the GP, neurologists, physiotherapists, occupational therapists, dieticians, and speech and language. Two interventions have been shown to be somewhat effective: riluzole and home oxygen'. ■

NOTES ON SPEECH FOR THE OSCE

Expressive dysphasia (Broca's aphasia)

Produced from a lesion in Broca's area, in the inferolateral frontal lobe. The speech centres are left sided in nearly 100% of right-handed people, and between 60-80% of left-handed people; the commonest syndrome is a left sided MCA stroke, usually involving Wernicke's area as well. The speech pattern is frustrated and hesitant, with difficulty producing speech. The patient is aware of the deficit and finds it very distressing. Expressive loss is present in written communication as well.

Receptive dysphasia (Wernicke's aphasia)

Produced from a lesion in Wernicke's area, in the posterior superior temporal lobe, in the left hemisphere as detailed above. Patients tend to speak in a mix of unintelligible words, a 'word salad', although a sentence structure is often present. The patient is usually unaware of the abnormal words being produced.

Conductive dysphasia

Produced from a lesion in the connection between speech centres – traditionally said to be damage to the arcuate fasciculus but this is controversial. Clinically, receptive function is intact, fluent speech can be produced, but repetitive function is impaired. This is rarely seen in isolation.

Nominal aphasia

Noun finding difficulty, generally arising from global deficit of cognition, such as in dementia, traumatic brain injury, or stroke.

02.9
EYE

INSTRUCTIONS Examine the eyes of this patient and present your findings as well as a differential diagnosis to the examiners.

STAGE	KEY POINTS AND ACTIONS	SCORE
	THE EXAMINATION	
Introduction	Introduce yourself. Elicit name, age, and occupation. Establish rapport.	0 1 –
Consent	Explain the examination to the patient and seek consent.	
Pain	Ask if the patient is in pain, and ensure they are otherwise comfortable.	0 1 –
	INSPECTION	
General	Note any other obvious co-morbidities that the patient may have (many systemic conditions can manifest in the eye; e.g. rheumatoid arthritis, diabetes).	0 1 –
Eyes	Look around the eye noting if the patient wears glasses (nasal indentations) or has any surrounding scars or lesions. Look at the eyes for asymmetry (proptosis, ptosis). Note if the eye is red and ask the patient to pull the eyelid down noting pallor or icterus (signs of systemic disease).	
	VISUAL ACUITY	
Assess	Ask the patient if they have noticed a change in their vision in either eye.	0 1 –
Snellen Chart	Mention that you would test visual acuity with the Snellen chart at 6 metres for each eye. Test each eye individually permitting the patient to wear spectacles (if they normally do so). If the vision is abnormal, correct any refractory errors by using a pinhole. Report acuity; e.g. 6/6 or 6/60.	0 1 2

STAGE	KEY POINTS AND ACTIONS	SCORE

Notation and Interpretation

6/6 (normal vision)
The first number denotes where the patient is standing (e.g. at 6 metres). The second number denotes the distance a person with normal vision could stand and read that letter.

		0 1 2

A
D F
H Z P
T X U D
Z A D N H
P N T U H X
U A Z N F D T
S P H T A F R D
S D F H T Z O R
D A U T D R O K N

6/60
Patient at 6 metres can only read what a person with normal vision could read at 60 metres.

6/12+2
Denotes how many letters beyond that line were read (+2) or how many were missed (-2).

PH	with Pinhole
OD	Right eye (Oculus Dexter)
OS	Left eye (Oculus Sinester)
CF	Count fingers
HM	Hand motion
LP/NLP	Light perception/No light perception (legally blind)
D	Distance
N	Near

Poor Vision

If acuity is worse than 6/60 or if the patient cannot read the Snellen chart, retest with patient brought forward to 3 metres and then to 1 metre. If acuity is worse than 1/60 then count fingers at 1 metre. If unsuccessful, test whether they can see hand movements and if still unsuccessful, test whether they can see light from a pen torch at 1 metre.

0 1 2

Near Sight

Mention that you would test nearsightedness using newsprint or a book.

Colour Vision – Ishihara Plates

Mention that you would test colour vision using Ishihara colour plates.

VISUAL FIELDS

Inattention

Test for visual neglect by simultaneously waggling a finger in both the patient's left and right visual fields. Normally both should be observed. Determine which finger, if not both, the patient saw. In a parietal lobe lesion, only the finger ipsilateral to the lesion is observed (as the contralateral visual field is neglected).

0 1 –

Confrontation

Test visual fields by confrontation. Sit directly opposite the patient and at the same level. Ask the patient to cover their right eye while you cover your left eye. Have the patient look straight toward you.

0 1 2

Test the patient's visual fields in all four quadrants by comparing them to your own. Request a red pin to perform this and move it from the periphery and into the patient's visual field, noting when the patient first notices the colour of the pin. Test central vision by moving the pin across the visual field. Move your waggling finger instead if a red pin is unavailable.

Using the pin, map out any visual defects and establish the presence of a hemianopia, scotoma, or enlarged blind spot.

STAGE	KEY POINTS AND ACTIONS	SCORE
Blind Spot – Map Defect	Find the patient's blind spot by first finding your own using the pin. Start laterally and bring the pin horizontally within the midplane. Determine when the pin disappears and reappears. An enlarged blind spot suggests papilloedema.	

PUPILLARY REFLEXES

Inspect	Inspect the pupil size, shape (irregular or regular), and the presence of ptosis (3rd nerve palsy, Horner's).	0 1 –
Reflexes	Ask the patient to fixate on an object in the distance. Only perform these tests if the patient's eyes have not been dilated for you.	0 1 2

Direct & Consensual: Shine a light directly at the pupil observing for pupillary constriction in that eye (direct). Illuminate one eye observing for pupillary constriction in the adjacent eye (consensual). Repeat for both eyes.

Swinging Light Test: Swing a light from one eye to the other observing for sustained pupillary constriction. Interrupted constriction suggests a relative afferent pupillary defect (optic neuritis).

Accommodation: Ask the patient to fixate on an object in the distance and then to look at a finger held close to the patient's face. Observe for any changes in pupillary size.

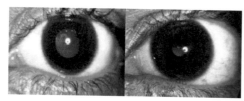

Fig. 2.9

Source: Shiv Shanker Pareek. *The Pictorial Atlas of Common Genito-Urinary Medicine.* London: Radcliffe Publishing; 2012.

EYE MOVEMENTS

Slow Pursuit	Ask the patient to keep their head fixed when following your finger with their eyes asking them to notify you if and when they experience any double vision or pain. Move your finger horizontally and vertically, then make a sign of an 'H' with your finger – keep your finger at an arm's length from the patient and not past 30 degrees of the midline. Ask the patient if they notice any double vision or pain at any time. Look for signs of nystagmus.	0 1 2

Dealing with double vision: Elicit whether the images are separated vertically or horizontally and in which direction the separation is maximal. Ask the patient to close one eye and note which image disappears (the outer or inner image).

Nerve Palsies That Can Affect Eye Movements

- **3rd nerve palsy** – Ptosis, pupillary dilatation, eye is found 'down and out' (posterior communicating artery aneurysm, DM)
- **4th nerve palsy** – Diplopia with downward gaze (superior oblique muscle – orbital trauma, DM, hypertension)
- **6th nerve palsy** – Abduction paralysed, diplopia on looking laterally (lateral rectus – cerebellopontine lesion, raised ICP)

FUNDOSCOPY

Explain	'I need to check your eyesight by having a look inside your eyes. I will be using an ophthalmoscope, which is simply a torch-light and magnifying glass allowing me to look into the back of your eyes. It is a simple procedure that will not hurt, but may feel a little uncomfortable'.

STAGE	KEY POINTS AND ACTIONS	SCORE
Handling	Ask the patient to fixate on an object in the distance. Switch the ophthalmoscope's light on and reset the ophthalmoscope to 0. Handle the ophthalmoscope competently by using your right eye to view the patient's right eye and using your finger to focus.	0 1 2
Red Reflex	Test and note the presence of the red reflex by focusing on the pupil 12 inches away from the patient's eyes. Absence of the red reflex suggests the presence of a cataract.	0 1 –
Optic Disc	Keep the beam of light pointing slightly nasally so that you can focus on the disc when looking at the fundi. Ensure that you are near enough to the patient when observing for the optic disc with steady fixation while using the ophthalmoscope. Note the following:	0 1 2

Signs to Observe in the Optic Disc

Margin	Indistinct neovascularisation	Optic disc oedema diabetic retinopathy
Colour	Pink Pallor	Normal optic disc Optic atrophy
Contour	Raised	Optic disc oedema
Cup-disc	**Ratio > 0.5** Possible glaucoma Ratio 0.3–0.5 Normal **Absence of cup** Papilloedema	

STAGE	KEY POINTS AND ACTIONS	SCORE
Periphery	Follow the blood vessels from the optic disc into the periphery. Then look at the four quadrants of the retina and finally at the macula. Examine the vessels for microaneurysms, venous beading, arteriolar narrowing, AV nipping, copper or silver wiring, haemorrhages, or exudates.	0 1 –
Quadrants	Observe all the quadrants of the retina, nasal and temporal to the optic disc.	0 1 –
Macula	Ask patient to look directly into the light in order to view the macula. Note its colour (pigmented – senile macular degeneration, pink – normal).	0 1 –
Repeat	Ask to examine the other eye and repeat the procedure from the red reflex.	0 1 –

ADDITIONAL POINTS

STAGE		SCORE
Finishing Off	Thank the patient and address any concerns.	0 1 –
Present	Present a structured, complete, and thorough presentation and offer your differential diagnosis with investigation and management (if appropriate). (*See* Chapter 2.31 for a useful structure.)	0 1 –

EXAMINER'S EVALUATION

Overall assessment of examination of eyes	0 1 2 3 4 5

Total mark out of 34

EXEMPLAR PRESENTATION

'Today I examined the eyes of Mrs X, a 52-year-old patisserie owner. Acuity was impaired at 6/12 in the right eye, with normal vision in the left. Fields were normal in left and right eyes. Direct, consensual and accommodation reflexes were intact. Eye movements were normal in slow pursuits and sacchades. On fundoscopy the left eye showed some exudates and microaneurysms. In the right eye there was neovascularisation at the disc, macular exudates, and haemorrhages and microaneurysms. These findings are most consistent with a diagnosis of proliferative diabetic retinopathy, predominantly in the right eye, with non-proliferative changes in the left.

I would like to complete a full neurological examination including peripheral nerves, dip the patient's urine, and send a full set of bloods including HBA1C and fasting glucose. Management for this patient would require laser phototherapy for the right eye and strict glucose control to prevent worsening retinopathy with annual slit-lamp examination in a multidisciplinary setting'. ∎

NOTES ON THE EYE FOR THE OSCE

Diabetic Retinopathy

Diabetic retinopathy is a complication of diabetes and is a leading cause of blindness.

It occurs when diabetes damages the blood vessels inside the retina. It is broadly classified as non-proliferative (background) or proliferative with or without macular involvement. Non-proliferative retinopathy is characterised by microaneurysms, hard exudates and cotton wool spots, dot and blot haemorrhages, and venous beading. Exudates involving the macula are known as clinically significant macular oedema (CMSO).

Proliferative retinopathy is characterised by these changes in addition to the formation of new friable blood vessels. These new vessels are defined as new vessels at disc (NVD) or new vessels elsewhere (NVE) and can bleed into the vitreous leading to floaters, increased ocular pressure and painful glaucoma.

Non-proliferative retinopathy

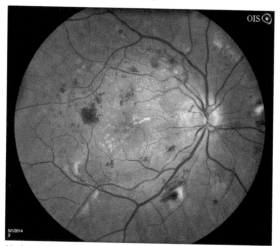

(Kindly reproduced from retinagallery.com- image attributed to Mayo Clinic Jacksonville, Florida)

Proliferative retinopathy

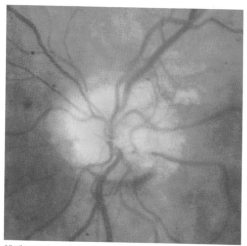

(Kindly reproduced from retinagallery.com- image not attributed)

Hypertensive Retinopathy

Hypertensive retinopathy is a complication of raised blood pressure and can lead to poor vision. It occurs when hypertension damages the blood vessels in the retina, causing them to thicken and narrow, reducing the blood supply to the retina and resulting in retinal damage.

Cotton wool spots

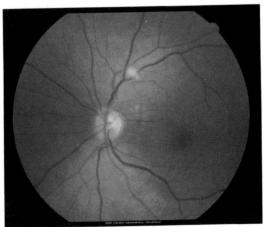

(Kindly reproduced from retinagallery.com- image attributed to Steven Cohen, Florida, US)

Hypertensive retinopathy Grade IV

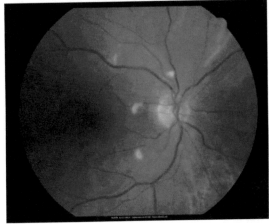

(Kindly reproduced from retinagallery.com- image attributed to Steven Cohen, Florida, US)

Stages of hypertensive retinopathy

Grade 1	Minimal arteriolar narrowing
Grade 2	AV nipping, silver wiring
Grade 3	As above + retinal haemorrhages and/or hard exudate and/or cotton wool spots (pictured)
Grade 4	As above + papilloedema (malignant hypertension) (pictured)

Senile Macular Degeneration

This is a gradual, age-related degeneration of the macula usually occurring bilaterally. It is the most common cause of blindness in the over 65s in the UK. There are two morphological types: non-disciform (dry type) and disciform (wet type), which has the worse prognosis. The disc may appear normal but there is drusen at the macula as seen below in dry ARMD and typically choroidal neovascularisation and in extremis haemorrhages in wet ARMD.

Dry macular degeneration

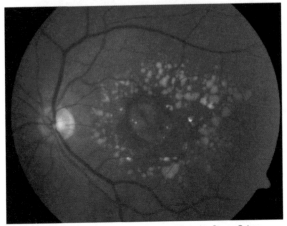

(Kindly reproduced from retinagallery.com- image attributed to Steven Cohen, Florida, US)

Wet macular degeneration

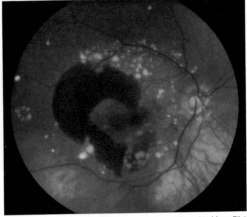

(Kindly reproduced from retinagallery.com- image attributed to Mayo Clinic Jacksonville)

Central Retinal Vein Occlusion

This is blockage of the retinal vein and is more common in diabetic and hypertensive patients. The fundus takes a 'stormy sunset' appearance with dilated, engorged veins with dot and blot haemorrhages alongside them. Cotton wool spots and papilloedema may also be apparent.

Papilloedema and Optic Atrophy

Papilloedema is congestion of the optic disc, usually associated with raised intracranial pressure. The disc is swollen and its margin may disappear. The retinal veins are often congested. In optic atrophy, the disc is grey and pale and the condition is associated with gradual loss of vision. It may be secondary to glaucoma, retinal damage, ischaemia, or poisoning.

CRVO

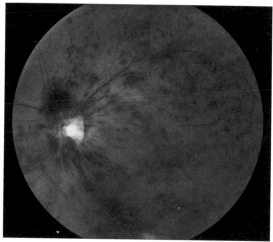

(Kindly reproduced from retinagallery.com- image attributed to Mayo Clinic Jacksonville)

Papilloedema

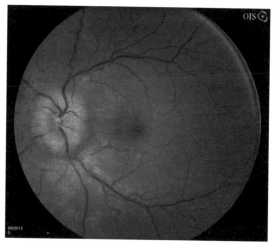

(Kindly reproduced from retinagallery.com- image attributed to Mayo Clinic Jacksonville)

02.10
EAR

INSTRUCTIONS Mr J, a beautician, has been complaining of hearing loss for the past four weeks. Examine his ear. Present your findings and diagnosis to the examiner.

STAGE	KEY POINTS AND ACTIONS	SCORE		
	THE EXAMINATION			
Introduction	Introduce yourself. Elicit name, age, and occupation. Establish rapport.	0	1	–
Consent	Explain the examination to the patient and seek consent.			
Pain	Always ask about pain. 'Before we begin, do you have any pain anywhere'?	0	1	–
	INSPECTION			
General	Look for hearing aids, dysmorphic features, or any evidence of trauma.	0	1	–
Ear	Note any sinuses, erythema, or discharge from the ear. Make a point of looking behind the ear at the mastoid area (this is where a mastoidectomy scar can be found).	0	1	2

Fig. 2.10 Pre-auricular dermoid cyst

Source: Tang T and Praveen B V. *MRCS Picture Questions Book 1*. London: Radcliffe Publishing; 2006.

STAGE	KEY POINTS AND ACTIONS	SCORE		
Palpation	Pinna tenderness may suggest otitis externa. Mastoid- press over the mastoid process in an attempt to elicit tenderness.	0	1	2
	ASSESSING HEARING			
Hearing	Ask the patient if they have any problems with hearing. Stand behind the patient and repeat a set of letters and numbers in each ear and ask the patient to recall them. Mask the non-examined ear by rubbing your finger and thumb together in front of it at the same time. Repeat three times if the patient makes a mistake.	0	1	2
Request	State that you would like to perform the Weber's and Rinne's tests using a 512Hz tuning fork and that you would examine the ears with an otoscope.			

STAGE	KEY POINTS AND ACTIONS	SCORE
Weber's	This tests for lateralisation. Strike the tuning fork sturdily and press the end of the instrument on the middle of the patient's forehead. Ask the patient where they hear the sound the loudest (in the centre or lateralised to one side). Normally, the sound is heard equally in both ears.	0 1 –
Rinne's	This test compares air conduction with bone conduction. Strike the tuning fork firmly and place the end on the mastoid. Tell the patient to indicate when they no longer feel the vibrations. Remove the butt from the mastoid process and place the tuning fork near the ear without touching it. Establish whether the tuning fork can be heard. Normally air conduction is more sensitive than bone conduction and the patient should be able to still hear the tone at the ear when they could no longer hear it at the mastoid. Repeat the test on the other side.	0 1 –

	Rinne's (R)	Rinne's (L)	Weber's
Conductive hearing loss - Right ear	Bone conduction > Air conduction	Air conduction > Bone conduction	Loudest in Right ear
Conductive hearing loss - Left ear	Air conduction > Bone conduction	Bone conduction > Air conduction	Loudest in Left ear
Sensorineural hearing loss – Right ear	Air conduction > Bone conduction (quiet/absent)	Air conduction > Bone conduction	Loudest in Left ear
Sensorineural hearing loss – Left ear	Air conduction > Bone conduction	Air conduction > Bone conduction (quiet/absent)	Loudest in Right ear

Easy way to remember this;
1. *Bone conduction should NEVER be louder than air conduction – wherever that is the case that ear is abnormal.*
2. *Weber's lateralises to the same ear in conductive hearing loss, and the opposite in sensorineural.*

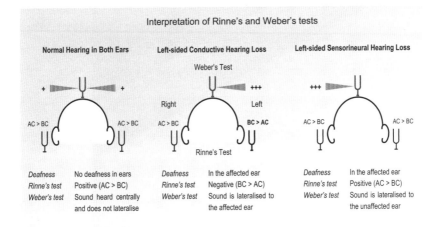

Interpretation of Rinne's and Weber's tests

	Deafness	Rinne's test	Weber's test
Normal Hearing in Both Ears	No deafness in ears	Positive (AC > BC)	Sound heard centrally and does not lateralise
Left-sided Conductive Hearing Loss	In the affected ear	Negative (BC > AC)	Sound is lateralised to the affected ear
Left-sided Sensorineural Hearing Loss	In the affected ear	Positive (AC > BC)	Sound is lateralised to the unaffected ear

OTOSCOPY

STAGE	KEY POINTS AND ACTIONS	SCORE
Explain	'I need to check your hearing by having a look inside your ears. I will be using an otoscope, which is simply a torch-light and magnifying glass. It is a simple procedure that will not hurt, but may feel uncomfortable'.	0 1 –
Technique	Hold the otoscope like a pen with your thumb and index finger, resting the ulnar border of your hand gently against the patient's cheek. Handle the otoscope competently by using your right hand to view the patient's right ear. Examine the good ear first. Choose a speculum size that is appropriate for the patient's ear canal.	0 1 2

STAGE	KEY POINTS AND ACTIONS	SCORE
Insert	Use the otoscope as a torch to inspect the surrounding structures of the ear. Warn the patient before inserting. Pull the pinna upward and backward and insert the otoscope into the ear canal. Inspect the pinna as well as the canal.	0 1 –
Canal	Look inside the ear canal for inflammation, foreign bodies, or debris (otitis externa).	
Tympanic Membrane	Note the following:	0 1 –

Observation of the Tympanic Membrane in the Ear

Membrane	Visible & intact/perforated/absent Visible blood vessels in the middle ear mucosa suggest a perforation (central/peripheral). A grommet can be seen in the anterior inferior quadrant of the tympanic membrane.
Colour	Pearly grey – Normal tympanic membrane Gold/blue – Fluid in the middle ear White – Tympanosclerosis (scarring)
Shape	Bulging (otitis media)/concave (normal)
Light Reflex	Present (normal) Absent (perforation)

OTHER

Structures	Inspect the surrounding structures in the ear, including the malleus, umbo, pars tensa and flaccida, and attic.	0 1 –
Malleus	Identify the malleus by following the narrower section of the light reflex.	
Pars Tensa	Inspect the pars tensa (below the short process of the malleus). Start in the posterosuperior quadrant and then move forward, downward, and backward until all 360° has been covered.	
Pars Flaccida	Inspect the pars flaccida (above the short process of the malleus).	
Attic	Inspect the attic within the pars flaccida (early cholesteatoma).	

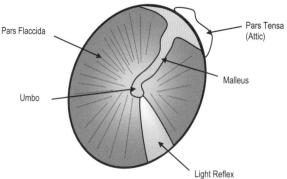

Repeat	Ask to examine the other ear and repeat the procedure from insert onward.	0 1 –
Finishing Off	Thank the patient.	0 1 –
Request	Request to complete a full ENT examination including nose and throat and to palpate for cervical lymphadenopathy.	

STAGE	KEY POINTS AND ACTIONS	SCORE
Present	Present a structured, complete, and thorough presentation and offer your differential diagnosis with investigation and management (if appropriate). (*See* Chapter 2.31 for a useful structure.)	0 1 –

EXAMINER'S EVALUATION	
Overall assessment of examination of ears	0 1 2 3 4 5
Total mark out of 25	

NOTES FOR THE OSCE

Hearing Loss

The causes of hearing loss can be divided into conductive and sensorineural:

Conductive hearing loss	Sensorineural hearing loss
Usually a result of impairment of sound transmission from the environment to the inner ear. **External canal** – blockage by wax, discharge or foreign body **Middle ear** – eardrum perforation due to trauma or infection **Conduction to the stapes** – otosclerosis and trauma	Results from damage to: **The neural receptors** of the inner ear (the hair cells, organ of Corti) **The nerve pathways to the brain** (notably the auditory nerve) **The auditory cortex** (rare) Causes include noise pollution, ototoxic **Senile deafness** (presbyacusis) **Drugs** – aminoglycosides; i.e. gentamicin **Infections** – mumps, German measles, influenza **Neoplasia** – acoustic neuroma **Ménière's disease**

Acoustic Neuroma

This is a benign tumour of the Schwann cells that surround the auditory nerve and grows in the middle ear. It is one of the most common types of benign brain tumour and causes of hearing loss. It is associated with neurofibromatosis and is usually diagnosed in those aged between 30 and 50 years. Common symptoms include dizziness, hearing loss, and tinnitus. If the tumour extends far enough, it may press on other nerves causing weakness and pain in the face.

Otosclerosis

This is a degenerative bone disease of the middle ear and is usually bilateral. Females have a 2:1 preponderance (rapidly worsening during pregnancy) with a large majority (up to 60%) having a positive family history. The most common symptom is a gradual (low-pitch) hearing loss often associated with dizziness and tinnitus.

Presbyacusis

Presbyacusis or senile deafness is a progressive sensorineural hearing loss that occurs with age. It is typically bilateral and symmetrical, and is common after 60 years of age. It is due to degeneration and loss of cochlea hair cells in the cochlea nerve. Characteristically, high-frequency hearing loss is noted causing words and speech to appear muffled.

02.11
NOSE

INSTRUCTIONS Mrs B, a 52-year-old, reports being unable to smell properly. Examine her nose and sense of smell.

STAGE	KEY POINTS AND ACTIONS	SCORE
	THE EXAMINATION	
Introduction	Introduce yourself. Elicit name, age, and occupation. Establish rapport.	0 1 –
Consent	Explain the procedure and gain consent.	
Pain	Always ask about pain. 'Before we begin, do you have any pain anywhere'?	0 1 –
	INSPECTION	
External	Inspect the external aspect of the nose anteriorly, superiorly, and from the side. Note any of the following:	0 1 2

Skin	Neoplasia – BCC, Melanoma
Discharge	Clear/coloured/blood-stained/watery/thick
Obvious deviation (best seen from standing behind the patient)	Congenital, post-trauma
Mucosal ulceration	Nasopharyngeal cancer, infection
Saddle-shaped	Trauma, granulomatosis with polyangiitis

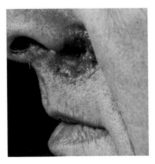

Fig. 2.11 **Basal cell carcinoma**

Source: Tang T and Praveen B V. *MRCS Picture Questions Book 1.* London: Radcliffe Publishing; 2006.

Then inspect the vestibule by raising the tip of the nose gently with your thumb. Look for cartilaginous collapse, as seen in cocaine use or repeated operations.

STAGE	KEY POINTS AND ACTIONS	SCORE		
Internal	Using a nasal speculum or an otoscope with a wide speculum attachment, inspect the inside of the nose. Inspect the nasal septum, inferior and middle turbinates, and the mucosa, noting any collapse, ulceration, active bleeding, perforation, or nasal polyp.	0	1	–
	PALPATION	0	1	2
Tenderness	Palpate the frontal and maxillary sinuses for sinusitis using your thumbs. Press over the supraorbital and infraorbital areas and gently percuss, eliciting any tenderness.			
	SPECIAL TESTS			
Alar Collapse	Ask the patient to inhale deeply through the nose and look for subtle collapse of the nostril on the affected side.			
Nasal Patency	Ask the patient to exhale through their nose over a cold metal tongue depressor. Condensation should form on the blade from both nostrils if they are patent.	0	1	–
Sense of Smell	Offer to use special odour bottles to test sense of smell.			
Finishing Off	Thank the patient.	0	1	–
Present	Present a structured, complete, and thorough presentation and offer your differential diagnosis with investigation and management (if appropriate). (*See* Chapter 2.31 for a useful structure.)	0	1	–

EXAMINER'S EVALUATION						
Overall assessment of examination of nose	0	1	2	3	4	5

Total mark out of 15

NOTES ON THE NOSE FOR THE OSCE

Loss of smell sensation

Unilateral loss of smell	Bilateral loss of smell
Neoplasia - Nasal polyps - Tumour	**Congenital** - Kallmann syndrome **Aquired** - Common cold (MOST COMMON) - Parkinson's (may be presenting symptom) - Trauma (damage to cribiform plate)

Nasal Deviation Acquired

The nasal septum consists of bone and cartilage. Although most nasal septums are mildly deviated, only when clinical symptoms are present should correction be offered. The most likely cause of this is post trauma but it may be developmental. The patient may also complain of long-standing unilateral nasal blockage post insult.

Rhinitis

Rhinitis is exceptionally common and is often divided into allergic, atrophic, infective, and non-allergic non-infective rhinitis. Allergic rhinitis may be perennial, all year round, or seasonal, such as in hayfever. Typical features include watery rhinorrhea, sneezing, and itchy eyes. Some patients may have a strong family history of atopy or themselves suffer from asthma and/or eczema. Infective rhinitis is usually virally mediated and self-limiting. Bacterial infection normally leads to purulent nasal discharge, headache, and facial pain (sinusitis).

Nasal Polyps

The most common cause of space occupying lesions of the nose, nasal polyps are usually bilateral. They are inflammatory in nature and arise from the lining of the paranasal sinuses of the nose. They are twice as common in males than females with an unclear aetiology (although infection and allergy have been implicated). Unilateral polyps should be biopsied to rule out malignancy.

Malignancy

There are a number of rarer cancerous lesions which may also present in the nose and lead to nasal obstruction, including papilloma, dermoid cyst, haemangioma, angiofibroma, dermoid cyst, squamous cell carcinoma, and adenocarcinoma.

Nasopharyngeal Carcinoma

[Mnemonic – **NOSE**]

- **N**eck mass
- **O**bstructed nasal passage
- **S**erous otitis media externa
- **E**pistaxis or discharge

02.12 ARTERIAL CIRCULATION

INSTRUCTIONS Examine this patient's arterial circulatory system. Present your findings and diagnosis to the examiner.

STAGE	KEY POINTS AND ACTIONS	SCORE
	THE EXAMINATION	
Introduction	Introduce yourself. Elicit name, age, and occupation. Establish rapport.	0 1 –
Consent	Explain the procedure and and gain consent from the patient.	
Pain	Ask if the patient is in pain and otherwise comfortable.	0 1 –
Position	Expose patient's legs and request them to lie down.	0 1 –
	INSPECTION	
	Stand at end of bed and observe for arterial changes to the legs. Also make sure to look for relevant scars (*see later*).	0 1 –

Signs to Observe in the Peripheral Arterial Examination

Colour	White/blue/purple/black
Trophic Changes	Shiny skin, hair loss, ulcers, thinning of the skin
Signs	Gangrenous patches, oedema, amputated toes, loss of subcutaneous fat
Pressure Points	Check the heel, malleoli, head of first metatarsal, lateral side of foot, toes (tips & between toes), dorsum of foot for ulcers
Ulcers	Describe in terms of size, shape, depth, edge, base

STAGE	KEY POINTS AND ACTIONS	SCORE
	PALPATION	
Temperature	Run the back of the hand along both limbs and soles of feet. Note the point when the temperature changes from warm to cold on both sides.	0 1 –
Capillary Refill	Press the tip of the nails on both first toes for 2 seconds and measure the time taken for the bland area to turn pink after pressure is released. Normal is <2 seconds from white to return to pink.	0 1 –
Pulses	Palpate the following peripheral pulses of the lower legs comparing both sides.	0 1 2

STAGE	KEY POINTS AND ACTIONS	SCORE

Location of the Peripheral Pulses

Dorsalis Pedis Artery	Feel along cleft between first two metatarsals with three fingers just lateral to the tendon of the extensor hallucis longus.
Posterior Tibial Artery	Draw an imaginary line between the medial malleolus and the insertion of the Achilles tendon. Place three fingers parallel to the leg at this spot (Pimenta's Point).
Popliteal Artery	Ask patient to bend their knee. Place your thumbs on tibial tuberosity, feel pulse with eight fingertips.
Femoral Artery	Found midway between symphysis pubis and ASIS.

AUSCULTATION

Bruits — Listen for bruits along the iliac, femoral, and popliteal arteries. Bruits suggest the presence of turbulent blood flow indicating narrowing of vessels at a higher point.   0 1 –

SPECIAL TESTS

Guttering — Elevate patient's legs about 15 degrees and look for venous guttering.   0 1 –

Buerger's Test and Angle — Elevate the leg further and look for the angle when it becomes pale (Buerger's angle). The leg of a normal individual remains pink even if the leg is raised to 90 degrees. A Buerger's angle of less than 30 degrees indicates severe ischaemia.   0 1 –

Reactive Hyperaemia — Sit the patient up and ask them to hang their legs over the bed, measuring the time it takes to refill and return to normal colour. Observe for redness of the leg suggestive of reactive hyperaemia (chronic lower limb ischaemia, 2–3 min to return to normal colour).   0 1 –

Ankle Brachial Pulse Index (ABPI)

Fig. 2.12 Ankle brachial pressure index (ABPI)

Source: Tang T and Praveen B V. *MRCS Picture Questions Book 1.* London: Radcliffe Publishing; 2006.

Finishing Off — Thank the patient and cover the legs.   0 1 –

Request — Offer to examine the rest of the peripheral vascular system as follows: feel the radial and carotid pulses, listen for a carotid bruit at the angle of the mandible, and palpate for radial-femoral delay (coarctation of aorta). Also request to perform a cardiovascular examination (to auscultate the heart) and an abdominal examination (to feel the abdomen for an aortic aneurysm).   0 1 –

EXAMINER'S EVALUATION

Overall assessment of examination of the arterial circulatory system   0 1 2 3 4 5

Total mark out of 19

NOTES ON THE ARTERIAL EXAMINATION

Intermittent Claudication

This is a cramp-like pain felt in the back of the calf, thigh, or buttocks that is precipitated by exercise but ceases after a couple of minutes of rest. It is due to moderate narrowing of the vessels due to atherosclerosis. The pain usually occurs after exerting oneself over a predictable fixed distance known as the claudication distance. The site of the pain can give an indication of the level of the arterial obstruction; e.g. foot pain – tibial or plantar artery obstruction, calf pain – obstruction of the femoral popliteal junction, thigh pain – occlusion of superficial femoral artery, buttock pain – occlusion in the bifurcation of the iliac artery. Peripheral pulses can be present in patients with intermittent claudication as opposed to critical ischaemia, where they are invariably absent.

Fontaine classification of chronic leg ischaemia

- **Stage I** Asymptomatic
- **Stage II** Intermittent claudication
- **Stage III** Ischaemic rest pain
- **Stage IV** Ulceration or gangrene, or both

Critical Ischaemia

This is a condition that presents as a continuous and aching pain in the leg at rest and normally affects males over 60 years of age. It is due to gross narrowing of the vessels due to atherosclerosis. The pain usually occurs when the foot is elevated (i.e. in bed), and to relieve the pain, patients usually hang their legs over the bed, bending their knees. Other symptoms may include pain in the foot and toes rather than in the calf muscle, ischaemic ulcers that are painful and appear punched out, pallor due to atrophic skin with a purple-blue cyanosed appearance, absent foot pulses, and gangrene. Buerger's sign (*see* above) is usually positive in critical ischaemia.

Signs and Symptoms of Acute Ischaemia

[Mnemonic—Six **P**s]

Painful, **P**ulseless, **P**allor (pale), **P**aralysis, **P**araesthesia (numbness), **P**erishingly cold

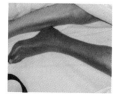

Fig. 2.13 Acute ischaemia

Source: Tang T and Praveen B V. *MRCS Picture Questions Book 1*.
London: Radcliffe Publishing; 2006.

Diabetic Foot

Foot ulcers are a significant complication of diabetes mellitus and are caused by neuropathy, trauma, and peripheral arterial disease. The patient often presents with ulcers at pressure points with either gangrenous or amputated toes. Pulses are often present with a warm foot. Gangrenous regions are often associated with infection and pus. It is important to perform a full lower limb neurological examination testing sensation, power, and reflexes and to check the patient's diabetic control.

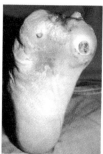

Fig. 2.14 Diabetic foot

Source: Tang T and Praveen B V. *MRCS Picture Questions Book 1*.
London: Radcliffe Publishing; 2006.

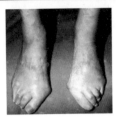

Fig. 2.15 Diabetic foot

Source: Tang T and Praveen B V. *MRCS Picture Questions Book 1*.
London: Radcliffe Publishing; 2006.

Abdominal Aortic Aneurysm

This is an abnormal dilatation of the arterial wall of the descending aorta in the abdomen. The abdominal aorta normally measures around 2 cm in size, with an aneurysm being anything larger than this. The exact aetiology is unknown, but it is associated with significant risk factors such as high blood pressure, raised cholesterol, smoking, and atherosclerosis. Although abdominal aortic aneurysms can occur at any age, they are more common in men aged between 40 and 70 years. The main complication is rupture, which is a surgical emergency. They can be detected on routine examination of the abdomen via palpation for an expansile pulsatility in the abdomen.

Causes of aneurysmal arteries

Most commonly due to atherosclerosis although other causes include:

- **Mycotic/infective** – Bacterial endocarditis, syphilis
- **Connective tissue disorders** – Marfan's, Ehlers-Danlos

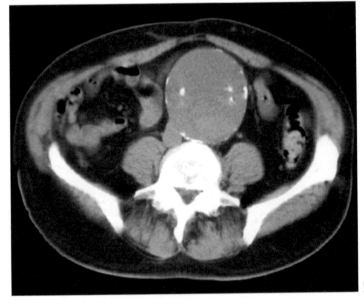

Fig. 2.16 CT showing large abdominal aneurysm

02.13 VENOUS CIRCULATION

INSTRUCTIONS Assess this patient's venous system.

STAGE	KEY POINTS AND ACTIONS	SCORE
	THE EXAMINATION	
Introduction	Introduce yourself. Elicit name, age, and occupation. Establish rapport.	0 1 –
Consent	Explain the examination to the patient and seek consent.	
Pain	Ask if the patient is in pain and otherwise comfortable.	0 1 –
Position and Exposure	Expose patient's legs and request them to stand.	0 1 –
	INSPECTION	
	Stand at the end of the bed and look for the following signs:	
Shape	Look for beer bottle shaped legs suggestive of oedema and venous compromise.	
Varicose Veins	Establish the location and distribution of any varicose veins. Look particularly along the long saphenous vein (groin to medial malleolus) and short saphenous vein (popliteal to lateral malleolus).	0 1 –

Skin

Venous stars	Fan shaped dilatation of superficial venules spreading from the ankle particularly below the medial malleolus
Eczema	Above the medial malleolus of lower calf
Ulcers	Over the medial malleolus (varicose ulcers)
Ankle swelling	Observe for evidence of oedema
Pigmentation	Brown discolouration (deposition of haemosiderin)
Thrombophlebitis	Hard inflamed and tender veins resembling thick cords
Lipodermatosclerosis	Fibrosis of skin and subcutaneous fat
Scars	From previous vascular surgery

STAGE	KEY POINTS AND ACTIONS	SCORE

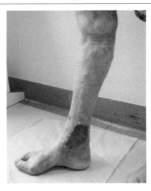

Fig. 2.17 Varicose vein with ulcer

Source: Tang T and Praveen B V. *MRCS Picture Questions Book 1*.
London: Radcliffe Publishing; 2006.

PALPATION

Temperature

Run the back of your hand along the patient's legs and soles of the feet. Feel along the medial side of the lower leg noting any temperature changes (warmness around the varicose veins) or tenderness (incompetent perforators).

0 1 –

Pitting Oedema

Palpate the skin of the lower leg feeling and looking for pitting oedema.

0 1 –

Veins

Feel along the long saphenous vein and short saphenous vein for tenderness (phlebitis) or hardness (thrombosis).

0 1 2

Distribution of the Long and Short Saphenous Veins
Long Saphenous Vein
Begins at the dorsal venous arch running anterior to the medial malleolus, then along medial aspect of the knee. Finally travels up the thigh to the saphenofemoral opening and into the femoral vein.

Short Saphenous Vein
Begins at the dorsal venous arch behind the lateral malleolus running up the midline of the calf and into the popliteal fossa, emptying into the popliteal vein.

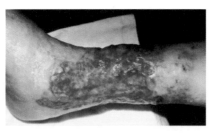

Fig. 2.18 Venous ulcer

Source: Tang T and Praveen B V. MRCS Picture
Questions Book 1. London: Radcliffe Publishing; 2006.

Junctions

Feel the **saphenofemoral junction** (4cm below and lateral to pubic tubercle) for a saphena varix (dilatation in the saphenous vein as it joins the femoral vein). Ask the patient to cough. If you feel an impulse it indicates saphenofemoral incompetence.

0 1 –

Feel the **saphenopopliteal junction** in the popliteal fossa and ask the patient to cough. If you feel an impulse it indicates saphenopopliteal incompetence.

AUSCULTATION

Bruits

Listen over a venous cluster for possible bruits (machine like murmur) indicating the possible presence of an arteriovenous fistula.

0 1 –

STAGE	KEY POINTS AND ACTIONS	SCORE
	SPECIAL TESTS	
Tap Test	Place the finger of one hand at the bottom of a long varicose vein and tap above this site with the other hand. Note the presence of an impulse (superficial vein incompetence).	0 1 –
Trendelenburg's	Perform the Trendelenburg's test by first asking the patient to lie flat. Next elevate their leg until all the superficial veins have collapsed. Occlude the saphenofemoral junction with two fingers and ask the patient to stand. Remove your fingers. Upon removal, if the superficial veins refill, this indicates incompetence at the saphenofemoral junction.	0 1 –
Tourniquet Test	Ask the patient to lie supine. Elevate their leg until the superficial veins are drained. Place a tourniquet tightly around the upper thigh then ask the patient to stand and observe below the tourniquet. Superficial veins filling below this level indicates incompetent perforators below the level of the tourniquet. Repeat the test down the leg. Keep on repeating the procedure until the veins below the tourniquet remain collapsed (i.e. do not fill). The venous segment with the incompetent perforators now lies above the level of the tourniquet.	0 1 –
Perthes' Test	Keep the tourniquet on the patient with the superficial veins emptied. Now ask the patient to stand on tiptoes up and down on the spot ten times and observe if the superficial veins refill (deep vein occlusion).	
Peripheral Pulse	Examine the peripheral pulses to assess arterial blood supply.	0 1 –
	FINISHING OFF	
Request	Offer an abdominal and pelvic examination (abdominal mass or pelvic mass may cause inferior vena caval obstruction). Also request a Doppler US probe to listen to flow in the incompetent valves.	
Thank	Thank the patient and cover legs. Acknowledge patient's concerns.	0 1 –
	EXAMINER'S EVALUATION	
	Overall assessment of examination of the venous system	0 1 2 3 4 5
	Total mark out of 20	

EXEMPLAR EXAMINATION

'I examined the venous system of the lower limbs of this 68-year-old llama farmer. On inspection there were visible varicosities in the distribution of both long and short saphenous veins, worse on the right leg. Skin changes included loss of hair, and venous stars. Of note there were no ulcers. Palpation revealed ankle swelling to the mid-calf bilaterally. There was no saphena varix at the saphenofemoral junction and there was no evidence of incompetence there. The tourniquet test showed the incompetence lies most likely at the level of the mid-thigh perforators. Perthe's test indicated no occlusion of the deep veins. All peripheral pulses were present. I would like to take a full history and examine using a Doppler US probe'. ∎

NOTES ON THE VENOUS EXAM FOR THE OSCE

Varicose Veins

Varicose veins are swollen, dilated, tortuous, irregularly shaped veins that commonly appear in the legs. They occur due to incompetence of the valves in the venous system. Although up to 20% of adults suffer from some form of varicose veins, typically older women are affected. They usually develop gradually and there may be a positive family history. Varicose veins are more apparent on standing and often cause the patient to experience a dull achy pain toward the end of the day. As a result, they commonly affect those who are required to stand for long hours such as conductors or guards.

Primary varicose veins are those in which a hereditary weakness in the vein walls causes dilatation and valvular incompetence causing retrograde flow (deep system should be normal on examination). Secondary varicose veins are those caused by the effect of deep vein thrombosis destroying the deep valves leading to reflux and a greater pressure in the deep system. They can also be caused by obstruction to venous outflow, such as with pregnancy, fibroids, and ovarian cysts or by the presence of a high-pressure flow such as an arteriovenous fistula. Chronic varicose veins can lead to venous insufficiency which causes venous eczema, skin pigmentation, and venous ulcers.

There are also rare genetic conditions such as Klippel-Trenaunay-Weber in which patients exhibit varicosities, port wine stains, and hemi-hypertrophy of the affected limb.

Explanation of the Tourniquet Test

Deoxygenated blood is carried up to the femoral vein via a system of veins that are both superficial and deep. The system is reliant on the presence of one-way valves and functioning calf muscles that act like a pump pushing the blood back to the heart. The deep system is under high pressure because the veins are surrounded by the calf, which pumps blood to the femoral vein. Blood in the superficial veins is shunted into the deep veins via perforators that also contain one-way valves. When the tourniquet is on, filling of superficial veins below this level indicates the presence of incompetent perforators below the level of the tourniquet. These incompetent perforators are allowing the blood to pool back into the superficial veins from the high-pressure system.

When the tourniquet is lowered with the superficial veins remaining collapsed, one can conclude that the incompetent perforators can be found at a site above the level of the tourniquet. And hence this helps to locate the approximate level of the defect.

Complications of Varicose Veins

- Haemorrhage
- Ulceration
- Lipodermatosclerosis
- Phlebitis
- Eczema
- Calcification of veins

Deep Vein Thrombosis

This is the formation of a blood clot in the deep venous system of the lower limbs and is usually due to prolonged immobility. A deep vein thrombosis only occurs when the blood clot partially or completely blocks blood flow in the vein. Risk factors include prolonged sitting, bed-rest, or immobilisation (long-haul flights), recent surgery, fractures (particularly hip and femur), and the use of hormones such as oestrogen and combined oral contraceptives. There is also an association with polycythaemia vera, malignant tumours, and inherited clotting disorders. Symptoms include a unilateral acutely painful swollen and hot leg. The clot may dislodge and travel via the bloodstream to the lungs causing a pulmonary embolus.

02.14
ULCERS

INSTRUCTIONS Examine this patient's foot ulcers. Present your findings and a possible differential diagnosis to the examiner.

STAGE	KEY POINTS AND ACTIONS	SCORE
	THE EXAMINATION	
Introduction	Introduce yourself. Elicit name, age, and occupation. Establish rapport.	0 1 –
Consent	Explain the examination to the patient and seek consent.	
Pain	Ask if the patient is in pain and otherwise comfortable.	0 1 –
Position & Exposure	Expose and position the patient's legs lying down.	0 1 –
	INSPECTION	
Site	Stand at the end of the bed and observe for the presence of any ulcers. Make sure you inspect the heels and between the toes.	0 1 –
	Note the exact location; i.e. whether it is the anterior, posterior, medial, or lateral surface and note the distance the lump is from the nearest bony prominence.	
Size	Measure both its width and length using a ruler.	
Shape	Describe the shape of the lump as circular, oval, or irregular.	
Ulcer Features	Describe features specific to the ulcer including its base, edge, depth, discharge, lymph nodes, and local tissues.	0 1 –
Base	Note the following:	

Features at the Base of an Ulcer

Colour	Pink/yellow/white
Penetration	Tendon/muscle/bone
Tissue	Granulation tissue/dead tissue/tumour (SCC)

STAGE	KEY POINTS AND ACTIONS	SCORE
Edge	The edge of the ulcer provides important information about its pathophysiology and takes the characteristic form of the underlying disease.	
	Flat sloping edge This indicates that epithelium is growing in from the ulcer edge in an attempt to heal it. Often these ulcers are venous ulcers. Note the skin around the ulcer is red-blue due to haemosiderin deposition.	
	Punched-out edge Punched-out edges indicate rapid death of a whole thickness of skin without the body making an attempt to repair it. This is usually caused by pressure on an insensible area of skin such as in diabetes and syphilis.	
	Undermined edge Occurs when an infection at an ulcer site destroys the subcutaneous tissues more than the superficial skin. Presents with reddish-blue overhanging skin and is often due to ulcers secondary to tuberculosis.	
	Rolled edge Occurs where there is slow growth of tissue at the ulcer edge and a necrotic centre and the peripheral tissue becomes heaped-up. This is classically seen in a rodent ulcer (basal cell carcinoma).	
	Everted edge The tissue at the edge of the ulcer is growing so fast that it overlaps the normal skin as it 'spills out' of the ulcer site. An everted edge is seen in squamous cell carcinoma and ulcerated adenocarcinoma.	
Depth	Measure the height in millimetres.	
Discharge	Can be serous, sanguineous, or purulent.	
Lymph Nodes	Feel lymph nodes for tenderness or enlargement (infection or malignancy).	
Local Tissues	Inspect the surrounding tissues and the rest of the legs for oedema, thickening, lack of hair, erythema, cracked skin, and dryness.	
	Also assess the local blood supply, by carrying out a limited arterial examination, and the local nerve supply, by testing sensation of the legs.	
	Blood Supply	
Temperature	Run the back of the hand along both limbs and soles of the feet. Note the point where the temperature changes from warm to cold.	0 1 –
Capillary Refill	Press the tips of the nails on both first toes for 2 seconds to assess capillary refill time. Normal capillary refill is when the nails go pink within 2 seconds.	0 1 –
Pulses	Palpate the peripheral pulses including the posterior tibial artery, dorsalis pedis artery, popliteal artery, and femoral artery, comparing strength between both sides.	0 1 –
Request	If any of the pulses are absent request to perform ABPI using Doppler.	0 1 –
	Nerve Supply	
Light Touch	Ask the patient for numbness or pain. If present ask them to demarcate the area. Test the dermatomes in the legs comparing both sides.	0 1 –
Pain Sensation	State you would like to test pain sensation by performing the pin prick test. Apply a pin to the sternum then to the dermatomes comparing both sides.	0 1 –
Proprioception	Assess joint position sense by starting at the DIPJ of the toes. Compare both sides. If unsuccessful move up to the MTPJ, followed by the medial malleolus and tibial tuberosity.	0 1 –
Vibration Sense	Apply a vibrating 128Hz tuning fork to the bony prominence on the toe. Compare both sides. If unsuccessful move to the MTPJ, followed by the lateral malleolus.	0 1 –

STAGE	KEY POINTS AND ACTIONS	SCORE
Finishing Off	Thank the patient and cover their legs. Acknowledge patient's concerns.	0 1 –
Request	Offer to assess if the patient is diabetic by performing a BM test or urinalysis, or to check diabetic control if diabetic via HbA1c levels.	0 1 –

EXAMINER'S EVALUATION	
Overall assessment of examination of the ulcers	0 1 2 3 4 5
Total mark out of 20	

Neuropathic Ulcers

These ulcers are secondary to spinal cord disease or peripheral neuropathy (diabetes).

They occur over pressure areas including the sole of the foot and beneath the heads of the metatarsals, and develop as a result of repeated trauma to an insensible part of the body. A diabetic ulcer is deep, painless and infected with a 'punched out' appearance. The surrounding tissues are warm and the peripheral pulses palpable due to an adequate blood supply. The ulcer is often accompanied by generalised sensory impairment.

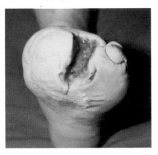

Fig. 2.19 Diabetic foot

Source: Tang T and Praveen B V. *MRCS Picture Questions Book 1*. London: Radcliffe Publishing; 2006.

Ischaemic Ulcers

These ulcers are caused by an inadequate or poor blood supply. There is usually underlying atherosclerosis or vasculitis. It predominantly affects the elderly but can be precipitated by injury at any age. In contrast to venous leg ulcers, ischaemic ulcers are extremely painful. The pain may interfere with sleep and there is often a history of claudication or rest pain. Also there is an absence of palpable peripheral pulses. An associated black eschar is often present. Ulcers are deep, painful, and coin shaped with a 'punched out' edge found at the pressure points or over the tips of the toes. The surrounding tissue is cold due to ischaemia with the base containing dead tissue and penetrating to the bone. Discharge is either serous or pus in nature.

Venous Ulcers

Incompetent venous valves result in an increase in capillary pressure with pooling of blood causing capillary damage, fibrosis, and easily damageable skin. These ulcers are found within the 'gaiter' area of the leg (particularly above the medial malleolus). They may be associated with lipodermatosclerosis and haemosiderin pigmentation. Ulcers are shallow and flat with an irregular pale purple or blue sloping edge. The base may penetrate to the tendons and bone and usually contains either fibrous or granulation tissue. Discharge is often seropurulent in nature.

Neoplastic Ulcers

Neoplastic ulcers comprise basal cell carcinomas and squamous cell carcinomas, both presenting with well-defined raised edges. They normally occur when the centre of the ulcer becomes necrotic with the surrounding edge continuing to grow. While a BCC has an ulcer with a rolled up edge and a pearly pink tinge to its base, an SCC has an everted edge with a deep reddish-brown appearance.

Marjolin's ulcer refers to a chronic ulcer which undergoes neoplastic change (to squamous cell carcinoma).

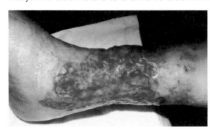

Fig. 2.20 Marjolin's ulcer

Source: Tang T and Praveen B V. *MRCS Picture Questions Book 1*. London: Radcliffe Publishing; 2006.

02.15
NECK LUMP

INSTRUCTIONS This patient has noticed a neck lump. Please examine this patient's neck and describe to the examiner what you are doing as you go along.

STAGE	KEY POINTS AND ACTIONS	SCORE		
	THE EXAMINATION			
Introduction	Introduce yourself. Elicit name, age, and occupation. Establish rapport.	0	1	–
Consent	Explain the examination to the patient and seek consent.			
Pain	Establish whether the patient is in pain.	0	1	–
Expose	Ask the patient to expose their neck.	0	1	–
	INSPECTION			
Neck	Observe the patient from the front and from the side. Look for scars, lesions, distended neck veins, goitre, or lumps.	0	1	–

Describing the Features of a Lump in the Neck

Site	Anterior/posterior triangle/midline Measure the distance to the nearest bony prominence
Size	Use a ruler to measure the lump's length and width
Shape	Circular/irregular; symmetrical/asymmetrical
Colour	Red/skin colour

STAGE	KEY POINTS AND ACTIONS	SCORE		
Sip Water	Ask the patient to sip some water, hold it in their mouth, then to swallow when asked to do so. If the lump moves on swallowing it may indicate a thyroid swelling, thyroglossal cyst, or lymph nodes.	0	1	–
Tongue Out	Ask the patient to stick their tongue out. If the lump moves on tongue protrusion it suggests a thyroglossal cyst (moves upward in the midline).	0	1	–
Look in Mouth	Inspect the oral cavity and throat using a pen torch for enlarged tonsils (infection or malignancy).	0	1	–
	PALPATION			
Feel	Stand behind the patient and palpate the lump. Place your hands on either side of the patient's neck and feel in the anterior and posterior triangles.	0	1	–

STAGE	KEY POINTS AND ACTIONS	SCORE
Lump	Feel the lump and note the following:	0 1 –

Features of a Neck Lump on Palpation

Temperature	Hot/cold/skin temperature
Tender	Tender (thyroiditis)/non-tender
Nodular	Solitary nodule/multi-nodular/diffusely enlarged
Surface	Smooth/rough/irregular
Consistency	Soft/spongy/rubbery/firm/stony hard
Mobility	Mobile/fixed (malignant)

STAGE	KEY POINTS AND ACTIONS	SCORE
Lymph Nodes	Palpate the anterior and posterior lymph nodes (malignancy).	0 1 –
Trachea	Feel for the tracheal position in the suprasternal notch. Note if the trachea is central or deviated.	0 1 –

PERCUSSION & AUSCULTATION

STAGE	KEY POINTS AND ACTIONS	SCORE
Percuss	Percuss down the midline of the neck and determine lower limit of the thyroid. A dull percussion note is suggestive of retrosternal extension.	
Auscultate	Ask the patient to hold their breath and then listen over the thyroid for any bruits (thyrotoxicosis).	0 1 –
Finishing Off	Thank the patient and acknowledge their concerns.	0 1 –

EXAMINER'S EVALUATION

Overall assessment of presenting correct physical findings		0 1 2 3 4 5

Total mark out of 18

DIFFERENTIAL DIAGNOSIS

Notes for the OSCE

Triangles of the Neck

Boundaries of Anterior Triangle	Boundaries of Posterior Triangle
Anteriorly – Line from the midchin to the jugular notch **Posteriorly** – Anterior border of the sternocleidomastoid **Base** – Lower border of mandible to mastoid process	**Anteriorly** – Posterior border of sternocleidomastoid **Posteriorly** – Anterior border of the trapezius **Base** – Middle 1/3 of clavicle

Branchial cyst
Appears from under the anterior border of the upper third of the SCM muscle

Carotid body tumour
Lies beneath the SCM muscle at the level of bifurcation of the common carotid artery

Cystic hygroma
Located in the posterior triangle

Thyroglossal cyst
Situated in the midline of the neck and is adherent to the larynx and trachea

Sternomastoid tumour
Located in the middle to lower third of the SCM muscle

Lumps in the Neck

Lymphadenopathy is the most common cause of neck swellings. Enlarged lymph nodes can be broadly classified into 4 categories, infective (TB, glandular fever, tonsillitis), metastatic (secondary deposits), lymphomas, and sarcoidosis.

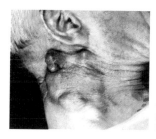

Fig. 2.21 **Metastatic lymphadenopathy**

Source: Tang T and Praveen B V. *MRCS Picture Questions Book 1*.
London: Radcliffe Publishing; 2006.

Branchial cyst is a remnant of the ectodermal pouch from the branchial cleft. It is located beneath the upper part of the SCM and presents as a painless cyst. It is a smooth cystic, ovoid shaped lump that is 5–10cm in diameter. It fluctuates but does not transilluminate light and cannot be compressed or reduced.

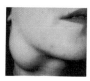

Fig. 2.22 **Branchial cyst**

Source: Tang T and Praveen B V. *MRCS Picture Questions Book 1*.
London: Radcliffe Publishing; 2006.

Carotid body tumour (chemodectoma) is a slowly growing painless lump. It is located at the bifurcation of the common carotid artery at the level of the upper border of the thyroid cartilage under the anterior border of the SCM muscle. It is a hard ovoid swelling that moves from side to side but not in the vertical plane. Transmitted pulsations are often present.

Fig. 2.23 **Angiogram showing a chemodectoma**

Source: Tang T and Praveen B V. *MRCS Picture Questions Book 1*.
London: Radcliffe Publishing; 2006.

Sternomastoid tumour is a firm solid swelling caused by trauma at birth. It is located at the middle third of the SCM muscle. Since the lump originates from the muscle only the anterior and posterior margins are distinct and may lead to torticollis in later life.

Cystic hygroma is a swelling of the jugular lymph sac and is situated at the base of the posterior triangle. The lump is a lobulated cyst and shows brilliant translucency.

Thyroglossal cyst is a cystic remnant of the thyroglossal duct that persists and is seen in early childhood. It is a hard well-defined spherical lump that is commonly found just above the hyoid bone and in the midline of the neck. Pathognomonic characteristics include moving on swallowing as well as on protrusion of the tongue.

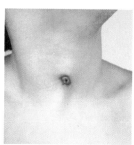

Fig. 2.24 **Fistulating thyroglossal cyst**

Source: Tang T and Praveen B V. *MRCS Picture Questions Book 1*.
London: Radcliffe Publishing; 2006.

For other causes of lumps originating from the thyroid gland *see* Thyroid chapter.

02.16 LYMPHATIC SYSTEM EXAMINATION

INSTRUCTIONS You will be asked to examine the lymphatic system of this patient. Please present your findings as well as a differential diagnosis to the examiners.

STAGE	KEY POINTS AND ACTIONS	SCORE
	THE EXAMINATION	
Introduction	Introduce yourself. Elicit name, age, and occupation. Establish rapport.	0 1 –
Consent	Explain the examination to the patient and seek consent. 'The examination will involve examining your hands, legs, neck, tummy, and groin. Would that be okay'?	
Position	Sit the patient at 45 degrees.	0 1 –
Expose	Ask the patient to remove their garments leaving on any underwear. Maintain the patient's dignity at all times as much as possible.	0 1 –
Question	Check the patient is comfortable and not in any pain.	0 1 –
Ask about B Symptoms	'Have you experienced weight loss, night sweats, or persistent fever in the past six months'?	0 1 –
	INSPECTION	

Signs in the Lymphatic Exam

Lymphadenopathy	Painless enlarged nodes
Acute lymphadenitis	Redness of overlying skin, oedema or tenderness
Lymphangitis	Observe for thin red streak marks leading to a group of nodes
Abdominal masses or distension	Massive hepato/splenomegaly
Cachexia	Late lymphoproliferative disease/TB
Haematological dysfunction	Pallor, breathlessness (anaemia)
	Easy bruising (thrombocytopenia)
Dilated subcutaneous veins, scars, sinuses, or ulcers	
Oedema in the upper or lower limbs	
Swellings or venous engorgement of the face and neck	SVC obstruction (large mediastinal mass)

STAGE	KEY POINTS AND ACTIONS	SCORE		
Hands	Check the pulse for tachycardia, collapsing pulse, and atrial fibrillation (hyperdynamic circulation; e.g. due to anaemia).	**0**	**1**	**–**
Face	Inspect for pallor of the conjunctiva (anaemia), old epistaxis (thrombocytopenia), and gum hypertrophy (acute myeloid leukaemia).	**0**	**1**	**2**
Palpation	Use the pulp of the fingertips to palpate the lymph node regions. Examine the lymph nodes of one half of the body and then compare with the other side.	**0**	**1**	**–**

If a swelling is detected in a lymph region, palpate it with the palmar aspects of three fingers. Note its site, size, number, consistency, tenderness, temperature, whether it is matted, and its mobility.

Describing the Features of a Lymph Node

Site	Symmetrical/asymmetrical distribution
Localized	Cervical, axillary, epitrochlear, inguinal popliteal
Generalized	Lymphoma, lymphatic leukaemia, viral (HIV, EBV, CMV), bacterial (TB, syphilis), toxoplasmosis, sarcoidosis, RA
Size	Measure dimensions using a ruler
Shape	Circular/irregular
Consistency	Soft – bacterial infection
	Firm – lymphatic leukaemia/syphilis
	Rubbery – Hodgkin's disease
	Stony hard – secondary carcinoma
Tenderness	Tender (infection)/non-tender (malignancy)
Matted	Matted – TB, acute lymphadenitis, malignancy
	Discrete – lymphoma, leukaemia
Mobility	Fixed to surrounding structures (malignancy)

STAGE	KEY POINTS AND ACTIONS	SCORE		
Cervical	To examine the cervical lymph nodes stand behind the patient with them seated. Use the pads of all four fingers of both hands to palpate both sides of the head simultaneously.	**0**	**1**	**2**

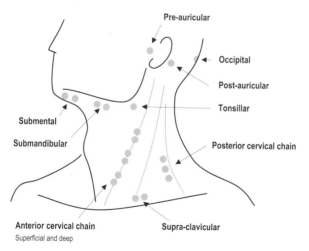

Pre-auricular
Occipital
Post-auricular
Tonsillar
Posterior cervical chain
Submental
Submandibular
Anterior cervical chain
Superficial and deep
Supra-clavicular

STAGE	KEY POINTS AND ACTIONS	SCORE

Examine in the following sequence:

1. Submental	Just below the tip of the mandible
2. Submandibular	Underside of the lower margin of the mandible
3. Tonsillar	Just below the angle of the mandible
4. Pre-auricular	In front of the ear
5. Anterior (superficial and deep) cervical chain	Lying both on top of and beneath the sternocleidomastoid muscles
6. Supraclavicular	Posterior cervical chain (lying anterior to the trapezius)
7. Post auricular	Over the mastoid process
8. Occipital nodes	Base of the skull posteriorly

Chest — Observe the JVP for any sign of SVC obstruction (*see* in large mediastinal lymphoma) – fixed and raised. Percuss retrosternally for mediastinal dullness. 0 1 2

Axilla — Examine the axillary lymph nodes by sitting in front of the patient. Support the patient's right elbow with your right hand while permitting the patient to rest their hand on your shoulder. Palpate the anterior, posterior, medial, central, and lateral axillary nodes with your free hand. Repeat for the opposite side. 0 1 2

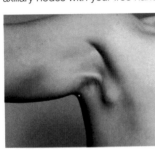

Fig. 2.25 Axillary lymphadenopathy

Source: Tang T and Praveen B V. *MRCS Picture Questions Book 1.* London: Radcliffe Publishing; 2006.

Epitrochlear — Palpate the epitrochlear lymph nodes with the elbow flexed at 90 degrees. Hold the patient's right wrist with the left hand and support his elbow with your other free hand. Palpate the right epitrochlear lymph region with the thumb of your right hand. 0 1 2

Abdomen — Inspect for obvious distension, especially in the left flank. Start palpating the spleen in the RIF and work slowly toward the left hypochondrium, feeling for splenomegaly. Percuss Traube's space, the 9th/10th ICS in the anterior axillary line, for dullness. Listen over the spleen for bruits, splenic rubs. 0 1 2

Palpate for Hepatomegaly — Examine the inguinal region for lymphadenopathy. 0 1 2

Inguinal — Have the patient lying flat on the couch before examining the inguinal lymph nodes. Palpate the horizontal chain, located just below the length of the inguinal ligament, and the vertical chain, found along the path of the saphenous vein. 0 1 2

Popliteal — Flex the patient's knees to 45 degrees in order to relax the popliteal fossa. Encapsulate the knee with your hands and palpate for enlarged lymph nodes with the fingers of both hands. 0 1 2

Causes of enlarged lymph nodes

Cervical region	Dental infections (submental), tonsillitis (tonsillar), middle ear infections, viral conjunctivitis (pre-auricular), outer ear infections (occipital), secondary syphilis (occipital), TB, glandular fever, secondary carcinoma, lymphoma, sarcoidosis
Axillary	Upper limb infections, breast infections (mastitis), secondary carcinoma
Epitrochlear region	Secondary syphilis, leukaemia, lymphoma
Inguinal region	Lower limb infections (ulcers), genital infections (primary syphilis, genital herpes)
Popliteal region	Infections of the foot and leg

Legs — Inspect for bruises, peripheral oedema (lymphoedema) and varicosities (abdominal malignancy). 0 1 2

STAGE	KEY POINTS AND ACTIONS	SCORE
Finishing Off	Thank the patient and offer to help them get dressed.	0 1 –
Request	Request to perform a full physical examination, take a full history and order some basic blood tests such as an FBC and LDH (for tumour load).	0 1 –
Present	Present a structured, complete, and thorough presentation and offer your differential diagnosis with investigation and management (if appropriate). (See Chapter 2.31 for a useful structure.)	0 1 –

EXAMINER'S EVALUATION

Overall assessment of examination of the lymphatic system	0 1 2 3 4 5

Total mark out of 35

EXEMPLAR PRESENTATION

'Today I examined the lymphatic system of Mrs F, a 23-year-old anthropology student. She was comfortable at rest, in no pain, and reported a six-week history of fever and night sweats. She was peripherally well perfused, with no pallor or obvious bruising. There was a large, 4-5cm, circular, rubbery, non-tender mass arising in the anterior cervical chain. There was also axillary and inguinal lymphadenopathy, several smaller, circular, rubbery and non-tender nodes were palpable at each site. The spleen was markedly enlarged, approximately 15cm below the subcostal margin. There was no peripheral oedema or varicosities. In summary this is a 23-year-old anthropology student with a large cervical lymph node and widespread lymphadenopathy with a six-week history of B symptoms. These findings are most consistent with a diagnosis of lymphoma, involving both sides of the diaphragm and therefore at least an Ann-Arbor stage III or greater. The differential includes other disseminated malignancy and TB. My initial management would be to ensure the patient is stable and comfortable, organise some basic blood tests including an FBC, U&E, and LDH to assess tumour load and arrange an excision biopsy of a safely accessible lymph node to gain a histological diagnosis, with staging imaging such as CT-PET chest/abdo/pelvis. Further management would be decided within the multidisciplinary team of a specialist unit'. ∎

DIFFERENTIAL DIAGNOSIS

Hodgkin's Disease

Hodgkin's disease is a malignant proliferation of lymphocytes with the presence of Reed-Sternberg cells. It is more common in males (2:1), especially before puberty, with a bimodal age incidence, and an early peak in young adulthood and another in advanced age. It normally presents as painless enlargement of the lymph nodes of the cervical group or occasionally in the axillary or inguinal region. Associated symptoms include weight loss, fever with rigors (Pel-Ebstein fever), and night sweats. On examination, the lymph nodes are ovoid in shape, smooth, discrete, and rubbery in consistency. Hepatosplenomegaly is also a feature of this condition.

Infectious Mononucleosis (Glandular Fever)

Glandular fever is a disease that frequently affects young adults. It is caused by the Epstein-Barr virus (EBV) and is spread by the transference of saliva (known as the 'kissing disease'), or water droplets. It causes generalised enlargement of the lymph nodes which are firm and slightly tender. It is associated with sore throats, fever, palatal petechiae, and splenomegaly with a positive Paul-Bunnell test.

Secondary Carcinoma

This represents metastases to local lymph nodes. These are slow growing, painless, stony hard, irregularly shaped lymph nodes that are fixated to surrounding structures. The site of the lymph node as well as the patient's symptoms gives an indication where the primary site of growth is; e.g. Virchow's node suggests the presence of a gastric carcinoma.

Tuberculosis Lymphadenitis

Tuberculosis lymphadenitis occurs in children and young adults especially amongst the immigrant population. Enlarged lymph nodes are detected by the patient most commonly in the cervical region but occasionally in the mesenteric and axillary regions. On examination, enlarged lymph nodes are noted in the deep cervical nodes. They are indistinct, firm masses that are matted together. After caseation, the lymph node becomes an abscess (collar stud abscess) which may open on to the surface via a central track and form a discharging sinus. This abscess is also found in the upper deep cervical lymph region. It is cold, tender, and rubbery in consistency with a mild reddish-purple discolouration to the overlying skin. If the abscess contains enough pus it may also fluctuate.

02.17 THYROID

INSTRUCTIONS Examine this patient's neck and then proceed as you see fit. Please present your findings as well as a differential diagnosis to the examiners.

STAGE	KEY POINTS AND ACTIONS	SCORE
	THE EXAMINATION	
Introduction	Introduce yourself. Elicit name, age, and occupation. Establish rapport.	0 1 –
Consent	Explain the examination to the patient and seek consent. 'I would like to examine a gland in your neck and its function – this will involve looking at your hands, head, and legs, listening and feeling the gland in the neck, and listening to your heart. Would that be okay'?	
Position	Sit the patient upright initially.	0 1 –
Question	Check the patient is comfortable and not in any pain.	0 1 –
Opening	Ask the patient an open question 'How did you get here today'? – assess for slow speech or hoarse voice (hypothyroidism).	0 1 –
	INSPECTION	
	Inspect the patient for appropriateness of clothing, visible tremor, and body habitus.	
Hands	**Hand signs in thyroid disease**	0 1 –

Hypothyroidism	Hyperthyroidism
Pallor of palmar creases (anaemia)	Fine tremor*
Carpal tunnel release scars	Thyroid acropachy (only seen in Graves')
Swollen hands	Tachycardia +/– atrial fibrillation
Bradycardia	Collapsing pulse (hyperdynamic circulation)

*Place a piece of paper across the outstretched hands to detect a tremor.

STAGE	KEY POINTS AND ACTIONS	SCORE
Arms	Check for proximal muscle weakness (seen in both hyper- and hypothyroidism).	0 1 –
Face	**Face signs in thyroid disease**	0 1 2

Hypothyroidism	Hyperthyroidism
Loss of outer ⅓ eyebrows (Queen Ann sign)	Proptosis
Dry skin	+/– Opthalmoplegia
Puffy, swollen face	Irritability
Pallor and hair thinning	Hair loss
Fatigued expression	

STAGE	KEY POINTS AND ACTIONS	SCORE
	Examine the patient from the front, and then stand behind and inspect the hair and observe for proptosis from above the patient looking down.	
	Examine the eye movements with one hand on the patient's head, and one finger an arm's length away, asking them to follow your finger with their eyes. Ask about pain and double vision.	
	Observe for opthalmoplegia (exclusively seen in Graves') and lid lag (hyperthyroidism – predominantly Graves').	
Neck	Inspect the neck with the patient's neck slightly tilted upwards. Look carefully for a goitre – a central, equally enlarged mass, firm, non-fluctuant that moves upward with swallowing but not with tongue protrusion. Give the patient a glass of water to swallow from and inspect the movement of the thyroid.	0 1 –
	Palpate the neck from behind; feel for a goitre. Again, ask the patient to swallow and protrude their tongue. Also palpate for cervical lymphadenopathy (seen in papillary carcinoma of the thyroid).	
	Percuss over the sternum for retrosternal extension of a goitre.	
	Listen for a bruit over the thyroid (pathognomonic for Graves' disease).	
Chest	Briefly auscultate the heart for flow murmurs (hyperthyroidism) and atrial fibrillation. If present, time the rate apically for one minute to establish the true heart rate.	0 1 –
Legs	Palpate the legs for thickened, brown discolouration – pretibial myxoedema (seen in Graves' exclusively).	0 1 –
	Ask the patient to cross their arms across their chest and stand observing for proximal myopathy.	
	Test the ankle jerk with the patient's knees on the chair facing away from you. Look for slow-relaxing reflexes (hypothyroidism).	
Finishing Off	Thank the patient and offer to help them get dressed.	0 1 –
Request	Request to perform a full cardiovascular examination, take some basic thyroid function tests and a full history.	0 1 –
Present	Present a structured, complete, and thorough presentation and offer your differential diagnosis with investigation and management (if appropriate). (See Chapter 2.31 for a useful structure.)	0 1 –

EXAMINER'S EVALUATION

Overall assessment of examination of the thyroid	0 1 2 3 4 5

Total mark out of 19

NOTES ON THE **THYROID** EXAM

Graves' Disease

This is an autoimmune condition typically seen in women, with more severe forms occurring in men and smokers. The pathognomonic features that favour Graves' over any other cause of hyperthyroidism are: thyroid acropachy, proptosis and ophthalmoplegia, thyroid bruit, and pretibial myxoedema. These signs are independent of biochemical thyroid function; they are thought to be caused by the underlying autoimmune process and not the overactive thyroid itself. Treatment depends on the severity of disease but the modalities of treatment are medical blockade – carbimazole and propylthiouracil, radiation – radioiodine treatment, or surgery – partial or total thyroidectomy and replacement. Smoking aggravates eye disease and it is extremely advisable to stop.

Other causes of hyperthyroidism

Multi-nodular goitre	Usually euthyroid but has the potential to bleed or form a toxic nodule (pictured below).
Toxic adenoma	Neoplastic production of thyroid hormone
De Quervains' thyroiditis	Also known as subacute thyroiditis, produces a transient hyperthyroid state and then a long hypothyroid state. Radio-labelled iodine scan shows globally decreased uptake despite hyperthyroid state. Occurs post-infection and post-pregnancy.
Drug-induced	Amiodarone can cause a hyper- or hypothyroid state.
Factitious hyperthyroidism	Levothyroxine is sometimes abused as an anti-weight gain medication in anorexic patients.
Struma ovarii	Ovarian teratoma produces thyroid hormone. Vanishingly rare.

Hypothyroidism

The commonest cause in this country is Hashimoto's, an autoimmune inflammatory condition associated with anti-TPO antibodies. In the developing world, iodine deficiency produces congenital hypothyroidism – this is known as cretinism. Severe, untreated hypothyroidism can present with profound peripheral oedema (anasarca), bradycardia, decreased consciousness, and hypothermia. This is known as myxoedema coma and is a medical emergency, if it is diagnosed in time. Mortality, even when treated, remains as high as 25-30%.

Thyroid Carcinoma

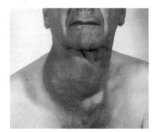

Fig. 2.26 Thyroid carcinoma

Source: Tang T and Praveen B V. *MRCS Picture Questions Book 1.*
London: Radcliffe Publishing; 2006.

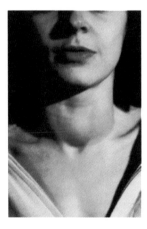

Fig. 2.27 Multinodular goitre

Source: Tang T and Praveen B V. *MRCS Picture Questions Book 1.*
London: Radcliffe Publishing; 2006.

02.18
BREAST

INSTRUCTIONS This patient is concerned about an abnormality in her left breast. Carry out a full examination of her breasts. The examiner will ask you for your findings and interpretation of them.

STAGE	KEY POINTS AND ACTIONS	SCORE
	THE EXAMINATION	
Introduction	Introduce yourself. Elicit name, age, and occupation. Establish rapport.	0 1 –
Consent	Explain the examination to the patient and seek consent.	
Chaperone	Inform the patient that you will request a chaperone.	0 1 –
Pain	Always ask about pain. 'Before we begin, do you have any pain anywhere'?	0 1 –
Expose	Ask the patient to undress to the waist and provide a blanket for her to cover herself with. Get the patient to sit on the edge of the bed with her arms by her sides.	
	INSPECTION	
General	Inspect the breasts with the patient's arms by her sides. Look for the following:	0 1 –

Signs to observe with patient's arms by her sides

Breast Symmetry	Symmetrical (same level)/asymmetrical
Contour	Shape deformity
Swellings	Fibrocystic changes, fibroadenoma, abscess, carcinoma
Nipple Inversion	Congenital, cancer
Nipple Discharge	Look for discharge on the patient's nipple or on clothes
Skin Changes:	
Peau d'orange	Dimpling of the skin (breast carcinoma)
Eczema around nipple	Paget's disease
Scars	Breast augmentation surgery, previous surgery

STAGE	KEY POINTS AND ACTIONS	SCORE

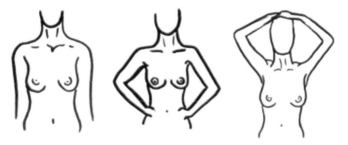

Inspect the breasts with the patient's arms elevated and placed on her head. Look for any indentation or tethering of any swellings (malignancy) and for asymmetrical contour of the breast. Inspect the breast with the patient's hands pressed firmly on her hips. Inspect axilla for enlarged lymph nodes or the presence of any scars.

Also note: Age (increased risk with age), body habitus (increased risk with obesity), and asymmetry in the arms (which may signify lymphoedema resulting from lymph node resection).

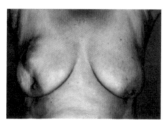

Fig. 2.28 Advanced breast cancer

Source: Tang T and Praveen B V. *MRCS Picture Questions Book 2*. London: Radcliffe Publishing; 2006.

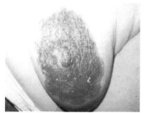

Fig. 2.29 Paget's disease of the breast

Source: Tang T and Praveen B V. *MRCS Picture Questions Book 2*. London: Radcliffe Publishing; 2006.

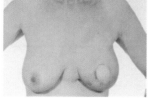

Fig. 2.30 Post breast reconstruction

Source: Tang T and Praveen B V. *MRCS Picture Questions Book 2*. London: Radcliffe Publishing; 2006.

PALPATION

Position | Lie the patient at a 45 degree angle with one hand behind her head. Before palpation, ask the patient if they have any breast tenderness or lumps. If there is, ask the patient to point toward it. Start palpating with the normal side first. | 0 1 –

STAGE	KEY POINTS AND ACTIONS	SCORE
Technique	Palpate all four quadrants of the breast with the flat of the fingers using the other hand to steady the breast. Use a rotary movement of the fingers when palpating and gently compress the breast tissue against the chest wall to feel for the presence of any swellings. Examine the breast in a concentric ring starting from the nipple and working outward. Examine the whole breast including its borders and then palpate the tail of Spence with the thumb and forefinger.	0 1 –
Lump	If a lump is present, establish the following:	0 1 –

Features of a breast lump to establish in examination

Site	Upper/lower, inner/outer quadrant
Size	Measure dimensions using a ruler
Shape	Circular/irregular
Consistency	Firm/rubbery/stony hard/spongy/soft
Temperature	Warm/cold
Mobility	Move the lump up and down and side to side: mobile/fixed/tethered

*Use this structure to describe the lump when presenting your findings.

STAGE	KEY POINTS AND ACTIONS	SCORE
Nipple	Ask the patient if they have ever noticed any discharge from the nipple and, if so, could they express it. Note the colour of the discharge and then state that you would smear and swab for cytology and microbiology.	

Types of Nipple Discharge
- **White** – Milk (Lactation)
- **Yellow** (exudate) – Fibroadenosis, abscess
- **Green** (cellular debris) – Fibroadenosis, duct ectasia
- **Red** (blood) – Duct carcinoma, duct papilloma

STAGE	KEY POINTS AND ACTIONS	SCORE
Axillae	Rest the patient's right elbow in your right hand, taking the weight of her forearm. With your spare hand, palpate the anterior, medial, posterior, and apex regions of the right axilla. Repeat on the other side.	0 1 –
Lymph Nodes	Stand behind the patient and palpate her cervical lymph nodes as well as the supraclavicular fossa. Feel for any nodes on the medial aspect of the humerus.	0 1 –
Repeat	Repeat the above examination on the other breast.	0 1 –
Finishing Off	Thank and cover the patient and acknowledge her concerns.	0 1 –
Request	Request to perform a full abdominal examination (looking for hepatomegaly and ascites), to auscultate the lungs, and to palpate the spine for any tenderness.	0 1 –

EXAMINER'S EVALUATION

Overall assessment of examination of breast	0 1 2 3 4 5

Total mark out of 17

EXEMPLAR PRESENTATION

'Today I performed a breast examination on Mrs X, a 26-year-old cartoonist complaining of an abnormality of her left breast. On inspection there were no scars or skin changes and the breasts were symmetrical in size and shape. The nipples appeared normal with no discharge. On palpation there was a discrete 1cm by 1cm palpable lump in the left upper quadrant of the left breast. It was round, with a rubbery consistency and mobile (with no tethering to the skin above or muscle below). I would like to proceed to take a full history from the patient. In this age group, the lump on examination is most likely to be a fibroadenoma'. ■

PEARLS FOR THE OSCE

Common Causes of Breast Lumps

Traumatic	Fat necrosis	Hard irregular lump with history of trauma
Infective	Pyogenic abscess	Tender lump with pus collecting in the abscess caused by bacterial infection
Physiological	Fibroadenosis	Fibrocystic change. Peak incidence above 35 years old
Neoplastic	Fibroadenoma	Benign tumour occurring in women below 35 years old
	Carcinoma	Malignant (primary/secondary)
	Phylloides tumour	Rare fibro-epithelial tumour
	Duct papilloma	Benign proliferation of epithelium in major ducts with bloody discharge in single nipple and swelling lateral to the areola

Breast Cancer

Breast cancer is the most prevalent cancer among women and accounts for a third of all female cancers in the UK.

The characteristics of breast carcinomas are firm, irregular masses that are rarely painful but often tethered or fixed to the skin. Accompanying features include nipple changes, localised oedema, lymphadenopathy, bloody discharge, and symptoms that correlate to metastatic disease (breathlessness, backache, jaundice, malaise, and weight loss). It is not uncommon to find a positive family history of breast cancer.

The 5 Modalities for the Treatment of Breast Cancer

Chemotherapy	**Adjuvant** – After surgery aimed at any residual disease **Neo-adjuvant** – Before surgery to shrink tumour
Surgery	**Breast conserving** – Lumpectomy, partial mastectomy, wide local excision **Mastectomy** – Removal of breast tissue and nipple **Lymph node surgery** – Sentinel lymph node biopsy guides extent of resection
Radiotherapy	Can be applied to the breast, chest wall, or lymph nodes
Hormonal therapies	For hormone receptor positive cancers in which progesterone and oestrogen stimulate their growth **Tamoxifen** – Oestrogen receptor antagonist Only for use in pre-menopausal women (oestrogen is still produced by ovaries): **Ovarian ablation** – Surgery or radiotherapy **Ovarian suppression** – Goserelin (LRH hormone antagonist) Only for use in post-menopausal women (oestrogen produced peripherally via an aromatase): **Aromatase inhibitors;** e.g. Anastrazole
Biological therapies	**Trastuzumab (Herceptin)** – Monoclonal antibody aimed at blocking HER 2 receptor which stimulates the growth of some cancers

Fibroadenoma

Fibroadenomas are the most common benign tumours of the female breast. They develop at any age but are more common in young women (25–35 years old) and are often mistaken for cancer. Fibroadenomas are rarely painful in nature but may be multiple in number. They are smooth in surface and rubbery hard in consistency. They are usually small (1–3cm in size), highly mobile (unlike breast carcinomas), and can occur in any part of the breast.

Fibroadenosis

Fibroadenosis or fibrocystic disease is the most common cause of breast lumps in women of reproductive age. The peak incidence is between 35 and 50 years of age. It is rare before 25 years. Patients usually present with single or multiple lumps in the upper outer quadrant of the breast, which are associated with cyclical breast pain, being at its greatest pre-menstrually. The lumps are often smooth and rubbery firm in texture and are usually bilateral in distribution. Sometimes there is nipple discharge which is either clear white or green in colour.

02.19
RECTAL

INSTRUCTIONS You are seeing Mr O, a 68-year-old man, who has presented with an abdominal mass and bleeding per-rectally. You have completed an abdominal examination and now wish to examine his back passage. Explain to the examiner what you would do, and then demonstrate on the model the procedure you would carry out.

STAGE	KEY POINTS AND ACTIONS	SCORE		
	THE EXAMINATION			
Introduction	Introduce yourself. Elicit name, age, and occupation. Establish rapport.	0	1	–
Explain	'Because of the symptoms you have presented with, I would like to examine your back passage to see whether there are any problems there. The examination may be slightly uncomfortable but will not be painful'.	0	1	–
Consent	Obtain consent.			
Chaperone	Request the presence of a chaperone, if appropriate.	0	1	–
Dignity	Keep the curtain drawn at all times to maintain privacy.			
Expose	Ask the patient to remove all their lower garments including any underpants.	0	1	–
Position	Have the patient lying on their left hand side with their buttocks at the edge of the bed and their knees drawn up to their chest.	0	1	–
Gloves	Wash your hands and don a pair of gloves.			
	INSPECTION			
Anus	Raise the uppermost buttock and inspect the anus as well as the surrounding skin. Look for scars, excoriations, skin tags, ulcers, fissures, polyps, prolapsed piles, or external haemorrhoids.	0	1	–

STAGE	KEY POINTS AND ACTIONS	SCORE

PALPATION

Lubricate Apply lubricant to the gloved index finger of your right hand.

Warn Warn the patient that you are about to enter the back passage. Ask them to first relax by breathing slowly and deeply and then to bear down as if they are trying to have a bowel movement. This helps to relax their external sphincter and should decrease discomfort.   `0  1  –`

Fissures may make the rectal examination extremely painful therefore cease and postpone until anaesthesia is made available.

Insert As the patient bears down gently insert your finger into the anus following through to the rectum. As your finger enters the anal canal, note for any pain, tenderness, or masses.

Sphincter Assess anal sphincter tone by asking the patient to tense and squeeze your index finger.   `0  1  –`

Rectum Palpate the entire rectum by rotating your hand clockwise and anticlockwise feeling for any masses. If a mass is detected, ask the patient to strain downwards in order to bring it closer to your finger.   `0  1  –`

Palpate the rectum noting if it is loaded with stool or if the rectum is collapsed or empty but inflated. Feel for the consistency of any faeces noting if they are hard or soft in nature.

Prostate In males, palpate the prostate gland noting for any tenderness, its size, shape, surface, consistency, and the presence of a midline groove.   `0  1  2`

Signs when Palpating the Prostate Gland

Size	Normal or enlarged
Shape	Regular (bilobed) or irregular
Surface	Smooth or uneven
Consistency	Firm/rubbery/hard
Central Sulcus	Present or absent
Rectal Mucosa	Mobile or fixed

Cervix In females, identify the uterine cervix and note its size and shape. Feel for the presence of any ovarian masses.

Withdraw Remove your index finger and examine the stool found on the glove. Note its colour and the presence of blood or mucus.   `0  1  –`

FINISHING OFF

Clean Wipe off any lubricant remaining on the anus and remove any faeces on the anal margin using a gauze or tissue.   `0  1  –`

Dispose Remove and dispose of the gloves along with any other waste safely.

Request Request a proctoscopy or sigmoidoscopy depending on your findings.

STAGE	KEY POINTS AND ACTIONS	SCORE
Thank the Patient	Acknowledge patient's concerns. Restore patient's clothing.	0 1 –
	Summarise your findings to the examiner.	

EXAMINER'S EVALUATION

Overall competence in performing the rectal examination	0 1 2 3 4 5

Total mark out of 19

DIFFERENTIAL DIAGNOSIS

A Normal Prostate

A normal prostate gland is between 2 and 3 centimetres in diameter with both lobes symmetrically arranged and divided by a shallow central sulcus. It has a smooth texture and is firm and rubbery in consistency. The rectal mucosa is mobile and is not fixed to any underlying tissue.

Benign Prostatic Hypertrophy

Benign prostatic hypertrophy is a condition caused by the benign hyperplasia of prostatic cells. It causes a generalised enlargement of the prostate with mild distortion to its shape. It presents as an enlarged, smooth, asymmetrically shaped prostate with a firm rubbery consistency. The midline groove is often present and is one of the last features to disappear. The rectal mucosa remains mobile and unfixed to the underlying tissues.

Prostate Carcinoma

Prostate carcinoma causes a hard, irregular, asymmetrical prostate gland that can be palpated on examination. Such features can be unilateral in nature affecting a single lobe. The central sulcus is often obliterated resulting in the loss of the midline groove. The rectal mucosa may be involved and may be tethered to the underlying gland.

02.20 INGUINAL SCROTAL

INSTRUCTIONS This patient has noticed a swelling in the groin. Carry out an appropriate examination. Present your findings to the examiner as you go along.

STAGE	KEY POINTS AND ACTIONS	SCORE
	THE EXAMINATION	
Introduction	Introduce yourself. Elicit name, age, and occupation. Establish rapport.	0 1 –
Consent	Explain the examination to the patient and seek consent.	
Expose & Position	Expose the patient's groin and external genitalia. Have the patient sitting at the beginning of the examination.	0 1 –
	EXTERNAL GENITALIA	
	Inspection	
Observe	Inspect the anterior aspect of the scrotum. Also examine the posterior aspect of the scrotum by pulling on posterior skin and not the patient's testes. Look for any skin changes or swellings in the inguinal or scrotal areas.	0 1 –
	Palpation	
Testis	Ask the patient if there is any pain or tenderness in the testis. An acute, tender, and enlarged testis is suggestive of torsion of the testis. Roll the testes between your thumb and index finger. Determine if both testicles are palpable. Note the absence of a testis (orchidectomy, undescended testis).	0 1 –
Epididymis	Locate the epididymis found above and posterior to the testes. Note any swellings (epididymitis).	0 1 –
Spermatic Cord	Feel along the spermatic cord found above the epididymis. Note any swellings (epididymal cyst).	0 1 –
	Differentials of Scrotal Swellings [Mnemonic—SHOVE IT] • **S**permatocele • **H**ydrocele/Haematocele • **O**rchitis • **V**aricocele • **E**pididymal cyst • **I**ndirect inguinal hernia • **T**orsion of the testis/Testicular tumour	

STAGE	KEY POINTS AND ACTIONS	SCORE
Lump	Feel the lump noting the following:	0 1 –

Describing the Features of a Scrotal Lump

Site	Testicular/separate (scrotum)
Size	Use a ruler to measure the lump's length and width
Shape	Circular/irregular
Consistency	Firm/rubbery/stony hard/spongy/soft
Transilluminate	No (solid) or Yes (cystic or hydrocele)
Upper Edge	If unable to palpate for upper border (Inguinoscrotal hernia)

Lymph Nodes	Suggest palpating Virchow's node (left superior clavicular node) and para-aortic nodes (testicular tumour).	0 1 –

Differential Diagnosis for Scrotal Lumps

Site & Transillumination	Diagnosis
Non-testicular & cystic	Epididymal cyst (spermatocele)
Non-testicular & solid	Epididymitis
Testicular & cystic	Hydrocele
Testicular & solid	Tumour, orchitis, granuloma

HERNIAS

Inspection

Inspection	Inspect for previous scars. Ask the patient to locate the lump. Ask them if they can stand for the remainder of the examination with their feet apart. Stand to the side of the patient whilst inspecting.	0 1 –

Palpation

Hernia	Locate the pubic tubercle and then locate the superficial ring (above and medial to it). Place one hand behind the patient and the examining hand over the swelling. Press firmly over the swelling. If no swelling is present, place your fingers over the superficial ring. Ask the patient if there is any pain and then press firmly over the superficial ring.	0 1 –
Lump	Feel the lump observing its site, size, shape, and consistency. Feel for its temperature as well as the presence of a cough impulse.	0 1 –

Describing the Features of a Hernia

Site	Describe the lump in relation to the pubic tubercle:
	Superior & medial: Superficial ring (Direct or indirect hernia)
	Inferior & lateral: Femoral ring (Femoral hernia)
Size	Use a ruler to measure the dimensions
Shape	Circular/irregular
Consistency	Firm/rubbery/stony hard/spongy/soft
Temperature	Hot (strangulated hernia)
Cough	Ask the patient to look away and to produce a cough. Positive cough impulse (inguinal hernia or saphena varix)

Reduce	Ask the patient to reduce the hernia. The patient may request to lie down to do this. While the hernia is reduced, place two fingers over the deep ring (1.5 cm above the femoral pulse).	0 1 2
State	Display anatomical knowledge of structures by stating that the inguinal ligament is the line between ASIS and the pubic tubercle and the deep ring is half way along this line (inguinal ligament's midpoint).	

STAGE	KEY POINTS AND ACTIONS	SCORE
Cough	Ask the patient to cough and feel for a cough impulse over the deep ring. If there is a cough impulse in the deep ring but an absence of a lump in the superficial ring, it suggests an indirect hernia. However, if there is no cough impulse over the deep ring but a lump appears in the superficial ring, it suggests a direct hernia.	
Percuss	Percuss the lump for a resonant percussion note (bowel involvement).	
Auscultate	Listen over the lump for bowel sounds (bowel involvement).	0 1 –
Lymph Node	Feel along the inguinal ligament (anterior superior iliac spine to the pubic tubercle) for the horizontal chain of nodes and over the medial thigh for the vertical chain of lymph nodes.	0 1 –
Femoral Artery	Palpate the femoral arteries and auscultate for bruits (femoral aneurysm).	0 1 –
Request	Suggest inspecting for saphenofemoral varix (disappears on lying down).	0 1 –
[Mnemonic:— 'Hernias **V**ery **M**uch **L**ike **T**o **S**well']	**Differentials for a Hernial Mass** • **H**ernias – Inguinal, femoral hernias • **V**ascular – Saphena varix, femoral aneurysm • **M**uscle – Psoas abscess • **L**ymph nodes – Inguinal lymph nodes • **T**esticle – Ectopic testis, undescended testis • **S**permatic cord – Lipoma, hydrocele	
Repeat	Repeat the examination on the other side.	0 1 –
	FINISHING OFF	
Thanks	Thank the patient and cover their legs. Acknowledge the patient's concerns. Restore patient's clothing.	0 1 –
Present	Wash your hands and summarise your findings to the examiner.	0 1 –
	EXAMINER'S EVALUATION	
	Overall assessment of examination of the inguinal scrotal	0 1 2 3 4 5
	Total mark out of 25	

NOTES FOR THE OSCE

Testicular Cancer

Testicular cancer is the commonest seen malignancy in young men.

There are generally two variants present, seminoma (30–50 yrs) and teratomas (20–30 yrs). It usually presents as a painless swelling of the testis. On examination, the lump is limited to the scrotum and may be difficult to feel discretely from the testis. It is often irregular, nodular, and large in size. The tumour is firm and hard with no evidence of fluctuation or transillumination. The para-aortic lymph nodes should be examined for secondary spread.

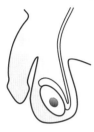

Hydrocele

A hydrocele is a collection of fluid within the tunica vaginalis. It is often classified into primary (idiopathic) and secondary (trauma, cancer, infection) hydroceles. On examination, a large swelling occupies one side of the scrotum (can be bilateral). The swelling is not tender (unless secondary), dull to percussion, fluctuant, and may have a fluid thrill. The fluid of the hydrocele envelops the testis often making it impalpable. If the swelling is not separate and distinct from the testis then a hydrocele can be ruled out.

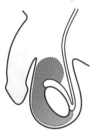

Epididymal Cysts

Epididymal cysts are fluid filled swellings located in the epididymis. On examination, a smooth multilocular cyst can be palpated, often bilaterally, in the scrotum. It is located above and behind the testis clearly distinct and separate from it. The cysts are fluctuant and brilliantly translucent as they contain clear fluid. Spermatoceles are unilocular cysts also found in the epididymis. Since they contain spermatozoa the fluid is grey and opaque and resembles barley water. As a result, transillumination is less pronounced than that of epididymal cysts.

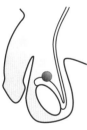

Epididymo-orchitis

Acute epididymo-orchitis is caused by infection of the epididymis which later spreads to the testis. It is caused by chlamydia (young), gonococcus (older) and E. coli. It normally presents with severe pain and swelling of the testis limited to one side of the scrotum. On examination the scrotal skin is red, hot, and oedematous with tenderness to the epididymis and testis on palpation. There may be enlargement of the whole testis.

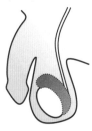

Varicocele

A varicocele is a collection of dilated veins in the pampiniform plexus. They appear tortuous and distended on standing and are often described as a 'bag of worms'. Classically, on lying down they disappear and become impalpable.

Lumps in the Groin

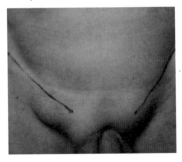

Fig. 2.31 Bilateral inguinal swelling

Source: Tang T and Praveen B V. *MRCS Picture Questions Book 1*. London: Radcliffe Publishing; 2006.

Inguinal hernias present as a lump in the groin or scrotum. They are the result of the herniation of the contents of the abdomen through the inguinal region. Both direct and indirect hernias pass through the superficial ring found above and medial to the pubic tubercle. Indirect hernias originate from the deep (internal) ring, travel obliquely along the inguinal canal and pass out through the superficial ring. They are the commonest type of hernia (80%) and often extend to the bottom of the scrotum.

This hernia can be reduced to the deep ring with a cough impulse felt if occluded with two fingers at this site. Direct hernias herniate through a weakness of the posterior wall of the inguinal canal and pass out through the superficial ring. They are less common (20%) and rarely extend to the bottom of the scrotum. If reduced, the hernia is not controlled by occlusion of the deep ring by a cough impulse and reappears through the superficial ring.

Femoral hernias are the herniation of the bowel through the femoral canal with their neck below and lateral to the pubic tubercle. They are more common in females and frequently strangulate.

02.21 GALS (GAIT, ARMS, LEGS, SPINE SCREEN)

INSTRUCTIONS You will be asked to examine the musculoskeletal system of this patient. Screen the patient systemically.

STAGE	KEY POINTS AND ACTIONS	SCORE
	THE EXAMINATION	
Introduction	Introduce yourself. Elicit name, age, and occupation. Establish rapport.	0 1 –
Consent	Explain the examination to the patient and seek consent. 'The examination will involve inspecting your joints and testing the movements in your arms, legs, spine, and hips. Would that be okay'?	
Expose	Ideally the patient should be wearing underwear only.	0 1 –
Position	Stand the patient up initially.	0 1 –
Questions	Do you have any pain or stiffness in any of your joints? Can you climb the stairs comfortably without any difficulty? Can you dress yourself completely without any difficulty?	0 1 –
	INSPECTION	
	Inspect the bedside for walking aids, wheelchairs, or braces.	0 1 –
	Inspect the patient from the front, sides, and back from head to toe for the following:	

Shoulders	Check for shoulder asymmetry and winging of the scapula
Arms	Check for a normal carrying angle, varus or valgus deformity, and fixed flexion deformity
Hands	Check for swelling of the wrists, obvious joint swelling, or deformity
Spine	Check for normal cervical lordosis, thoracic kyphosis and lumbar lordosis, and spinal scoliosis
Pelvis	Check for alignment of the iliac crests
Legs	Check for wasting of the quadriceps
Knees	Check for knee swelling or deformity, valgus or varus deformity of the knees, fixed flexion deformity, popliteal fossa swelling
Lower legs	Check for calf wasting, ankle swelling, forefoot abnormalities, pes cavus or pes planus deformity

STAGE	KEY POINTS AND ACTIONS	SCORE
	GAIT	
Sitting	Observe the patient whilst they are sitting. Look for any postural abnormality or instability (truncal ataxia). Ask the patient to cross their arms over their chest while sitting and see if this exacerbates imbalance.	

STAGE	KEY POINTS AND ACTIONS	SCORE
Rising	Ask the patient to stand up from the chair. Note any difficulty sitting up or standing up. If they are unsteady, make sure that you are in a position capable of supporting them if they fall.	
Walking	Ask the patient to walk to the end of the room, turn round, and return. Permit the patient to use a walking aid if they normally do so. Observe each stage of their gait including the start, rate, type of gait, arm swinging, and how they turn around.	0 1 2

Observing each stage of the patient's gait

- **Start** – Hesitation with shuffling – Parkinsonism
- **Rate** – Fast/Slow – Slow (Parkinsonism)
- **Gait**

Trendelenburg	Weakness of gluteus maximus muscle on opposite side to the sag
Antalgic (reduced stance phase)	Typically due to arthritis in the hip/knee
Scissoring gait	Spastic diplegia – CP/MS
Wide based	Ataxic gait (cerebellar disorder)
Festinant	Parkinsonism
Stamping	Proprioceptive loss (peripheral neuropathy)
High-stepping	Common peroneal nerve injury with foot drop
Circumduction	Pyramidal distribution of weakness with hyperextended leg (hemiparetic)

- **Arms** – Absent arm swing – Parkinson's
- **Turn** – Difficult in turning – En bloc in Parkinson's

STAGE	KEY POINTS AND ACTIONS	SCORE
Heel to Toe	Ask the patient to walk a straight line, putting the heel of one foot directly in front of the toe of the other, as if on a tightrope. Observe if the patient veers over to one side (cerebellar lesion) or has a wide based gait and generalised loss of balance (truncal ataxia).	0 1 –
Romberg's Test	Have the patient stand in one place with their eyes open, feet together, and arms by their sides. Ask them to close their eyes. Reassure the patient that you are in position to support them if they fall.	0 1 2

Negative – No difference to stability with eyes open or closed (even if they continue to be unstable)

Positive – If the patient is less stable with eyes closed (dorsal column disease, loss of proprioception)

STAGE	KEY POINTS AND ACTIONS	SCORE
Arms	Look for joint swelling in the hands, check muscle bulk in the thenar and hypothenar eminences of the hands. Feel for joint tenderness in the wrist and metacarpophalangeal joints (MCPs).	0 1 2
Movements	Ask the patient to bring their arms behind their head, and then behind their back (assess functional use of arms).	0 1 –

Ask the patient to make a power grip and then to touch each finger to each thumb.

Ask the patient to undo a button and hold a pen (fine pincer movements).

LEGS

Lie the patient down.

STAGE	KEY POINTS AND ACTIONS	SCORE
Look	Look for any deformities, muscle wasting, fasciculations or scars.	0 1 –

Check the soles of the feet for ulcers, deformities, or callouses.

STAGE	KEY POINTS AND ACTIONS	SCORE
Feel	Feel for normal quadriceps muscle bulk.	0 1 2
	Check for crepitus in the knee joint with one hand on the knee as it is flexed.	
	Check for knee effusion by firstly milking the suprapatellar bursa into the joint with a downward motion of one hand, and sharply tapping the patella with the index finger.	
	A positive test will see the patella sink and then bounce up again. This detects moderate effusions.	
	Feel across the metatarsophalangeal joints for pain.	
Move	Ask the patient to raise their leg straight off the bed without pain.	0 1 2
	If they have pain, test for sciatica by flexing their knee, flexing the hip further, and then extending the knee again (patients with sciatic nerve impingement will have a relief of pain when the knee is flexed and return of pain when it is extended again).	
	Assess internal and external rotation flexing the patient's hip and knee with one hand and holding their foot in the other. Lateral movement of the foot in this position produces internal rotation of the hip, while medial movement of the foot produces external rotation.	
Spine	Look for items in the table under INSPECTION.	0 1 –
Feel	Feel lumbar spine flexion.	0 1 2
	Stand at the patient's side. Place two fingers on the lumbar vertebrae with the patient standing and ask them to touch their toes. Your fingers should move apart by 4-6cm and then return.	
	MOVE	
C-Spine	Ask the patient to touch their chin to their chest and then look at the ceiling (cervical flexion and extension).	0 1 2
	Ask the patient to touch each ear to each shoulder (lateral cervical flexion).	
	Ask the patient to turn their head to face each shoulder (cervical rotation).	
	Assess for pain and limitation in range of movement.	
	FINISHING OFF	
Thanks	Thank the patient and offer to help them get dressed.	0 1 –
Request	Request to fill out the score sheet for GALS exam; offer to fully examine any area identified as abnormal.	0 1 –
Present	Present a structured, complete, and thorough presentation and offer your differential diagnosis with investigation and management (if appropriate). (*See* Chapter 2.31 for a useful structure.)	0 1 –
	EXAMINER'S EVALUATION	
	Overall assessment of GALS examination	0 1 2 3 4 5
	Total mark out of 31	

NOTES ON THE GALS EXAM

This is designed to screen a patient systemically in 1-2 minutes for an orthopaedic or rheumatological abnormality. In your exams it may be a prelude to performing a further regional examination, so it is worth learning to perform it thoroughly but also quickly.

Patients are scored 1 point for the appearance of each modality (e.g. 1 for Gait, 1 for Arms, etc.) and 1 point for movement (gait excluded) plus 1 for each 'yes' answer at the beginning, to give a total of 10 points. This is recorded in a table as below.

	Appearance	Movement
Gait	Normal	n/a
Arms	Normal	Normal
Legs	Normal	Normal
Spine	Normal	Normal

Further reading:

http://www.arthritisresearchuk.org/health-professionals-and-students/student-handbook/the-msk-examination-rems.aspx

CLINICAL SKILLS

03.1 HAND WASHING

INSTRUCTIONS Explain to the examiner how you would wash your hands prior to examining a patient.

STAGE	KEY POINTS AND ACTIONS	SCORE
	INTRODUCTION	
Introduction	Introduce yourself and explain who you are.	0 1 –
Jewellery	Remove all jewellery including watches, rings, and bracelets.	0 1 –
Sleeves	Roll up sleeves.	0 1 –
	THE PROCEDURE	
Preparation	Turn on the hot and cold water taps ensuring optimal temperature.	
Wet Hands	Wet both hands and apply 5mL of disinfectant on the palm of one hand.	0 1 –
Technique	Mention that you would rub hands together vigorously until a soapy lather appears and continue this for at least 15 seconds (up to 1 minute). Wash hands with a six-stage hand-washing technique.	0 1 2

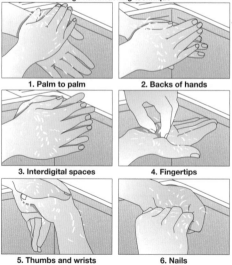

Six stage handwashing technique

1. Palm to palm
2. Backs of hands
3. Interdigital spaces
4. Fingertips
5. Thumbs and wrists
6. Nails

STAGE	KEY POINTS AND ACTIONS	SCORE		
Position	Position hands such that arms are not contaminated when washing.	0	1	–
Rinse	Rinse both hands under the running warm water. Avoid splashing water onto clothes or the floor.	0	1	–
Dry	Dry hands using paper towels from dispenser. Dry each hand thoroughly.	0	1	–
Taps	Switch taps off using elbows or by using a towel acting as a hand barrier.	0	1	–
Dispose	Dispose of the towels in the appropriate yellow clinical waste container.	0	1	–
Technique	Hand washing performed quickly and effectively.			

QUESTIONS

Alcohol	When asked by the examiner, be able to explain how applying alcohol antiseptic differs from hand washing; i.e. leave alcohol to air dry and should not use alcohol with patients suspected of C. Difficile.	0	1	–
Importance	Be able to provide two reasons as to why hand washing is important; i.e. reduce spread of infection to other patients and to prevent spread of infection to self.	0	1	2
Scenario	Be able to name the five WHO moments of hand washing http://www.who.int/gpsc/tools/Five_moments/en/	0	1	2

EXAMINER'S EVALUATION

Overall assessment of hand washing technique   0 1 2 3 4 5

Total mark out of 21

03.2
VENEPUNCTURE

INSTRUCTIONS You are the foundation year House Officer on call in Medicine. Mr R has been admitted to your ward with a chest infection and acute renal failure. You have been asked to take bloods to assess response to treatment.

STAGE	KEY POINTS AND ACTIONS	SCORE		
	INTRODUCTION			
Introduction	Introduce yourself. Elicit name, age, and occupation. Establish rapport.	0	1	–
Explain	'In order to check how well you are responding to treatment, I need to take some blood from you. This will involve initially placing a band around your arm and then inserting a thin needle into your vein. You may feel a small scratch when the needle is inserted. It is a simple and quick procedure that is routinely done. Do you have any questions'?	0	1	–
Consent	Obtain consent to proceed and check patient's ID, date of birth, and full name before commencement.	0	1	–
Position	Ensure that the patient is either sitting or lying comfortably.			
Equipment	Collect and set up the equipment.			
	THE EQUIPMENT			
	Equipment tray/kidney dish Pair of gloves 21G (green) needle or 23G (blue) needle Disposable tourniquet Syringe (10mL) or vacutainer EDTA (usually purple/lavender) bottle and SST or Lithium Heparin (usually yellow or light green top) blood bottles Sharps box Cotton bud and alcohol street			
	THE PROCEDURE			
Wash Hands	Wash hands using six-stage technique and with appropriate disinfectant.			

STAGE	KEY POINTS AND ACTIONS	SCORE		
Gloves	Put on non-sterile gloves.	0	1	–
Position	Correctly position the patient with his arm horizontal and fully extended.			
Tourniquet	Apply the tourniquet above the antecubital fossa.	0	1	–
Select Vein	Choose an appropriate vein by palpation. Mention techniques that may help reveal a vein such as gentle percussion or making and releasing a fist.	0	1	–
Clean	Clean the area with one swipe of an alcohol steret and allow to air dry.	0	1	–
Insertion	Retract the skin inferiorly to stabilize the vein and insert the needle at an angle between 15 and 30 degrees.	0	1	2
Blood Bottles	Using a 20mL syringe, draw blood and fill the appropriate blood bottles (haematology and biochemistry bottles) or, using a vacutainer, insert appropriate bottles atraumatically without losing the vein. Wait until bottles are appropriately full.	0	1	2
Release	Release the tourniquet.	0	1	–
Needle	Remove needle and place cotton bud on the wound site.	0	1	–
	CLOSING UP			
Sharps	Dispose of the needle in the yellow sharps container.	0	1	–
Waste	Dispose of the gloves and any soiled material appropriately.	0	1	–
Labels	Label the blood bottles clearly with the surname, first name, date of birth, hospital number, and date taken.	0	1	–
Form	Offer to complete a blood request form and complete all relevant sections, including clinical details, accurately and legibly.	0	1	–
Finishing Off	Thank the patient and ask if they have any questions.			

	EXAMINER'S EVALUATION						
	Overall assessment of blood taking skills	0	1	2	3	4	5
	Total mark out of 22						

Commonly used blood bottles

This will vary trust to trust.

Blood Bottle	Additive	Common Tests
Purple or lavender	EDTA	FBC, ESR (requires full bottle), blood film
Light green	Lithium Heparin	Electrolytes, ammonia, liver function tests
Yellow	SST	Electrolytes, ammonia, liver function tests
Blue	Sodium citrate	Clotting studies

03.3
CANNULATION

INSTRUCTIONS You are the foundation year House Officer on call in Medicine. Mr R has been admitted to your ward with a chest infection and acute renal failure. You have been asked to insert a cannula to give IV fluids. Explain to the examiner what you are doing as you go along.

STAGE	KEY POINTS AND ACTIONS	SCORE
	INTRODUCTION	
Introduction	Introduce yourself. Elicit name, age, and occupation. Establish rapport.	0 1 –
Explain	'I have been asked to insert a cannula so we can give you some fluids. It is a simple procedure involving inserting a thin, plastic tube into a vein on the back of your hand. The tube will then be connected to a bag containing fluid. You may feel a small scratch when inserting the needle. Do you have any questions'?	0 1 –
Consent	Obtain consent before beginning the procedure.	
Equipment	Collect and set up the equipment.	

THE EQUIPMENT

Pair of gloves
Tourniquet
Sharps box
Cannula (18G green, 20G pink, 23G blue)
Cannula adhesive dressing
Alcohol swabs or skin disinfectant (varies with hospital)
10mL syringe
0.9% NaCl 10mL flush
Green needle
Cannula extension set or adapter
OPTIONAL – spare 10mL syringe or vacutainer with cannula adapter

STAGE	KEY POINTS AND ACTIONS	SCORE		
	CANNULATION			
Wash Hands	Wash hands using six-stage technique and with appropriate disinfectant.	0	1	–
Prepare	Attach the green needle to the 10mL syringe and draw up the NaCl 0.9% flush. Make sure there are no bubbles in the syringe. If using an extension set, flush each line with the saline to remove air; clamp each line after use to ensure no air enters after flushing.	0	1	–
	Ask patient to roll up sleeve or remove clothing to get clear sight of area.			
Tourniquet	Wear gloves. Apply tourniquet. Request patient to clench fist. Identify vein. Clean area with swab. Remove cannula from wrapping and take off the cap.	0	1	–
Sharp Scratch	Warn patient of impending 'sharp scratch'. Stabilise vein by retracting hand via palmar flexion. Introduce cannula at a shallow angle and watch for flashback. Advance cannula and needle by 2mm. Keep needle stationary and advance plastic cannula only. Remove tourniquet. Press over vein above cannula to control bleeding.	0	1	–
Sharps Bin	Remove needle and dispose into the sharps bin.	0	1	–
	OPTIONAL			
Taking Blood	Attach a 10mL syringe or vacutainer with cannula adapter to the cannula and gently aspirate 10mLs of blood. Press over vein once more to control bleeding.	0	1	2
Secure Cannula	Cap the cannula by using the provided cap or attaching the extension set or the adapter to the cannula end. Apply the adhesive dressing to the cannula thereby securing it.	0	1	–
Flush	Flush the cannula with 10mL of normal saline 0.9%.	0	1	–
Document	Inform examiner that you would record the date inserted on the cannula dressing and the drug chart.	0	1	–
Finishing Off	Thank the patient and throw away any remaining waste.			

EXAMINER'S EVALUATION

Overall assessment of inserting an IV cannula	0	1	2	3	4	5

Total mark out of 17

03.4
IV INFUSION

INSTRUCTIONS Set up a normal saline drip into this model arm using the cannula provided. Explain to the examiner what you are doing as you go along.

STAGE	KEY POINTS AND ACTIONS	SCORE		
	INTRODUCTION			
Introduction	Introduce yourself. Elicit name, age, and occupation. Establish rapport.	0	1	–
Explain	'I have been asked to give you some fluids. The cannula in your hand will be connected to a bag containing fluid. Do you have any questions'?	0	1	–
Consent	Obtain consent before beginning the procedure.			
Equipment	Collect and set up the equipment.			
	THE EQUIPMENT			
	Correct fluid bag Giving set Alcohol swabs			
	THE PROCEDURE			
Wash Hands	Wash hands with six-stage technique and appropriate disinfectant.			
	Fluid Bag			
Chart	Inform the examiner you would check the fluid prescription chart to ensure you are using the correct fluid solution and there are no allergies. State that you would want to check the patient's renal function and electrolytes before administering fluids.	0	1	–
Integrity	Check the integrity of the fluid bag looking for any holes or contaminants.	0	1	–
Check	Check expiry date, solution type, and concentration.	0	1	–
Prepare	Remove fluid bag from cover and hang on stand. Remove giving set (put in off position by pushing roller down fully) and insert into fluid bag (remove blue winged part and pass through portal).	0	1	2

STAGE	KEY POINTS AND ACTIONS	SCORE
Run Through	Run through to remove air (by putting giving set in open position) and squeeze on tube-like compartment to half fill the chamber with fluid. Switch tap to closed position once complete.	0 1 –
	Drip	
Open Clamp	Attach the end of giving set to cannula and switch the tap on. Ensure drip rate is appropriate.	0 1 –
Drip Calculation	Each giving set will have information on the set that gives you the drops per mL for that set – this will vary with IV giving sets but is usually 15, 20, or 60 drops per minute.	0 1 2

The calculation is:

$$\frac{\text{Total volume to be given (mLs)}}{\text{Total time for infusion (mins)}} \times \frac{\text{Drops per mLs}}{1} = \text{drops per minute}$$

e.g.

$$\frac{1000}{360} \times \frac{15}{1} = 41 \text{ drops per minute or 7 drops per 10 seconds}$$

Extravasation	Make sure there is no swelling over point where cannula was inserted. Secure to arm.	0 1 –
Document	Inform examiner that you would record on fluid chart the date and time, and sign when fluids were commenced. State that you would observe the patient for anaphylaxis.	0 1 –
Finishing Off	Thank the patient and throw away any remaining waste.	

EXAMINER'S EVALUATION

Overall assessment of setting up IV fluids and drip	0 1 2 3 4 5

Total mark out of 18

03.5 BLOOD TRANSFUSION

INSTRUCTIONS Ms Brown has had shortness of breath on exertion for two weeks. A recent blood test revealed a haemoglobin of 7g/dL. She has been written up for three units of blood to be transfused. Give one unit of blood.

NOTE: Failure to observe correct procedure may result in death. This is a catastrophe that is largely preventable if the following recommendations are always observed.

STAGE	KEY POINTS AND ACTIONS	SCORE
	INTRODUCTION	
Introduction	Introduce yourself. Elicit name, age, and occupation. Establish rapport.	0 1 —
Explain	'Your blood test has shown that you are anaemic and require a top-up of blood. We would like to give you some blood via the drip in your hand. Do you have any objections to receiving blood products? Do you have any questions'?	0 1 —
Consent	Obtain consent and check patient's ID before beginning the procedure.	0 1 —
Equipment	Collect and set up the equipment on the trolley.	
	THE EQUIPMENT	
	Pair of gloves Blood transfusion giving set Adhesive plaster Sharps box Syringe containing saline flush 1 blood unit from blood bank Tourniquet Alcohol swabs Calculator	

STAGE	KEY POINTS AND ACTIONS	SCORE

THE PROCEDURE
Confirm Details

Check

Have two people check the patient's identity with at least one being a qualified health professional; i.e. a registered nurse or a doctor.

0 1 –

Patient's Details

Confirm the patient's details such as full name, gender, hospital number, and date of birth on a number of different sources such as patient's wrist band, medical notes, verbal check, prescription chart, blood compatibility report, and on the blood unit label.

0 1 2

Blood Group

Check the patient's blood group on the blood compatibility report against the blood unit label and the laboratory reports.

0 1 –

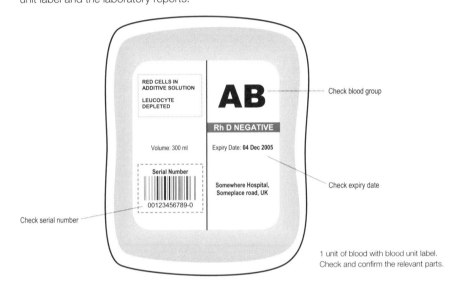

1 unit of blood with blood unit label.
Check and confirm the relevant parts.

Expiry Date

Check the serial number of the unit and the expiry date on the blood unit label and compatibility report. If any discrepancy is noted the blood must not be administered. Query any discrepancy with laboratory staff.

0 1 –

ADMINISTERING THE BLOOD

Inspection

Inspect the blood bag for evidence of leaks, discolouration, turbidity, or clots.

0 1 –

Giving Set

Connect the giving set to the blood bag for transfusion. Infusion of blood must be through a blood administration set with an integral filter (double barrel set).

0 1 –

Drip Rate

Set an appropriate drip rate for the volume of blood as outlined in the IV transfusion chapter. One unit of blood is typically 300mL. Administration is between 2 and 3.5 hours maximum. Remember packed red cells cannot be out of the fridge for longer than 4 hours due to infection risk.

0 1 –

Reaction

Ensure that the nurse commences observations for adverse reactions to the transfused blood on 0 minutes, 15 minutes, 30 minutes and then hourly. Assess BP, pulse, temperature, and airway patency and ask patient if they feel an itch or notice a rash.

0 1 –

STAGE	KEY POINTS AND ACTIONS	SCORE
Document	Record the date and time of the transfusion on the prescription chart and blood compatibility report. Include the signatures of both witnesses on the forms.	
	Document the details of the transfusion into the patient's notes, specifying the total number of units given, blood group, the rate of infusion, and presence or absence of adverse reactions.	
Finishing Off	Thank the patient and ensure that they are comfortable. Answer any possible questions.	

EXAMINER'S EVALUATION

Overall competence in giving blood transfusion	0 1 2 3 4 5

Total mark out of 17

TRANSFUSION REACTIONS

	Reaction Type	Features	Treatment
Haemolytic reactions	**ABO incompatibility**	-Nearly immediate onset -Rigors, lumbar pain, breathlessness, hypotension	-Stop blood transfusion -Resuscitate patient (e.g. with IV fluids) -Send all blood back to lab
	Non-ABO incompatibility	-Similar but not as severe as ABO reactions	As above
Non-haemolytic reactions	**Non-haemolytic febrile transfusion reaction**	-Early onset -Fevers -Otherwise well	-Slow rate of infusion -Give paracetamol
	Sepsis (shock)	-Sometimes subacute -Rare, more common with platelets -Fevers, hypotension, positive cultures	-Stop infusion -IV fluid resuscitation -Antibiotics
	Transfusion Related Acute Lung Injury (TRALI)	-Maybe late onset (within 6 hours) -Breathlessness, hypoxemia, critically unwell, frothy sputum -X-ray shows multiple perihilar nodules with lower lung field infiltration	-Supportive treatment -May require HDU/ITU care
	Fluid overload	-Raised JVP -Peripheral oedema -Breathlessness, hypoxaemia	-IV diuresis -Careful fluid management
	Anaphylaxis	-Shock, urticaria, and rash -Bronchospasm, chest pain, nausea	-Slow transfusion -Give antihistamines -Stop if very severe

Source: http://www.patient.co.uk/doctor/blood-transfusion-reactions

03.6 INTRAVENOUS INJECTION

INSTRUCTIONS You are a foundation year House Officer. Your SHO has asked you to give Mr Dane 10mg of metoclopramide as an IV injection via the cannula. Demonstrate how you would carry out this procedure using the arm and the equipment provided. Explain the procedure to the examiner as you proceed.

STAGE	KEY POINTS AND ACTIONS	SCORE		
	INTRODUCTION			
Introduction	Introduce yourself. Elicit name, age, and occupation. Establish rapport.	0	1	–
Explain	'I have been asked to give you an anti-sickness drug (metoclopramide) which is a drug that will ease the sickness and uneasy feeling you are experiencing. For it to work quickly it must be administered through the drip in your arm in the form of an injection. Do you have any questions'?	0	1	–
Consent	Obtain consent and check patient's ID before beginning the procedure.	0	1	–
Side Effects	Warn the patient of any possible side effects of the drug.	0	1	–
	THE PROCEDURE **Check the Drug**			
Drug Allergies	Check for a history of drug allergy asking specifically about this drug. You may need to read the patient's drug chart and ask them directly for an allergy.	0	1	–
Check BNF	Check the BNF regarding the dosage information of the drug and for its potential side effects. BNF: Slow IV injection [vial 5mg/mL] over 1-2 mins.	0	1	–
Equipment	Collect and set up the equipment.			

STAGE	KEY POINTS AND ACTIONS	SCORE

THE EQUIPMENT

Syringe (5mL)
Ampoule of sterile water for injection
Ampoule of drug
Pair of gloves
21 G green needle
Alcohol swab x 2
Tourniquet
10mL normal saline flush 0.9%
10mL syringe

Stage	Key Points and Actions	Score
Syringe	Wear gloves and then select an appropriate syringe size such as a 5mL syringe and an appropriately sized needle; i.e. 21 G green needle.	0 1 –
Check Drug	Confirm the name of the drug you are administering on the ampoule, the strength, and expiry date with a nurse or another staff member (or examiner).	0 1 –
Draw Drug	After checking the drug, prepare to give the injection. Attach the green (21 G) needle to the syringe and draw up the appropriate amount of drug (2mL).	0 1 –
	Draw up the saline flush 0.9% in the same fashion into a 10mL syringe.	
	Powder mixture: Check the name, strength, and expiry date of sterile water. Dilute the drug with the appropriate amount according to manufacturer's or BNF instructions. Inject the water into the ampoule and shake until all solid has dissolved.	

ADMINISTER THE DRUG

Stage	Key Points and Actions	Score
Expel Air	Hold the syringe vertically with the needle pointing upward. Tap the syringe allowing the lingering air bubbles to collect at the top. Slowly squeeze the plunger of the syringe, expelling the air bubbles while containing the drug in the barrel.	0 1 –
Change Needle	Discard the needle in the sharps bin.	0 1 –
Check the Cannula Site	Tell the examiner you would check the date the cannula was inserted and for any skin breakdown or erythema around the site.	0 1 –
Administer the Drug	Wear gloves and use a sterile alcohol swab to cleanse the cannula port.	0 1 –
Speed	Administer the medication at the correct speed and rate as defined by the BNF (over 1 to 2 minutes).	0 1 –
Flush	Flush the cannula with 10mL normal saline. Ask about pain as it is administered.	0 1 –
Document	Record the time the drug was administered on the drug chart and sign.	0 1 –
Dispose	Dispose of sharps appropriately.	0 1 –
Finishing Off	Thank the patient and throw away any remaining waste.	

EXAMINER'S EVALUATION

Overall assessment of administering IV drug injection	0 1 2 3 4 5
Total mark out of 22	

03.7 INTRAMUSCULAR INJECTION

INSTRUCTIONS You are a foundation year House Officer. Mr West has been suffering from severe renal colic. He has been written up for diclofenac 75mg IM. Demonstrate how you would carry out this procedure using the manikin arm and the equipment provided. Explain the procedure to the examiner as you proceed.

STAGE	KEY POINTS AND ACTIONS	SCORE		
	INTRODUCTION			
Introduction	Introduce yourself. Elicit name, age, and occupation. Establish rapport.	0	1	–
Explain	'I have been asked to give you some medication. For it to work quickly it must be administered as an injection into the arm. You may feel a sharp scratch when the needle enters the muscle. Do you have any questions'?	0	1	–
Consent	Obtain consent and check patient's ID before beginning the procedure.	0	1	–
Contraindications	Ascertain if the patient has any contraindications to the medication such as previous gastric bleeds, renal failure, or severe heart failure.	0	1	–
Side Effects	Warn the patient of any possible side effects of the drug.	0	1	–
	THE PROCEDURE **Check the Drug**			
Drug Allergies	Check for a history of drug allergy asking specifically about this drug. You may need to read the patient's drug chart or ask them directly for allergy.	0	1	–
Check BNF	Check the BNF regarding the dosage information of the drug (diclofenac) and for its potential side effects. BNF: vial 25 mg/mL.	0	1	–
Equipment	Collect and set up the equipment.			

STAGE	KEY POINTS AND ACTIONS	SCORE

THE EQUIPMENT

Syringe (5mL)
21 G green needle for drawing up
23 G needle for injecting
Ampoule
Alcohol swab and gloves

Syringe	Wear gloves and then select an appropriate syringe size such as a 5mL syringe and an appropriately sized needle; i.e. 21 G green needle.	0 1 –
Check Drug	Confirm the name of the drug on the ampoule as well as the strength and expiry date with a nurse or another staff member (or examiner).	0 1 –
Draw Drug	After checking the drug, prepare to give the injection. Attach the green (21G) needle to the syringe and draw up the appropriate amount of drug (3mL).	0 1 2

For Powder: Check name, strength, and expiry date of sterile water dilute. Dilute the drug with the appropriate amount according to BNF or manufacturer's instructions. Inject the water into the ampoule and shake until all the solid has dissolved.

| **Choose Site** | Choose an appropriate site for the intramuscular injection. | |

Possible Sites for Intramuscular Injections

Muscle	Notes
Mid deltoid	This site is good for low volume injections such as those less than 5mL. Because of its good blood supply it has the most rapid rate of uptake of all the intramuscular sites. It is also the most accessible.
Gluteals	Upper outer quadrant of the buttock. Excellent site for large volume injections. However, risk of sciatic nerve and vessel injury in addition to muscle wastage in the elderly.
Rectus femoris	Anterior lateral aspect of the thigh (vastus lateralis). Good for most injections especially oil based (depots), sedatives, and narcotics.

Administer the Drug

Expel Air	Hold the syringe vertically with the needle pointing upward. Tap the syringe allowing the lingering air bubbles to collect at the top. Slowly squeeze the plunger of the syringe, expelling the air bubbles while containing the drug in the barrel.	0 1 –
Change Needle	Discard the needle in the sharps bin and attach the 23G needle before administering the medication.	0 1 –
Enter Muscle	Use a sterile alcohol swab to cleanse the site. Identify landmarks to avoid such as likely nerve and vascular routes. Pinch the skin at the injection site (gluteal) and inform the patient of a sharp scratch when the needle pierces the skin. As you inject the patient with the medication, ensure that the syringe is at 90 degrees to the patient's skin and is inserted in a swift dart-like motion to 2–3mm below the hilt.	0 1 2
Drawback	Attempt to draw back blood into the syringe to ensure that the needle is not in a blood vessel. If blood is aspirated select a different site. Administer the drug slowly according to BNF guidelines.	0 1 –

STAGE	KEY POINTS AND ACTIONS	SCORE
Withdraw	Withdraw the needle and apply compression to the injection site using cotton wool and a plaster.	0 1 –
Dispose	Dispose of sharps appropriately.	0 1 –
Document	Record the time the drug was administered on the drug chart and sign.	0 1 –
Finishing Off	Thank the patient and throw away any remaining waste.	

EXAMINER'S EVALUATION

Overall assessment of administering IM drug injection	0 1 2 3 4 5

Total mark out of 24

Common IM Medications

Drug	Site	Contraindications
Most Vaccines	Typically deltoid	Intercurrent illness, immunosuppressed for live vaccines (MMR, BCG, Yellow Fever, Varicella)
Ceftriaxone	Typically deltoid, usually where no IV access available	Anaphylaxis to cephalosporins and penicillins (10% chance of cross-reaction)
Cyclizine	Typically deltoid, sometimes gluteal	Previous abnormal reactions

03.8 MALE CATHETERISATION

INSTRUCTIONS You are a foundation year House Officer in Urology. Mr J has presented with acute urinary retention. You decide he needs urinary catheterisation to relieve his symptoms. Explain to the patient what you will do and insert the catheter with the equipment provided. Explain to the examiner what you are doing as you proceed.

STAGE	KEY POINTS AND ACTIONS	SCORE
	INTRODUCTION	
Introduction	Introduce yourself. Elicit name, age, and occupation. Establish rapport.	0 1 –
Explain	'Because of the symptoms you are having, I am going to insert a flexible plastic tube through your penis into your bladder to relieve the pressure. It should not be painful but may feel a little uncomfortable. Do you have any questions or concerns'?	0 1 –
Consent	Obtain consent before beginning the procedure.	
Equipment	Collect and set up the equipment on the trolley.	
	THE EQUIPMENT	
	Catheterisation pack Foley catheter 16 or 18 Catheter bag Antiseptic solution Sterile gloves 10mL sterile water filled syringe Lignocaine gel (Instillagel or equivalent) Three plastic prongs 10mL saline solution	

STAGE	KEY POINTS AND ACTIONS	SCORE
	THE PROCEDURE **Trolley**	
Preparation	Put on an apron, clean the trolley using bactericidal spray, and wash hands.	0 1 –
Patient	Expose the patient and ask him to retract his foreskin.	0 1 –
Sterile Field	Peel the outer plastic covering of the catheterisation pack and slide the pack onto the trolley. Unwrap the paper covering, touching only the outside of the paper, and form a sterile area. Stick the yellow disposable bag onto the side of the trolley. Place the above equipment sterilely into the area. Pour the sterile water into a small bowl with swabs (found in catheter pack).	0 1 2
Gloves	Don a pair of sterile gloves.	0 1 –
	Patient	
Drape & Gauze	Make a hole in the drape and place it on the patient such that his penis passes through the hole. Wrap a gauze around the shaft of the penis and grasp this gauze with your left hand. Keep this hand (left) fixed in place.	0 1 –
Clean Penis	Holding one wet swab with a plastic prong, wipe the left half of the glans once only. Dispose of the swab and prong. Taking a newly soaked swab and prong, wipe the right half of the glans once only then dispose of the swab and prong. Finally, take a new wet swab and prong and wipe the meatus of the penis once only. Dispose of as previously.	0 1 –
Anaesthetic	If there has been any contact between the gloves and the non-sterile area whilst cleaning, it is important to wear a second pair of sterile gloves before inserting anaesthetic. Hold the shaft of the penis with a sterile glove, insert the LA (lignocaine 2%) by squeezing a small amount (5mL) into the urethra while the penis is held vertically. Apply gentle pressure to the shaft of the penis with your left hand in order to occlude the urethra. Hold for between 3 and 5 minutes giving time for the anaesthetic to work. Be careful not to break the sterile field by touching the penis directly. Place the remainder of the anaesthetic solution into the cardboard receptacle.	0 1 –
	Catheter	
Preparation	Place the catheter, still in the inner plastic covering, into the cardboard receptacle and put it between the patient's legs. Rip open the end of the catheter covering and massage the end of the catheter out of it by a few centimetres.	0 1 –
Lignocaine	Dip the tip of the catheter into the LA jelly previously deposited in the receptacle.	
Insert Catheter	Hold the penis vertically and insert the catheter into the urethra, touching only the plastic covering and not the catheter directly. Keep the end of the catheter over the receptacle to catch any sudden flow of urine. When encountering resistance, lower the penis to a horizontal position to negotiate the prostate.	0 1 –
Inflate Balloon	Inflate the catheter balloon with 1mL of sterile water. Request the patient to say if they feel any pain. Continue filling slowly with the remaining 9mL, asking the patient if they are in any pain. Tug on the catheter to make sure that the balloon becomes lodged in the neck of the bladder.	0 1 –

STAGE	KEY POINTS AND ACTIONS	SCORE
Catheter Bag	Attach the drainage bag to the end of the catheter and replace the foreskin (or request the patient to do so) to avoid a paraphimosis.	0 1 –
Dispose	Dispose of waste appropriately.	0 1 –
Document	Document in the notes the size of catheter used and the residual volume of urine initially collected. Place the catheter sticker in the notes if available.	0 1 –
	Send the urine for microscopy and culture and document its appearance in the notes.	
Finishing Off	Thank the patient, cover them, and throw away any remaining waste.	

EXAMINER'S EVALUATION

Overall assessment of urinary catheter insertion   0   1   2   3   4   5

Total mark out of 21

03.9 NASOGASTRIC INTUBATION

INSTRUCTIONS You are a foundation year House Officer in Geriatrics. Mrs T has had difficulty in swallowing after a left sided CVA and has been made nil by mouth. Please demonstrate how you would insert a nasogastric tube for feeding on the model provided. Explain the procedure to the examiner as you proceed.

NOTE: Indications   Aspiration (GI surgery, intestinal obstruction) and feeding
Contraindications   Base of skull fracture, history of oesophageal stricture
Does not pass down   Pharyngeal pouch, volvulus of stomach

For feeding and medications a fine bore tube (8G gauge + guide wire) is used since it is more comfortable and causes less oesophageal inflammation and stricture formation and can remain longer in place (more than a week). For aspiration use a 16F gauge NG tube.

STAGE	KEY POINTS AND ACTIONS	SCORE		
	INTRODUCTION			
Introduction	Introduce yourself. Elicit name, age, and occupation. Establish rapport.	0	1	–
Explain	'Because of your problems swallowing, I have been asked to insert a nasogastric tube into your stomach. It is a simple procedure involving passing a small, flexible tube into your stomach through your nose. This tube will allow us to give your body food and medicines directly'.	0	1	–
Consent	Obtain consent before beginning the procedure and check patient's ID.	0	1	–
	THE EQUIPMENT			
	Xylocaine spray NG tube (Ryle's tube) A glass of water KY jelly Gloves + pH paper Receptacle Adhesive tape Spigot or bag to attach to tube			

STAGE	KEY POINTS AND ACTIONS	SCORE
	THE PROCEDURE	
Position	Ask the patient to sit upright on a chair or on the edge of the bed. Wash your hands and don a pair of non-sterile gloves.	0 1 –
Equipment	Collect and set up the equipment on a trolley.	
Measure	Measure the distance from the tip of the patient's nose to the ear lobe and from the ear lobe to two finger breadths above the umbilicus. Mark the distance on the tube with some tape or using the gradations on the tube.	0 1 –
Nose	Inspect the nose for nasal deviation or obstruction. Ask the patient if they suffer with nasal polyps or are on any medication (warfarin). Spray the nostrils with Xylocaine spray.	0 1 –
Insert Tube	Squirt jelly onto a gauze and lubricate the end section of the tube. Pass the tube into the patient's nostril and along the floor of the nose into the nasopharynx. Warn the patient to inform you when they are aware of the tube in the back of the throat. When they do, ask the patient to tilt their head forward and take sips of water through a straw. Each time the patient swallows advance the tube a few centimetres (so that the epiglottis is closed whenever the tube is advanced). Stop inserting the tube once you have reached the desired length.	0 1 2
Coughing	Mention that if the patient begins to cough violently, you would pull the tube back a few centimetres before restarting.	0 1 –
Check	Attempt to withdraw liquid stomach contents using a bladder syringe and confirm acidity using pH paper (pH <5.5 is safe to use).	0 1 2

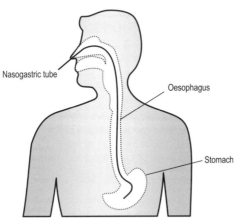

Nasogastric tube
Oesophagus
Stomach

Inserting a Nasogastric Tube

STAGE	KEY POINTS AND ACTIONS	SCORE
Bile Bag	Connect to a bile bag. Tape the tube to the patient's nose and to the side of the face.	0 1 –
X-Ray	Request a chest x-ray to confirm appropriate placement of the tube before commencing feeds.	0 1 –
Document	Write in notes the time, date, tube size, and how much was drained.	0 1 –
Finishing Off	Thank the patient and throw away any remaining waste.	

EXAMINER'S EVALUATION

Overall assessment of inserting nasogastric tube   0   1   2   3   4   5

Total mark out of 19

03.10 SURGICAL GOWN AND SCRUB

INSTRUCTIONS You are the surgical foundation year House Officer on call. Your SHO is busy in A&E clerking patients and you have been called into theatre to help the Registrar perform a total hip replacement operation. Explain to the examiner how you would ready yourself for theatre.

STAGE	KEY POINTS AND ACTIONS	SCORE		
	INTRODUCTION			
Introduction	Introduce yourself and explain who you are.	0	1	–
Jewellery	Request to remove all jewellery including watches, but may keep wedding band on.	0	1	–
Equipment	Collect and set up the equipment.			
	THE EQUIPMENT			
	Scrub brush Theatre gown Pair of sterile gloves Mask and cap Theatre shoes Scrubs			
Theatre Scrubs	Explain that you would change into theatre scrubs and put on theatre shoes.	0	1	–
Cap & Mask	Wear an appropriate theatre cap (non-sterile) ensuring that all hair is concealed within it. Also wear an appropriate theatre mask (non-sterile), covering nose and mouth fully.	0	1	–
	THE PROCEDURE			
Preparation	Open the gown pack, sterile gloves, and scrub brush and place in sterile field aseptically.	0	1	–
Taps	Turn on the hot and cold water taps ensuring optimal temperature.	0	1	–
Wash	Correctly wash your hands (palm, dorsum, and in between fingers) with appropriate disinfectant, lathering up to the elbows on both arms. Ensure you lather soap from hand down toward elbow.	0	1	2

STAGE	KEY POINTS AND ACTIONS	SCORE

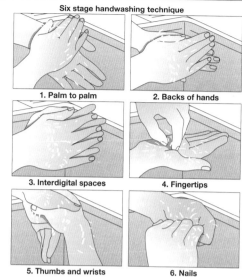

Six stage handwashing technique

1. Palm to palm
2. Backs of hands
3. Interdigital spaces
4. Fingertips
5. Thumbs and wrists
6. Nails

STAGE	KEY POINTS AND ACTIONS	SCORE
Disinfectant	Be able to name two disinfectant solutions (Hibiscrub or Betadine) when asked by the examiner which disinfectant you would use.	0 1 2
Brush	Take the nail cleaner from the brush and clean thoroughly under the fingernails for about 1 minute. Use the brush side of the scrub brush to concentrate on the hand areas.	0 1 –
Sponge	Place disinfectant on the sponge side of the brush using your elbows to release soap solution from the container. Scrub down from the fingertips, palm, and dorsum of hand to the elbow on one arm and then proceed to the other. Spend 3 minutes on each arm in total and 1 minute on the hands.	0 1 2
Explain	Be able to explain correctly why we do not use the brush side on the forearms when requested to do so by the examiner; i.e. to prevent bringing out deeper organisms in the hair follicles to the surface.	0 1 –
Rinse	Rinse both arms starting from hands down to the elbows correctly, ensure water is running downward to elbows. Switch off taps using elbows.	0 1 –
Dry	Dry your hands using sterile towels provided in the gown pack. Dry each arm with an individual towel, starting from the hand, moving down toward the elbow. Dispose of the towels appropriately.	0 1 –
Gown	Pick up the gown from the reverse side and shake to open out without touching the outer surface. Pass right and left hands through the gown leaving the cuffs covering the hands. Do not allow the gown to touch the floor and maintain aseptic technique.	0 1 2
Gloves	Pick up the internal part of the gloves through the gown cuffs without touching the outside surface.	0 1 2
	Wear the gloves aseptically either through reverse placement or any other technique.	
Tie Gown	Swivel anticlockwise whilst requesting an assistant to tie the sash of the gown. Tie the remaining bow on the gown by yourself.	0 1 –
Technique	Whole technique performed aseptically. Hands kept above elbows throughout gowning and aseptic field maintained.	0 1 –

EXAMINER'S EVALUATION

Overall assessment of surgical gowning technique	0 1 2 3 4 5

Total mark out of 27

03.11 TAKING BLOOD CULTURES

INSTRUCTIONS You are a foundation year House Officer in Medicine. Ms G has been admitted with lower lobe pneumonia and has spiked a temperature of 40 degrees. You wish to take some blood cultures. Explain to the patient what you have to do and take some blood cultures with the equipment provided.

STAGE	KEY POINTS AND ACTIONS	SCORE
	INTRODUCTION	
Introduction	Introduce yourself. Elicit name, age, and occupation. Establish rapport.	0 1 –
Explain	'I have been asked to take a sample of blood from your arm as you have had a raised temperature. The procedure is the same as taking blood for a blood test and will help us identify and treat the type of infection you have. Do you have any questions'?	0 1 –
Consent	Obtain consent and check patient's ID before beginning the procedure.	0 1 –
Equipment	Collect and set up the equipment on the trolley.	
	THE EQUIPMENT	
	2x Culture bottles (anerobic and aerobic bottles) 20mL syringe 21G needle (green) x 3 Pair of gloves Sharps box Tourniquet Cotton bud and alcohol swab	
	THE PROCEDURE **Venepuncture**	
Prepare	Wash your hands with disinfectant and don non-sterile gloves.	0 1 –
Position	Correctly position the patient with their arm horizontal and fully extended.	0 1 –
Tourniquet	Apply the tourniquet above the antecubital fossa.	0 1 –
Vein	Choose an appropriate vein by palpation and clean the area with one swipe of an alcohol steret and allow to air dry.	0 1 –

STAGE	KEY POINTS AND ACTIONS	SCORE
Syringe	Attach a 21G green needle onto the 20mL syringe.	0 1 –
Insertion	Retract the skin inferiorly to stabilise the vein and insert the needle at an angle of between 15 and 30 degrees.	0 1 2
Venesect	Remove 20mL of blood from the site.	
Tourniquet	Release the tourniquet.	0 1 –
Haemostasis	Remove the needle and place cotton bud on the wound site.	0 1 –

BLOOD CULTURE BOTTLES

Sterile Needle	Discard old green needle into the sharps box while replacing it with a new sterile 21G green needle.	0 1 –
Prepare	Prepare the bottles by removing the caps and cleansing each rubber top with an alcohol swab. This is to ensure sterile access to culture medium. Never use a blood culture bottle that has had its cap already removed.	0 1 –
Transfer	Transfer blood from the syringe to the blood culture bottles by injecting between 8 and 10 mL of blood into each. Avoid inoculating air into the anaerobic bottle – if using a closed venepuncture system (e.g. vacutainer) inoculate blood into the aerobic bottle first; this allows any air to be removed by running blood through the system. If using a needle and syringe, inoculate the anaerobic bottle first and then the aerobic bottle to avoid inoculating the air at the end of the syringe.	0 1 2

FINISHING OFF

Waste	Dispose of the needles and syringe into the yellow sharps container. Dispose of gloves and any soiled material appropriately.	0 1 –
Labels	Label the blood culture bottles clearly with the surname, first name, date of birth, hospital number, and date and time taken.	0 1 –
Form	Fill in a microbiology request form ticking the box MC&S (microscopy, culture, and sensitivity) and complete all the relevant sections including clinical details accurately and legibly. Send bottles in plastic bag to the microbiology laboratory.	0 1 2
Thank	Thank the patient and ask if they have any questions.	

EXAMINER'S EVALUATION

Overall assessment of taking blood for blood cultures	0 1 2 3 4 5

Total mark out of 25

Notes on Taking Blood Cultures

Blood cultures need to be taken very carefully in order to maximise the diagnostic yield in the laboratory; a missed bacteraemia in a very unwell septic patient is disastrous.

    a. Always inoculate as much blood as possible; this maximizes the chances of detecting the organism in the lab.

    b. NEVER repalpate the area with your fingers, and clean it thoroughly; this avoids skin contaminants creating false results, and sometimes masking the true pathogen.

    c. The relationship between fever and bacteraemia is not as straightforward as fever=bacteraemia. The evidence suggests there isn't much relationship between the two. Therefore if you suspect infection in a patient there is no value in taking cultures only if they spike a temperature. Take them immediately.

    d. Additionally a fever requires a sufficient immune response to infection. In the immunosuppressed and the elderly this may not occur; take cultures in anyone in these categories with a suspicion of infection.

    e. One culture is rarely sufficient to catch a significant bacteraemia. Ideally two should be taken from different sites at different times in patients with significant sepsis.

    f. Most importantly, when considering starting antibiotics make sure that cultures of blood (and urine) have been taken. If the patient is very unwell do not delay antibiotic administration but take all measures to get the cultures ASAP.

03.12 TAKING A BLOOD PRESSURE

INSTRUCTIONS You have been asked to see Mr G who has had his blood pressure measured by a friend. He was told he had a high reading and is concerned. Please measure the blood pressure and explain to the patient what the results mean.

NOTE: It is important to select the appropriate cuff size to determine the patient's blood pressure. Cuffs that are too large for the patient's arm may result in a lower than expected blood pressure while cuffs that are too small may give a falsely elevated reading. The cuff bladder should have a width equal to at least 40% of the upper arm circumference.

STAGE	KEY POINTS AND ACTIONS	SCORE		
	INTRODUCTION			
Introduction	Introduce yourself. Elicit name, age, and occupation. Establish rapport.	0	1	–
Explain	'I understand that you are here for me to check your blood pressure. What I would like to do first is get you to sit up straight and remove your jumper. I will place a blood pressure cuff around your arm and inflate it. This may feel a little uncomfortable. I will then place my stethoscope on your arm and take your pressure. Do you understand what I have just told you'?	0	1	–
Confirm	Check that the patient has rested for at least five minutes.	0	1	–
Consent	Ask the patient if he is happy to proceed.			
	THE PROCEDURE			
Cuff	Choose the appropriate cuff size for the patient from a choice of two – larger cuff for obese patient, smaller one for paediatric patient.	0	1	–
BP Machine	Check that the cuff is fully deflated and attached correctly.			
Position	Correctly position the patient with his arm horizontal and fully extended. Place the BP machine approximately in line with the level of the heart.	0	1	–
Placement	Palpate the brachial artery and place the BP cuff neatly and securely around the arm with the arterial point over the brachial artery.	0	1	2
Check	Check the approximate systolic level by palpating the radial/brachial artery once the cuff is inflated.	0	1	–

STAGE	KEY POINTS AND ACTIONS	SCORE		
Procedure	Auscultate over the brachial artery and deflate the cuff slowly, watching the BP reading closely. Listen for the Korotkoff sounds.	0	1	–

Korotkoff sounds

Sound	Interpretation
1	The first tapping sound heard as the pressure cuff falls – this is the systolic pressure
2	The blood flow murmurs between systolic and diastolic murmurs
3	Loud, crisp tapping sound
4	Thumping noise nearing diastolic – this is diastolic blood pressure in pregnancy
5	Once all noises disappear fully – this is the diastolic pressure in non-pregnant adults

STAGE	KEY POINTS AND ACTIONS	SCORE		
Repeat	Take at least two BP measurements.	0	1	2
Accuracy	Ensure that the BP reading is measured to within 2mmHg of the correct value.	0	1	2

FINISHING OFF

Explain	Appropriately explain the results to the patient. 'I have taken your BP reading today and the result is slightly raised. Normally we take the reading on two or three separate occasions as simple things like exercise and anxiety may falsely increase the reading. I suggest we repeat your BP in two weeks' time to confirm whether your pressure is in fact high'.	0	1	–
Concerns	Deal with patient's concerns appropriately and allay any fears.			
Documents	Request the patient's notes to document the blood pressure reading.	0	1	–
Thank	Thank the patient and ask if they have any questions.			

EXAMINER'S EVALUATION

Overall assessment of measuring blood pressure	0	1	2	3	4	5

Total mark out of 20

03.13 BLOOD GLUCOSE

INSTRUCTIONS You are a foundation year House Officer in Endocrinology. Mr B has been diagnosed as a new diabetic. He is to be discharged from the ward and it is your job to explain to him how to use his new BM machine to monitor his diabetes.

STAGE	KEY POINTS AND ACTIONS	SCORE		
	INTRODUCTION			
Introduction	Introduce yourself. Elicit name, age, and occupation. Establish rapport.	0	1	–
Understanding	Confirm the patient knows that he is diabetic and check his understanding of diabetic monitoring.	0	1	–
Explain	'As you know you have been diagnosed as having diabetes. In order to check how well you are responding to treatment, you need to monitor the sugar levels of your blood. I am here today to show you how to use this BM meter. Do you have any questions'?	0	1	–
Consent	Obtain consent to proceed and check patient's ID before commencement.	0	1	–
Position	Ensure that the patient is sitting in a warm room.			
Equipment	Collect and set up the equipment.			
	THE EQUIPMENT			
	BM meter BM test strip Pair of gloves Lancet Cotton bud Sharps box			
	THE PROCEDURE			
Check Meter	Ensure that the diabetic meter is working and check calibration.	0	1	–
Test Strip	Open a new test strip and check expiry date on box. Ensure that the BM test strip is compatible with the meter by comparing codes.	0	1	–

STAGE	KEY POINTS AND ACTIONS	SCORE
Gloves	Wash hands and wear a pair of non-sterile gloves.	0 1 –
Wash Hands	Advise the patient to wash their hands with warm water.	
Prepare Meter	Place the strip in the meter and load the lancet with a pricker.	0 1 –
Take Blood	Choose a finger in the non-dominant hand and 'milk' blood proximal to distal along the finger. Prick the side of the finger and not the pulp. Try and obtain sufficient blood for BM reading with only a single prick of the lancet. Give patient cotton bud to achieve haemostasis.	0 1 –
Meter Reading	Take enough blood for the meter to deliver an accurate reading.	0 1 –
Disposal	Safely dispose of sharps into sharps box and soiled materials appropriately.	0 1 –

EVALUATION

Assessment	Correctly read the reading from the blood glucose meter.	0 1 –
Record	Record the reading in the BM diary or the patient's notes.	0 1 –
Check	Check that the patient has understood the procedure.	0 1 –

EXPLANATION

Level of BM	Explain to the patient what blood glucose concentration to aim for.	0 1 –
	'The target we aim for in diabetics is a blood glucose of around 5-8mmol/L before feeding and two hours after eating'.	
Importance	Explain to the patient the importance of good glycaemic control.	0 1 –
	'It is important for you to understand that keeping your glucose within these tight limits will reduce the risk of further complications of diabetes such as affecting your sight, sense of feeling, and kidneys'.	
Regularity	Explain how often the blood glucose should be checked.	0 1 –
	'As you are a newly diagnosed diabetic, I would initially advise you to check your blood glucose levels up to three or four times a day to ensure that your medications are working well and not sending your sugar too low. I would advise that you check your levels before breakfast, 2 hours after lunch and before you sleep at night. When your doctor is happy with your control they may reduce how frequently you check your levels'.	
Confirm	Confirm that the patient has understood what you have explained to them.	0 1 –
Finishing Off	Thank the patient and ask if they have any questions.	

EXAMINER'S EVALUATION

Overall assessment of explaining and using BM machine	0 1 2 3 4 5
Total mark out of 23	

03.14 URINE DIPSTICK

INSTRUCTIONS You are a foundation year House Officer in Accident & Emergency. Ms C has presented with burning when passing urine. Explain to the patient how to provide a urine specimen, test it using the sticks provided, and explain to the patient the findings.

STAGE	KEY POINTS AND ACTIONS	SCORE		
	INTRODUCTION			
Introduction	Introduce yourself. Elicit name, age, and occupation. Establish rapport.	0	1	–
Brief History	Elicit patient's symptoms of burning when passing urine, increased frequency of going to the toilet, and lower abdominal pain.	0	1	2
	EXPLANATION			
Fresh Sample	Explain the importance of providing a fresh sample in the sterile container provided.	0	1	–
Cleaning	Explain the need to clean the genitalia thoroughly before providing a sample.	0	1	–
Mid-Stream	Explain to the patient how to deliver a mid-stream urine specimen and the importance of this.	0	1	–
	'Because of the symptoms you are describing I wish to carry out a urine test. This involves you providing me with a fresh specimen of urine in this sterile container. So that we do not get any misleading results it is important that you follow what I say as closely as you can. Before providing the sample of urine, it is important that you clean and wash the area down below well. Do not allow your skin or body to touch the bottle when passing urine. When you begin to pass urine, do not collect the initial part, but when you are mid-stream fill the container from then onward. Once you are done please return the bottle to me'.			
	TESTING THE URINE			
Wear Gloves	Wash hands and wear a pair of non-sterile gloves.	0	1	–
Test Strip	Take a test strip from box and check expiry date.	0	1	–
Dip	Place the whole stick in the urine for one second ensuring that all testing areas are covered. Tap away any excess urine and hold the strip horizontally.	0	1	–

STAGE	KEY POINTS AND ACTIONS	SCORE

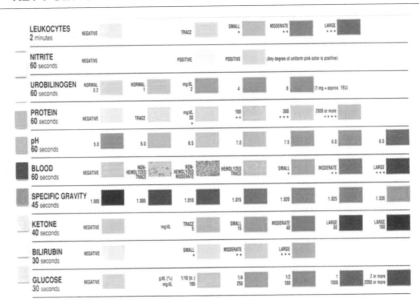

Results	Read the stick correctly after 60 seconds have passed or as long as the box indicates.	0 1 –
Disposal	Dispose of the soiled material and gloves in yellow bag.	0 1 –

EVALUATION

Protein	Explain the finding of protein in the urine and its significance to the patient.	0 1 –
Blood	Explain the finding of blood in the urine and its significance to the patient.	0 1 –
Nitrites	Explain the finding of nitrites in the urine and its significance to the patient.	0 1 –
Identify	Correctly advise the patient of the likelihood of a urine infection and the need for antibiotic cover.	0 1 –
Laboratory	Discuss with the patient the need to send the specimen to the laboratory to confirm the presence of bacteria.	0 1 –

'I have tested your urine sample and would like to explain to you what the results mean. There was protein, blood, and nitrites in your urine. Although each of these on their own could signify some damage to your kidneys, when they are all present together the most likely cause is a urinary tract infection. On some occasions the urine sample may be contaminated and therefore the results may be incorrect. To confirm the presence of bacteria and what kind it is, we will have to send the specimen to the laboratory. The results should be available for your GP to follow up. However in the meantime, we strongly advise that you take some antibiotic treatment which I will be happy to prescribe. Do you have any questions'?

STAGE	KEY POINTS AND ACTIONS	SCORE
Check	Confirm that the patient has understood what you have explained to them.	
Finishing Off	Ask patient if they have any questions or concerns.	

EXAMINER'S EVALUATION

Overall assessment of urinary dipstick testing	0 1 2 3 4 5

Total mark out of 21

CLINICAL CASE

You are a foundation year House Officer in Medicine. Mr B, a 25-year-old man, has had nocturia and frequency of urine for the past two weeks. Explain to the patient how to provide a urine specimen, test it using the sticks provided, and explain to the patient the findings.

Follow the breakdown as above, but replace the evaluation section as below:

EVALUATION

Stage	Key Points and Actions	Score
Glucose	Explain the finding of glucose in the urine and its significance to the patient.	0 1 –
Symptoms	Elicit additional symptoms from the patient such as weakness, tiredness, and increased thirst.	0 1 2
Identify	Correctly advise the patient of diabetes being a likely diagnosis.	0 1 –
Blood Test	Explain the need to send a blood glucose sample to the laboratory to confirm the urine result.	0 1 –
Check	Confirm that the patient has understood what you have explained to them. Ask the patient if they have any questions or concerns.	0 1 –

'I have tested your urine sample and would like to explain to you what the results mean. We found the presence of glucose in your urine. Although this may be entirely innocent, we cannot exclude the possibility that you may suffer from diabetes. I understand that this may be a lot to take in now. However, I must stress that to confirm or negate this, we must send a blood sample to the laboratory. Can I take the time now to briefly ask what do you understand by diabetes? Do you have any questions you wish to ask me'?

03.15 BASIC LIFE SUPPORT

INSTRUCTIONS You are leaving your busy medical outpatient clinic when suddenly a man in the waiting area collapses in front of you. Nobody else is available for help. Assess the situation and commence resuscitation.

STAGE	KEY POINTS AND ACTIONS	SCORE
	THE PROCEDURE **Assessment [Mnemonic–SSSS]**	
Safe	Ensure your own safety by confirming that it is safe to approach the patient. Ensure there is no immediate danger from the surrounds such as electricity, gas, or chemical spillage.	0 1 –
Shout	Check the responsiveness of the victim by shouting, 'Are you alright'?	0 1 –
Shake	Gently shake his shoulders to see if there is a physical response.	0 1 –
Shout for help	If there is no response shout for help. Shout, shake, and shout for help.	0 1 –

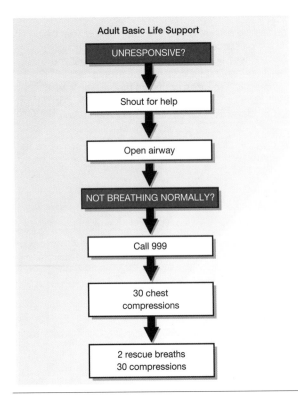

Adult Basic Life Support

UNRESPONSIVE?

Shout for help

Open airway

NOT BREATHING NORMALLY?

Call 999

30 chest compressions

2 rescue breaths
30 compressions

STAGE	KEY POINTS AND ACTIONS	SCORE

AIRWAY

Position

If necessary turn the patient on to his back and then open his airway by gently tilting his head back and lifting his chin. If you suspect a cervical spine injury then open the airway by jaw thrust only.

0 1 2

Obstruction

Inspect the mouth and remove any visible obstructions (using finger sweep method) such as dislodged dentures, vomit, or foreign bodies, but leave in place any well-fitting dentures.

0 1 –

Only attempt to remove any further objects if suction or McGill forceps are available to safely do so.

Breathing

Keeping the airway open, bring your ear to the victim's mouth and observe for signs of breathing. Look for chest movements, listen for breath sounds, and feel for breathing against your cheek for a maximum of 10 seconds.

0 1 2

Assistance

If the patient is breathing, turn him into the recovery position, checking for continued breathing, and send for help or if alone, go and seek assistance.

0 1 –

If the patient is not breathing, leave the side of the patient and seek assistance by telephoning the emergency number for help – if with someone ask them to go and to bring back a bag-valve mask and automated external defibrillator if possible, in the meantime begin chest compressions.

Dial 2 2 2 2 (or equivalent depending on the crash system in your local hospital). State the following clearly and slowly.

'Adult cardiac arrest, medical outpatients department, Clinic A, Level 1. Please put out a crash call'.

CPR

Deliver 30 chest compressions at a ratio of 30 compressions: 2 breaths.

0 1 2

Identify the costal margin and the xiphisternum. After interlocking your fingers, place the heels of your hands two finger breadths above the xiphisternum and apply chest compressions, 1/3 of the depth of the patient's chest or 5-6cm, at a rate of 100–120 BPM. Ensure that you are positioned vertically above the patient with your arms straight and with your shoulders above your wrists.

If there is more than one person present, change CPR giver every 1-2 minutes.

Ventilate

For in-hospital arrests use a bag-valve mask to ventilate.
One-person technique – only if sufficiently competent – use one hand to create a seal over nose and mouth with the mask and the other to squeeze the bag. If available this bag should be connected to oxygen as soon as possible.

0 1 –

If with another person use a two-person technique – one person creates a two-handed seal with the mask and the other ventilates with the bag. Two, slow, well-controlled squeezes are sufficient – ensure the patient's chest rises and falls and if not, consider adjusting their airway.

Maintain the airway by ensuring that the head is tilted, chin is lifted, and nose is pinched closed.

If no bag-valve mask immediately available, use a mouth-to-mouth technique. Use a one-way face-mask valve if available. Take a normal breath and then place your lips around the patient's lips and ensure a good seal is available. While pinching the patient's nose, blow for two seconds, watching the chest rise and fall as above. Repeat a second time and then continue CPR.

Recheck

Stop to recheck for signs of circulation only if the patient makes a movement or takes a spontaneous breath. Otherwise, continue until help arrives, the patient shows signs of life, or you feel exhausted.

0 1 –

Instructions

The Resuscitation team arrives with an automated external defibrillator (AED).

STAGE	KEY POINTS AND ACTIONS	SCORE		
Pads	Attach pads to correct location on patient (as marked on either pad, it does not matter if the pads are reversed) with one on the right upper chest next to the sternum and the other in the anterior axillary line, mid-chest (over the V6 chest electrode position) and free of breast tissue.			
	Ensure CPR is still ongoing during the process.	0	1	–
Defibrillator	Switch on the AED and follow the instructions. Ensure no one is touching the patient when the AED is analysing the rhythm. (In BLS you would not be expected to be able to use a manual defibrillator.)	0	1	–
	If the AED suggests a shock, make sure no one is touching the patient and any oxygen is removed. Deliver the shock while watching the patient to make sure this remains the case as the shock is delivered.			
CPR	Continue CPR for another 2 minutes before checking for a pulse again (the AED will instruct you to do this).	0	1	–

EXAMINER'S EVALUATION

Overall assessment of performance of basic life support	0	1	2	3	4	5	

Total mark out of 22

03.16 OXYGEN THERAPY

INSTRUCTIONS Mr Hopkins is a 65-year-old man with a history of COPD and presents to A&E with breathlessness. Manage him with oxygen as appropriate.

STAGE	KEY POINTS AND ACTIONS	SCORE		
	INTRODUCTION			
Introduction	Introduce yourself. Elicit name, age, and occupation. Establish rapport.	0	1	–
Explain	'Because of your breathing problems we need to check your oxygen saturation which will tell us how well your lungs are functioning. If necessary we may need to commence you on oxygen therapy which will be delivered by a face mask. Do you have any questions'?	0	1	–
Consent	Obtain consent and check patient's ID before beginning the procedure.	0	1	–
	THE EQUIPMENT			
	Oxygen cylinder			
	Venturi valves (blue, white, yellow)			
	Venturi mask			
	Hudson non-rebreathing mask			
	Pulse oximeter			
	THE PROCEDURE			
Monitor	State you would like to monitor the patient's oxygen saturation. Attach a pulse oximeter correctly to the end of the patient's finger, ensuring there is no nail varnish present on the nail which may result in a false reading.	0	1	2
	Turn the machine on and interpret the oxygen saturation value. O_2 saturation <90%: Patient is hypoxic and requires oxygen therapy.			
Face Mask	Select the Venturi mask and assemble with tubing correctly. Connect the mask to an oxygen supply such as an oxygen cylinder. Apply the mask gently to the patient's face and tighten the elastic gently.	0	1	2
	Select the appropriate Venturi valve to attach to the face mask and apply the appropriate flow rate to deliver oxygen to the patient.			
	Select the blue Venturi valve delivering oxygen at 24% with 2L/min flow rate.			

STAGE	KEY POINTS AND ACTIONS	SCORE
ABG	After supplying the appropriate concentration of oxygen to this COPD patient, request to perform an arterial blood gas sample. This is to accurately assess the patient's carbon dioxide and oxygen concentrations.	0 1 –
Interpret	The examiner supplies you with a card containing the ABG results:	0 1 2

	1	2	3
pH	7.4	7.29	7.31
PaO_2	7.1kPa	6.8kPa	10kPa
PCO_2	4.0kPa	7.6kPa	7.3kPa
Interpretation	Type I respiratory failure	CO_2 retention, respiratory acidosis – type II respiratory failure	CO_2 retention, adequate oxygenation
Action	Increase oxygen therapy – change up to 28% via Venturi – aim sats 94%. Monitor for retention.	Urgent optimization of medical treatment – may require NIV if not improving	Reduce oxygen therapy – switch to nasal cannulae – aim sats 88-92%.

	Interpret the results and correctly alter the oxygen therapy accordingly.	
Reinterpret	After changing the oxygen therapy, wait 1 hour to allow alteration of the patient's saturation levels and metabolic status. Repeat the process and interpret a range of ABG results while adjusting the oxygen delivery accordingly.	0 1 2

Different Venturi Valves

Colour	Conc.	Flow Rate
Blue	24%	2 L/min
White	28%	4 L/min
Yellow	35%	6 L/min
Red	40%	8 L/min
Green	60%	12 L/min

Finishing Off	Thank the patient and throw away any remaining waste.

EXAMINER'S EVALUATION

Overall assessment of setting up oxygen therapy	0 1 2 3 4 5

Total mark out of 17

Further reading:
https://www.brit-thoracic.org.uk/document-library/clinical-information/oxygen/emergency-oxygen-use-in-adult-patients-guideline/emergency-oxygen-use-in-adult-patients-guideline/

SELECTING THE RIGHT MASK
Nasal Cannulae

Use a nasal cannula for a patient who has adequate ventilation and tidal volume but needs more oxygen. The nasal cannula gives the patient more freedom than a mask, which may make them feel claustrophobic. It is ideal for patients with normal vital signs or with slightly low oxygen saturations.

Face Masks

The simple face mask is indicated for a patient who needs a little higher concentration. The higher flow rate keeps them from rebreathing exhaled carbon dioxide (CO_2).

Hudson Mask

Normally comes with a non-rebreathing bag that fills with oxygen. It contains two small, one-way valves that allow expired CO_2 to leave the mask. These masks are considered low-flow devices, but can deliver higher oxygen concentrations than a simple face mask. This mask is ideal in severe asthma, acute left ventricular failure, pneumonia, or trauma patients.

Venturi Masks

Venturi masks that contain a Venturi valve attachment are said to be high-flow masks that can provide a stream of oxygen at fixed concentrations, ideal for patients with chronic respiratory failure such as COPD. In practice, BTS guidelines recommend prescribing a target saturation for oxygen, not a fixed rate of oxygen, allowing nursing staff to switch between delivery methods to achieve this target.

03.17 SETTING UP A NEBULISER

INSTRUCTIONS You are a foundation year House Officer in Medicine. Ms S, a lady with a background of asthma, has been referred by a local GP suffering with an audible wheeze and dyspnoea. She has had an ABG. You have seen her and decide that she needs salbutamol nebulisation. Set up the nebuliser machine, explaining to the patient what you are doing, and deliver the appropriate medication.

STAGE	KEY POINTS AND ACTIONS	SCORE		
	INTRODUCTION			
Introduction	Introduce yourself. Elicit name, age, and occupation. Establish rapport.	0	1	–
Explain	'As a result of the breathing problems you are experiencing I am going to give you some medication (salbutamol) via a nebuliser. A nebuliser is a device which helps deliver medication to the lungs where they will work to relax your breathing tubes and help you breathe easier. The machine will be connected to oxygen and you will have to wear a mask. Because it uses a pump to deliver medication, the machine may make an unpleasant noise when in use. Do you have any questions'?	0	1	–
Consent	Obtain consent and check patient's ID before beginning the procedure.	0	1	–
	THE PROCEDURE			
Assemble	Correctly assemble the nebuliser and attach it to the oxygen supply.	0	1	–
Check	Check the drug chart and ascertain the drug to be administered and its dose. Confirm that the drug is to be nebulised.	0	1	–
Drug	Choose the right drug, salbutamol (5mg) for nebulisation and check its expiry date. Confirm the details with another colleague, such as a nurse.			
	Carefully separate a new vial from the strip. Open the vial by twisting the top off. Never use one that has already been opened.	0	1	2
Chamber	Unscrew the cap from the mixing chamber and squeeze the contents of the plastic vial into the outer chamber of the nebuliser. Reattach the cap and attach the nebuliser to either a mouthpiece or mask as preferred by the patient.	0	1	–
Check Device	Turn on the compressor and check for a steady mist emerging from the mask. If there is no mist, check all tubing connections and confirm that the compressor is working properly.	0	1	–

STAGE	KEY POINTS AND ACTIONS	SCORE
Apply Mask	Place the mask to the patient's face and gently tighten the elastic cord.	0 1 –
Flow Rate	Set the airflow rate at 5–7L/min. Use oxygen as the driving gas with patients with acute asthma or air if the patient is retaining carbon dioxide; i.e. COPD patient.	0 1 –
Breathe	Ensure that the patient is resting comfortably in an upright position and ask them to breathe normally into the mask. They should continue to breathe into the mask until there is no longer any mist produced.	0 1 –
Document	Sign the drug chart that the nebulised drug has been administered.	0 1 –
Cleaning	Give advice about cleaning the mask and chamber in order to reduce the risk of infection. Disassemble the nebuliser and wash all parts (except tubing) with warm soapy water. Rinse thoroughly with warm water and shake. Dry the nebuliser parts with a clean cloth.	0 1 2
Finishing Off	Thank the patient and answer any questions.	

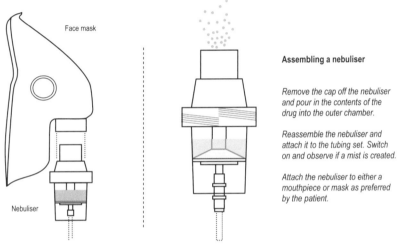

Face mask

Nebuliser

Assembling a nebuliser

Remove the cap off the nebuliser and pour in the contents of the drug into the outer chamber.

Reassemble the nebuliser and attach it to the tubing set. Switch on and observe if a mist is created.

Attach the nebuliser to either a mouthpiece or mask as preferred by the patient.

EXAMINER'S EVALUATION

Overall assessment of setting up nebuliser device   0 1 2 3 4 5

Total mark out of 20

03.18 ARTERIAL BLOOD SAMPLING

INSTRUCTIONS You are the medical House Officer on call. Mr G was admitted under your care two days ago for infective exacerbation of COPD. The nurse in charge has bleeped you stating that Mr G's health is deteriorating and he is having difficulty in breathing. Demonstrate to the examiner how you would take an arterial blood sample on the manikin provided. Explain to the examiner what you are doing as you go along.

STAGE	KEY POINTS AND ACTIONS	SCORE
	INTRODUCTION	
Introduction	Introduce yourself. Elicit name, age, and occupation. Establish rapport.	0 1 –
Explain	'I understand that you are having some difficulty in breathing. In order to check how things are progressing, I need to take some blood from your wrist. Although this procedure can be quite painful, I can reassure you that it is a quick procedure that is essential for your further management. Do you have any questions'?	0 1 –
Consent	Obtain consent to proceed and check patient's ID before commencement.	0 1 –
Position	Ensure that the patient is either sitting or lying comfortably.	
Equipment	Collect and set up the equipment on a trolley.	
	THE EQUIPMENT	
	Pre-heparinised syringe Arterial gas needle Local anaesthetic: Lignocaine 1% (optional) Pair of non-sterile gloves Alcohol swabs Sharps box Cotton wool/gauze	
	THE PROCEDURE	
Prepare	Wash hands with disinfectant and don a pair of gloves.	0 1 –

STAGE	KEY POINTS AND ACTIONS	SCORE
Position	Have the patient lying down or sitting with their arm well supported. Position the patient's arm with the palm facing up and the wrist hyper-extended resting on a rolled up towel.	
Identify Artery	Locate the radial pulse with the index finger and middle finger of your non-dominant hand. Palpate the artery to determine its size, depth, and direction. Avoid using your thumb since it has its own pulse and may be confused with the patient's.	0 1 –
Anaesthetic (offer to the patient)	Clean the skin with an alcohol swab and infiltrate the skin with lignocaine 1% local anaesthetic at the proposed sample site. Enter with the needle at 10 degrees to the surface of the skin. Pull back slightly on the plunger with each infiltration to check if a vein has been punctured. Warn the patient of a short stinging sensation and then wait between 1 and 2 minutes for the anaesthetic to take effect. (BTS guidelines recommend the routine use of local anaesthetic for all patients except in emergency situations, unconsciousness, or anaesthesia.)	0 1 –
Drape	Prepare a drape over the sample area.	
Syringe	Hold the pre-heparinised syringe and attach an ABG needle. Expel the excess heparin. Be careful not to aspirate any air back into the syringe. Hold it in the dominant hand as you would hold a pencil.	0 1 –
Insertion	Re-identify the radial pulse and introduce the needle at 45 degrees with the bevel facing toward the patient. As you insert the needle, a flash of blood will appear in the hub of the needle. Stop advancing the needle further and allow the blood to fill the syringe under arterial pressure. Spontaneous filling of the syringe confirms that an artery has been successfully accessed. Aspirate gently if needed. If you missed the artery, slowly withdraw the tip of the needle and re-insert. Do not probe with the needle as repeated puncture of a single site increases the likelihood of haematoma, scarring, or laceration of the artery.	0 1 2
Aspirate	Aspirate (if needed) approximately 2mL of blood and withdraw the needle.	0 1 –
Pressure	Place a gauze or cotton wool over the site and apply firm pressure for 5 minutes. If required, ask the patient to press firmly on the wound site.	0 1 –
Haematoma	Inspect for an enlarging haematoma and if necessary apply further pressure.	0 1 –
Expel Air	Expel any air from the syringe and cap it with a rubber or latex square.	0 1 –
	FINISHING OFF	
Waste	Dispose of the used needle into the yellow sharps container and dispose of any gloves and soiled material safely.	0 1 –
Labels	Label the specimen clearly with the surname, first name, date of birth, hospital number, and date taken.	0 1 –
Analyser	The sample should be analysed swiftly in a blood gas analyser within 5 minutes if possible.	
	EXAMINER'S EVALUATION	
	Overall assessment of arterial blood sampling	0 1 2 3 4 5
	Total mark out of 20	

03.19 ANKLE BRACHIAL PRESSURE INDEX (USING A DOPPLER)

INSTRUCTIONS You are a foundation year House Officer in Vascular Surgery. Mr R, a smoker of 30 years, has been experiencing pain in the back of the calves when walking 30 yards.

You suspect he has claudication and wish to measure his ankle brachial pressure index. Explain to the patient what you wish to do and measure his ABPI.

STAGE	KEY POINTS AND ACTIONS	SCORE
	INTRODUCTION	
Introduction	Introduce yourself. Elicit name, age, and occupation. Establish rapport.	0 1 –
Explain	'Because of the symptoms you have, I wish to measure the blood pressure in your arms and legs. I will be using a small Doppler device which allows measurement of flow in a blood vessel using sound waves, and a blood pressure cuff. It is a simple procedure and is not painful. Do you have any questions'?	0 1 –
Consent	Obtain consent and check patient's ID before beginning the procedure.	0 1 –
Equipment	Collect and set up the equipment.	
	THE EQUIPMENT	
	Continuous wave Doppler unit Sphygmomanometer Lubricating jelly Calculator	
	THE PROCEDURE	
Position	Ensure the patient is lying flat and feels comfortable and relaxed. Ask them to expose their feet and arms for this procedure. Allow the patient to rest for 20 minutes to ensure that any pressure changes noted are not caused by the patient moving around but are due to arterial disease.	0 1 2

STAGE	KEY POINTS AND ACTIONS	SCORE
	Brachial	
Pulse	Place an appropriately sized cuff around the arm.	0 1 –
	Locate the brachial pulse on the medial anterior surface of the antecubital fossa and apply ultrasound contact gel over the skin.	
Probe	Hold the probe at a 45 degree angle to the direction of blood flow in the artery. Move the Doppler probe around gently until you get a good signal.	0 1 2
Cuff	Inflate the cuff until the signal disappears, then slowly release the pressure from the cuff until the signal returns. Cuff deflation must proceed slowly (no greater than 2mmHg per second) in order to accurately obtain the pressure at which blood flow returns.	0 1 2
Document	Record this pressure (brachial systolic) then repeat for the other arm. Use the higher of the two values to calculate the ABPI.	0 1 –
	Ankle	
Placement	Place the same sized cuff around the ankle immediately above the malleoli.	0 1 –
Pulse	Locate the dorsalis pedis pulse with your fingertips or the Doppler probe and apply ultrasound contact gel. Take the (ankle) systolic pressure as described for the brachial and record the result.	0 1 –
Repeat	Repeat the measurement for the posterior tibial pulse and if required the peroneal pulse. Use the highest reading obtained between the pulses to calculate the ABPI for that ankle. Repeat for the other leg.	0 1 –
	Additional Points	
Finishing Off	Wipe the ultrasound contact gel away from skin of the patient as well as from the head of the handheld Doppler probe and wash your hands. Offer to restore the patient's clothing.	0 1 –
	THE EVALUATION	
Calculate	Calculate the ankle brachial pressure index by using the following equation. You should obtain two separate values for either leg. Do not forget to use the highest reading between the dorsalis pedis and posterior tibial pressure for each leg and the highest reading of brachial pressure in both arms.	0 1 –
Interpret	Interpret the ankle brachial pressure index and explain its significance.	0 1 2
	Interpreting Ankle Brachial Pressure Index ABPI > 1.0 Normal ABPI 0.4–0.8 Claudication ABPI 0.1–0.4 Critical Ischaemia * In diabetics, the ABPI can be falsely elevated due to vessel wall calcification.	
Thanks	Thank the patient and answer any possible questions.	

EXAMINER'S EVALUATION	
Overall assessment of presenting correct physical findings	0 1 2 3 4 5

Total mark out of 23

THE ANKLE BRACHIAL PRESSURE INDEX

The ABPI is the most common diagnostic test for diagnosing peripheral arterial disease. It is a measurement of blood flow through the peripheral arteries and assesses for narrowing or blockage of the leg arteries. Healthy individuals usually have an ABPI of between 0.97 and 1.1. Values less than 0.97 identify patients with a degree of peripheral artery disease or complete stenoses. Most patients with symptoms of claudication will have an ABPI between 0.4 and 0.8 and those with critical ischaemia usually have values less than 0.4.

ABPIs can often produce misleading results. A normal ABPI at the level of the ankle may suggest adequate blood flow at that point, but it does not account for the possibility of a distal occlusion due to emboli, micro-emboli, and atherosclerotic plaques. In diabetics, the ABPI of the ankle may be falsely elevated. This is because of calcification of the walls of the blood vessel, which offers greater resistance to compression.

$$\frac{\textit{Highest ankle Doppler pressure (for each leg)}}{\textit{Highest brachial Dopple pressure (of two arms)}} = ABPI$$

03.20 CONFIRMATION OF DEATH

INSTRUCTIONS You are a foundation year House Officer in Vascular Surgery. The nurses bleep you to confirm the death of a palliative care patient in side room 4. Demonstrate to the examiner how you would do this.

STAGE	KEY POINTS AND ACTIONS	SCORE
	INTRODUCTION	
Introduction	Introduce yourself to the nurse. Establish the name, date of birth, and hospital number of the patient.	0 1 –
DNAR	Check that the patient has a do not attempt resuscitation in place.	0 1 –
Observe	Observe the patient for respiratory effort and spontaneous movements. Look for additional signs suggestive of the time of death, such as rigor mortis.	0 1 –
Response	Attempt to elicit a verbal response from the patient	0 1 –
Pain Response	Check response to painful stimuli by supraorbital notch pressure or supraclavicular pinch. Note the temperature of the body.	0 1 –
Pupils	Check that the pupils are fixed and dilated to light bilaterally. This is indicative of brainstem death.	0 1 –
Feel	For two central pulses for a total of 5 minutes (carotid and femoral for example).	0 1 –
Auscultate	For heart sounds for a total of 5 minutes For breath sounds for a total of 5 minutes In practice the above can be done simultaneously while observing the patient for 5 minutes for any spontaneous effort. If no sign of life, confirm the death.	0 1 –
Record in the Notes	- No response to pain or verbal stimulus - Pupils fixed and dilated - No heart or lung sounds for 5 minutes - No respiratory effort for 5 minutes - No central pulses for 5 minutes - Record the time of death as the time you confirmed the death	0 1 2

STAGE	KEY POINTS AND ACTIONS	SCORE

In hospital this can be supplemented by an ECG showing asystole.

Finishing Off   Sign the death certificate if appropriate.

EXAMINER'S EVALUATION

Overall assessment of confirmation of death   0   1   2   3   4   5

Total mark out of 15

03.21 RECORDING AN ECG

INSTRUCTIONS Mr Philips has been experiencing chest pain since 9am this morning. You wish to carry out an ECG tracing of his heart. Explain to the patient what this entails and record his ECG.

STAGE	KEY POINTS AND ACTIONS	SCORE
	INTRODUCTION	
Introduction	Introduce yourself. Elicit name, age, and occupation. Establish rapport.	0 1 –
Explain	"I have been asked to perform an ECG tracing of your heart. This is simply a device that records the rhythm and electrical activity of the heart and involves attaching small patches on the arms, legs and chest which are connected to the ECG machine. It is a simple procedure that will not shock or cause pain."	0 1 –
Consent	Obtain consent and check patient's ID before beginning the procedure.	0 1 –
Expose	Lay the patient on the couch and expose the patient's arms and chest.	0 1 –
	THE PROCEDURE	
Limb Leads	Attach the limb leads to the dorsal aspect of the forearms and on the outer aspect of the lower limbs, above the ankles. Ensure good contact between the electrode sticky pads with their adjacent leads. The limb leads are colour co-ordinated and are usually longer than the chest leads. Attach them in a clockwise fashion to the limbs in accordance with the colour of the traffic lights [or via the Mnemonic – 'Ride Your Green Bike'] starting from the right arm (red), left arm (yellow), left leg (green) and finally the right leg (black).	0 1 2
Chest Leads	Attach the remainder of the leads to the chest from V1 to V6. Ensure that there is good contact with the electrode.	0 1 2
Positions of the Chest Leads	V1 4th intercostal space, right sternal edge V2 4th intercostal space, left sternal edge V3 Halfway between V2 and V4 V4 5th Intercostal space, mid-clavicular line V5 5th Intercostal space, anterior axillary line V6 5th intercostal space, mid-axillary line	0 1 2
Print	Turn the machine on and press 'filter' and then 'start' to print the ECG.	0 1 –
Document	Write down the patient's name, DOB, hospital number and the time and date when the ECG was taken on the actual ECG.	0 1 –

	EXAMINER'S EVALUATION	
	Overall assessment of recording of the ECG	0 1 2 3 4 5
	Total mark out of 17	

MANAGEMENT OF THE ACUTELY UNWELL PATIENT

04.1 GENERAL SCHEMATA

As a foundation year doctor you will be expected to undertake the initial management of acutely unwell patients. Increasingly, medical schools are testing the ability to take a structured logical approach to this task. Whilst initially practicing in such a manner may seem unnatural the value of having an ingrained system such as the one below cannot be underestimated for finals and beyond.

A typical instruction for such a station may be 'You are a foundation year house officer covering the ward at night. Mr F has increasingly abnormal observations over the past hour. Please examine and manage this acutely unwell patient in a structured manner'.

The aim is to be able to take a DR ABCDE approach as demonstrated below. The scenarios are designed to be used as role-play aids. They can either be read through as a systematic exemplar assessment of a patient, or used as a role-play tool; one person takes the role of candidate and conducts the assessment, on a dummy, patient, or imagined other, and the other person takes the role of examiner. Using the prompts under each section to respond to the candidate, give the examination findings and feedback.

The following is a general schemata for the basic assessment which should be applied in any scenario.

Danger	• Check around the bedside for potential hazards; e.g. spills, wires, blood.
Response	• Introduce yourself. Ask a simple question.
	'Hello, I hear you are not feeling very well. Can you tell me more about it'?
Airway	If the patient is talking this indicates the airway is patent.
Look	• Look for signs of airway obstruction; such as paradoxical abdominal breathing, distress, or blue lips.
	• Look for swollen lips and tongue and blotchy skin in anaphylaxis.
	• Look inside the mouth for any obstruction.
Listen	Listen for gargling or snoring obstructive sounds and look in the mouth.
Treat	• Suction if there are visible secretions or blockage. Remove any obstructing material with McGill forceps.
	• Head-tilt chin lift. Consider the need for airway adjuncts if not managing own airway. Place in the recovery position if appropriate.
	• High-flow oxygen if appropriate — 15 litres via non-rebreathe mask.
Breathing	
Look	• Peripherally: cyanosis
	• Centrally: blue lips, respiratory distress, visible chest expansion, tracheal, and intercostal recession
Feel	• Chest expansion
	• Percussion

Listen	• Auscultate front and back
Measure	• Respiratory rate (normal 10-20)
	• Saturations (Healthy individual > 95%, COPD or background lung disease > 88%)
	• Consider arterial blood gases
	• Consider chest x-ray if relevant
Treat	• Sit patient up
	• High-flow oxygen if appropriate
Re-assess	• Re-assess patient

Circulation

Look	• Peripherally: cap refill, cyanosis
	• Centrally: conjunctival pallor, hydration status
	• JVP
Feel	• Peripheral pulses, apex beat
Listen	• Auscultate heart
Measure	• Urine output
	• Temperature
	• Capillary refill
	• Heart rate and rhythm
	• Blood pressure
Treat	• Insert two wide-bore cannula in each anterior cubital fossa and send bloods as needed.
	• Consider IV fluid challenge; e.g. 500mL crystalloid STAT.
	• Obtain a 12-lead ECG.
Reassess	• Re-assess patient.

Diability

Pupils	• Check that pupils are equal and reactive to light.
GCS / AVPU	• Score the patient on the GCS or AVPU scale.
	• AVPU: **A**lert, responds to **V**oice, responds to **P**ain, **U**nresponsive
	• GCS: 3-15/15 (see below)
	• A score of P on the AVPU scale is equivalent to a GCS of 8 or less.
Capillary BM	• Check the patient's glucose level.
Pain	• Check if the patient is in pain and give analgesia if not already done so.
Treat	• Treat any blood sugar < 4 (see Hypoglycaemia chapter).
	• Consider airway adjuncts and even intubation in any GCS < 8.
Re-assess	• Re-assess patient.

Exposure

Fully expose the patient and examine them from head to toe.

Head	• Check for Raccoon eyes or Battle's sign indicative of base of skull fracture.
	• Check for rhinorrhea or otorrheoa to check for CSF leak.

Chest	• Check the skins for rashes, lacerations, or bruising, especially over ribs suggestive of fractures.
	• Check for pacemaker/ICD sites (very important if peri-arrest).
Abdomen	• Look for Grey-Turner's and Cullen's sign of retroperitoneal bleeding and rashes.
	• Feel for tenderness, distension, or peritonism.
	• Listen for bowel sounds.
	• Consider a PR if relevant.
Back	• Same as for chest.
Legs	• Look for rashes, bruising, signs of DVT.
	• Check the peripheral pulses.

AMPLE HISTORY

If the patient is able you should attempt to gather a relevant history—we would recommend doing this at the bedside as part of the on-going resuscitation of an acutely unwell patient, but do not delay the immediate steps to talk to the patient.

When able, use the mnemonic [AMPLE].

Allergies: Check, if possible, before administering ANY drug (including but not limited to chlorhexidine, colloid fluids, and any antibiotic).

Medications:

Past medical history: Concisely - any heart problems, lung problems. Ask especially about asthma, COPD, and angina.

Last meal: Very important for any patient with trauma or acute abdominal pain.

Events: Establish time course of the events leading to presentation.

MANAGEMENT

Explain to the patient what the working diagnosis is and what will happen next in simple terms. Use this to present your differential to the examiner and what you would do next.

Mention specifically:

-The leading diagnosis and the differential

-Any further investigations you would want to perform

-Your immediate management

-Senior involvement

-The next person you would involve

-Handover to that person using a structured format (e.g. RSVP or SBAR)

-Mention you would not leave the patient

EXEMPLAR PRESENTATION

'Mr F is a 65-year-old recruitment consultant presenting with acute onset, left sided, crushing central chest pain. His airway is patent and he is alert and awake. His lungs are clear and his saturations >95% in air. He is peripherally well perfused, with a cap refill of <2 secs, urine output of >50mL/hour and blood pressure of 120 systolic. Heart sounds are normal and JVP is not raised. His ECG shows >4mm ST elevation in leads V1-V4 with reciprocal inferior depression. This is in keeping with an acute ST-Elevated myocardial infarction. I have given him 300mg aspirin PO, 300mg clopidogrel PO, a trial of GTN spray, and 2.5mg of IV morphine which made him much more comfortable. In line with current BTS guidance on oxygen in acute MI, I have withheld oxygen while his saturations are above 95%. I would like to notify the registrar on-call to come up and review the patient but I would also handover using a SBAR technique to the cardiology registrar on-call to perform urgent percutaneous coronary intervention if local or immediate transfer to a unit that can. I would not leave the patient until a senior arrived and I handed over to him or her'. ■

Now try the following scenarios for practice—use the mark scheme to assess the candidate and the examiner response column to provide findings and feedback.

04.2
PALPITATIONS

INSTRUCTIONS You are a foundation year House Officer on the wards when the nursing staff ask you to see Mrs G, a 24-year-old with sudden onset palpitations. Please examine and manage this acutely unwell patient in a structured manner.

STAGE	KEY POINTS AND ACTIONS		SCORE
	SCORE SCHEME	**EXAMINER RESPONSE**	
Danger	• Check around the bedside for potential hazards; e.g. spills, wires, blood.	'Safe to approach'.	0 1 –
Response	• Introduce yourself. Ask a simple question.	*'My heart is racing doctor'.* *Follow-up information: no chest pain, had previous episodes, in hospital for a mole removal.*	0 1 –
Airway	• Recognise airway patency as patient is speaking.		0 1 –
Breathing			
Look	• Look for signs of respiratory distress. • Be able to state signs (*see* table above).	*'Looks well, no respiratory distress'.*	0 1 –
Feel	• Check chest expansion. • Percuss chest.	*'Chest expansion – equal, bilateral; Percussion – resonant throughout'.*	0 1 –
Listen	• Auscultate front and back.	*'No crackles, rubs or wheezes, good breath sounds throughout, bases clear'.*	0 1 –
Measure	• Respiratory rate • Saturations • Consider arterial blood gases • Consider chest x-ray if relevant	*'Respiratory rate – 24 Saturations – 99% in air ABG results (if asked for) – pH 7.48 pCO2 3.0kpa PO2 15kpa Lac 0.3 Glu 5 BE 1 Bicarbonate 27 (Correct interpretation; minor respiratory alkalosis secondary to hyperventilation) CXR: arranged – will take some time to return'.*	0 1 –
Treat	• Sit patient up. • High-flow oxygen.		0 1 –

STAGE	KEY POINTS AND ACTIONS		SCORE		
Re-assess	• State 'I would re-assess patient'.	*'No change'.*	0	1	–
Circulation					
Look	• Peripherally: cap refill, cyanosis Centrally: conjunctival pallor, hydration status • JVP	*'Peripherally: cap refill < 2 seconds, warm, and well perfused* *Centrally: looks well, JVP not raised'.*	0	1	–
Feel	• Peripheral pulses, apex beat	*'Peripheral pulses: Heart rate is 150 and regular, good volumes* *Apex: non-displaced'.*	0	1	–
Listen	• Auscultate heart.	*'Tachycardia, no murmurs'.*	0	1	–
Measure	• Urine output • Temperature • Capillary refill • Heart rate and rhythm • Blood pressure	*'Urine output – 45mL/hr (patient weighs 60kg)* *Temperature – 36.6 C* *Capillary refill – as above* *Heart rate and rhythm – as above* *Blood pressure – 136/80 mmHg'.*	0	1	–
Treat	• Insert two wide-bore cannula in each anterior cubital fossa and send bloods: FBC, U&E, Mg, calcium, and phosphate. • IV fluid challenge – 500mL crystalloid STAT. • Ask for a 12-lead ECG. • State 'I would initiate SVT treatment' (*see* below).	*'ECG shows sinus tachycardia with narrow complexes'.*	0	1	–
Reassess	• State 'I would re-assess patient'.	*'No change with fluids'.*	0	1	–
Diability					
Pupils	• Check that pupils are equal and reactive to light.	**'Equal and reactive'.**	0	1	–
GCS / AVPU	• Score the patient on the GCS or AVPU scale.	**'GCS 15/15'.**	0	1	–
Capillary BM	• Ask for BM.	**'BM 5'.**	0	1	–
Pain	• Ask if patient is in pain.	**'Patient is pain free'.**	0	1	–
Treat	Nil required		0	1	–
Exposure					
	• State 'I would fully expose the patient and examine them from head to toe'.	'Normal head Normal chest Soft, good bowel sounds Soft calves, no sign of DVT'.	0	1	–
	• State 'I would seek senior help at appropriate time'.		0	1	–

STAGE	KEY POINTS AND ACTIONS	SCORE

AMPLE HISTORY

When able, use the mnemonic—AMPLE.
Allergies: *No allergies.*
Medications: *OCP only, no new medications.*
Past medical history: *Previous palpitations, nil else.*
Last meal: *Had a coffee and toast at breakfast.*
Events: *Started 30 minutes ago.*

VIVA ON MANAGEMENT OF ARRYTHMIAS

SVT in haemodynamically stable patients

First line:
Vagal manoeuvres – e.g. carotid sinus massage (contraindications - known carotid artery stenosis or carotid bruit; auscultate first), Valsava manoeuvre (contraindications – severe coronary artery disease).

Second line:
IV adenosine 6mg (Contraindications: asthma, COPD) – reassess if no response;
IV adenosine 12mg – reassess, if no response;
IV adenosine 12mg – reassess, if no response.

SVT in unstable patients (shock, syncope, myocardial ischaemia, heart failure)

First line: Synchronized DC cardioversion with sedation
What you need to do: fast-bleep the medical registrar or cardiology registrar and an anaesthetist.

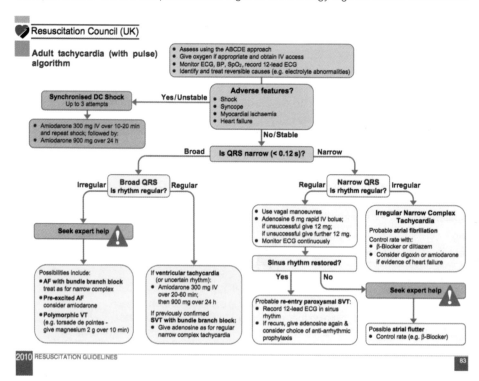

Reproduced with kind permission from the Resusciation Council (UK).

STAGE	KEY POINTS AND ACTIONS	SCORE

EXAMINER'S EVALUATION

Overall assessment of palpitation management   0   1   2   3   4   5

Total mark out of 27

EXEMPLAR PRESENTATION

'Mrs G is a 24-year-old marine biologist presenting with a 30-minute history of palpitations. She is bright and alert, the airway is patent. Her lungs are clear and her saturation is >99% in air with a slightly high respiratory rate of 25 and a correspondingly normal ABG. Her heart rate is 150 and regular. An ECG shows a narrow complex tachycardia. She is pain free. Blood pressure is 136 systolic and urine output is adequate for her weight. BM is normal, GCS 15/15, and the rest of the examination is also normal. She has a history of palpitations but is otherwise healthy. There are no signs of venous thromboembolic disease. The diagnosis is supraventricular tachycardia, the differential is a spontaneous event, or secondary to another cause; e.g. underlying venous thromboembolism, sepsis, alcohol use, or underlying heart disease. My immediate management would be carotid sinus massage or valsava if there were no contraindications. I would then seek senior help to administer 6mg adenosine IV with cardiac monitoring. The next steps would be to administer a further 12mg adenosine and then a further 12mg again. I would like to notify the registrar on-call to review and cardiology. I would hand the patient over using an SBAR technique and not leave the patient until a senior arrived'. ∎

04.3 PULMONARY EMBOLISM

INSTRUCTIONS You are a foundation year House Officer on the wards when the nursing staff ask you to see Mrs K, an 80-year-old with sudden onset shortness of breath and chest pain. Please examine and manage this acutely unwell patient in a structured manner.

STAGE	KEY POINTS AND ACTIONS		SCORE
	CANDIDATE	**EXAMINER RESPONSE**	
Danger	• Check around the bedside for potential hazards; e.g. spills, wires, blood.	'Safe to approach'.	0 1 –
Response	• Introduce yourself. Ask a simple question.	*'I feel breathless, my chest hurts'. Follow-up information: chest pain worst on inspiration, began one hour ago very suddenly, in hospital for elective hip replacement 2 days previously. Not on any anticoagulants.*	0 1 –
Airway	Recognise airway patency as patient is speaking.		0 1 –
Breathing			
Look	• Look for signs of respiratory distress. • Be able to state signs (*see* table above).	*'Looks unwell, respiratory distress, no lips or tongue swelling'.*	0 1 –
Feel	• Check chest expansion. • Percuss chest.	*'Chest expansion – equal, bilateral Percussion – resonant throughout No chest tenderness'.*	0 1 –
Listen	• Auscultate front and back.	*'No crackles, rubs or wheezes, good breath sounds throughout, bases clear'.*	0 1 –

STAGE	KEY POINTS AND ACTIONS		SCORE
Measure	• Respiratory rate • Saturations • Consider arterial blood gases • Chest x-ray	'*Respiratory rate – 40 Saturations – 83% in air (> 91% on 15L of oxygen) ABG results in air (if asked for) – pH 7.51 pCO2 1.8kPa PO2 6.8kPa Lac 1.2 Glu 6.6 BE 6 Bicarbonate 27 ABG results on 15L oxygen – pH 7.50 pCO2 1.9kPa PO2 7.5kPa Lac 1.0 Glu 6.2 BE 4 Bicarbonate 25 (Correct interpretation; severe type I respiratory failure with a respiratory alkalosis) CXR: NAD'.*	0 1 –
Treat	• Sit patient up. • High-flow oxygen via non-rebreathe. Administer treatment dose low-molecular weight heparin (if no contraindications, *see* below). • Arrange CT pulmonary angiogram to confirm diagnosis.		0 1 –
Re-assess	• State 'I would re-assess patient'.	'*Saturations improve to 91% on oxygen'.*	0 1 –
Circulation			
Look	• Peripherally: cap refill, cyanosis Centrally: conjunctival pallor, hydration status • JVP	'*Peripherally: cap refill < 2 seconds, warm and well perfused, no peripheral cyanosis Centrally: looks well, JVP 3-4cm'.*	0 1 –
Feel	• Peripheral pulses, apex beat	'*Peripheral pulses: Heart rate is 110 and regular, good volumes Apex: non-displaced'.*	0 1 –
Listen	• Auscultate heart.	'*Tachycardia no murmurs'.*	0 1 –
Measure	• Urine output • Temperature • Capillary refill • Heart rate and rhythm • Blood pressure	'*Urine output- 50mL/hr (patient weighs 55kg) Temperature – 36.6 C Capillary refill – as above Heart rate and rhythm – as above Blood pressure – 120/80 mmHg'.*	0 1 –
Treat	• Insert two wide-bore cannula in each anterior cubital fossa and send bloods: FBC, U&E, CRP • IV fluid challenge - 500mL crystalloid STAT • Ask for a 12-lead ECG.	If candidate asks for D-Dimer challenge them on when it is appropriate (*see* below). '*ECG- shows sinus tachycardia with narrow complexes rate 110'.*	0 1 –
Reassess	• State 'I would re-assess patient'.	*No change*	0 1 –
Diability			
Pupils	• Check that pupils are equal and reactive to light.	'*PEARL*'	0 1 –

STAGE	KEY POINTS AND ACTIONS		SCORE
GCS / AVPU	• Score the patient on the GCS or AVPU scale.	'GCS 15/15'	0 1 –
Capillary BM	• Ask for BM.	'BM 6.3'	0 1 –
Pain	• Ask if patient is in pain.	'Mild pain in chest'.	0 1 –
Treat	• Simple analgesia	*'Improves with paracetamol'.*	0 1 –
Exposure	Fully expose the patient and examine them from head to toe.		
	• State 'I would fully expose the patient and examine them from head to toe'.	*'Soft abdomen, good bowel sounds* *Right leg swollen, hip scar intact* *Right calf swollen, tense and painful'.*	
	STATE 'I WOULD SEEK SENIOR HELP AT APPROPRIATE TIME'.		0 1 –

AMPLE HISTORY

When able, use the mnemonic—AMPLE.
Allergies: *Penicillin allergy*
Medications: *Anastrazole, aspirin, lansoprazole*
Past medical history: *Breast cancer 5 years previously, right hip replacement 2 days previously, GORD*
Last meal: *Had lunch*
Events: *Started one hour ago, tender right calf for 1 day post-op*

MANAGEMENT

Acute PE in high-risk patient

No cardiovascular compromise;	Cardiovascular compromise;
High-flow oxygen Senior involvement Treatment dose low molecular weight heparin (typically given prior to radiological diagnosis if no contraindications) – dose by weight as per BNF Confirm diagnosis with CT Pulmonary angiogram	(decreased BP, right heart failure, cardiac arrest) Peri-arrest call Thrombolysis (if no contraindications)

EXAMINER'S EVALUATION

Overall assessment of pulmonary embolism management   0 1 2 3 4 5

Total mark out of 26

EXEMPLAR PRESENTATION

'Mrs K is an 80-year-old retired beekeeper presenting with a 60 minute history of breathlessness. She is awake and alert, but looks unwell and the airway is patent. Her lungs are clear, her respiratory rate is 40, and saturations were 83% in air, improving to only 91% on 15L oxygen via non-rebreathe mask. An ABG showed severe type I respiratory failure with a PaO2 of 7.4 on 15L and a corresponding respiratory alkalosis. Heart rate was 110 and systolic blood pressure was 120, the ECG showed a sinus tachycardia only. She showed no signs of cardiovascular compromise. BM is 6.6 and GCS is 15. On exposing the patient there was a swollen right leg with painful, tense, swollen calf. The surgical wound was intact. She has a history of breast cancer on anastrozole, takes aspirin and lansoprazole, and underwent elective hip replacement 2 days ago. The leading diagnosis is acute pulmonary embolism. The differential is spontaneous pneumothorax and acute myocardial infarction and angina. My immediate management would be to give high-flow oxygen, administer treatment dose low molecular weight heparin, and arrange an urgent CTPA. I would send bloods including troponin and U&E to check renal function prior to CTPA. I would like to notify the registrar on-call to review and handover the patient using an SBAR technique and not leave the patient until a senior arrived.' ■

Well's Score

The likelihood of pulmonary embolism can be scored using the Well's criteria for PE. (NOTE: there are separate scores for PE and for DVT.)

	No	Yes
Clinical signs and symptoms of DVT	0 points	3 points
PE is most likely diagnosis	0 points	3 points
Tachycardia (> 100 BPM)	0 points	1.5 points
Immobilization or surgery in the previous 4 weeks	0 points	1.5 points
Previously diagnosed DVT or PE	0 points	1.5 points
Hemoptysis	0 points	1 point
Active malignancy	0 points	1 point
Total	0-1 points	Low probability
	2-6 points	Intermediate probability
	>7 points	High probability

D-Dimer

The role of D-Dimer in the diagnosis of VTE is *only* to exclude a thrombus in patients at low risk. It has a good negative predictive value but no other utility. In the above scenario, a D-Dimer is not indicated, as she would score 10 points and therefore high probability.

04.4
SEPSIS

INSTRUCTIONS You are a foundation year House Officer in A&E when the nursing staff ask you to see Mr B next, a 62-year-old with raised temperatures. Please examine and manage this acutely unwell patient in a structured manner.

STAGE	KEY POINTS AND ACTIONS		SCORE
	SCORE SCHEME	**EXAMINER RESPONSE**	
Danger	• Check around the bedside for potential hazards; e.g. spills, wires, blood.	'Safe to approach'.	0 1 –
Response	• Introduce yourself. Ask a simple question.	*'I feel terrible doctor'. Follow-up information: feverish, no appetite, feels shivery. ONLY IF ASKED – some right flank pain and dysuria, no cough or breathlessness, no photophobia or headache*	0 1 –
Airway	• Recognise airway patency as patient is speaking.		0 1 –
Breathing			
Look	• Look for signs of respiratory distress. • Be able to state signs (*see* table above).	*'Looks unwell, pale, clammy'.*	0 1 –
Feel	• Check chest expansion. • Percuss chest.	*'Chest expansion – equal, bilateral Percussion – resonant throughout'.*	0 1 –
Listen	• Auscultate front and back.	*'No crackles, rubs or wheezes, good breath sounds throughout, bases clear'.*	0 1 –
Measure	• Respiratory rate • Saturations • Consider arterial blood gases • Consider chest x-ray if relevant	*'Respiratory rate – 26 Saturations – 98% in air ABG results (if asked for) – pH 7.33 pCO2 4.5kPa PO2 14.8kPa Lac 3.9 Glu 4.1 BE -2 Bicarbonate 21* **(Correct interpretation;** *mild metabolic acidosis secondary to a high lactate, borderline hypoglycaemia)* CXR: NAD'.*	0 1 –
Treat	• *Nil*		0 1 –
Re-assess	• State 'I would re-assess patient'.	*'No change'.*	0 1 –

STAGE	KEY POINTS AND ACTIONS		SCORE
Circulation			
Look	• Peripherally: cap refill, cyanosis; Centrally: conjunctival pallor, hydration status • JVP	*'Peripherally: cap refill 5 seconds, cool peripheries* **Centrally: looks well, JVP absent'.**	0 1 –
Feel	• Peripheral pulses, apex beat	*'Peripheral pulses: Heart rate is 119 and regular, weak pulses* *Apex: non-displaced'.*	0 1 –
Listen	• Auscultate heart.	**'Tachycardia no murmurs'.**	0 1 –
Measure	• Urine output • Temperature • Capillary refill • Heart rate and rhythm • Blood pressure	*'Urine output – 10mL/hr (patient weighs 100kg)* *Temperature – 38.6 C* *Capillary refill – as above* *Heart rate and rhythm – as above* *Blood pressure – 90/54 mmHg'.*	0 1 –
Treat	• Insert two wide-bore cannula in each anterior cubital fossa and send bloods: FBC, U&E, LFTs, CRP and 2 sets of blood cultures. • IV fluid challenge - 500mL crystalloid STAT. • Ask for a 12-lead ECG. • Request chest x-ray and urine dip.	*'ECG- shows sinus tachycardia with narrow complexes rate 119'.*	0 1 –
Reassess	• State 'I would re-assess patient'.	*'Blood pressure post-fluids 101/60mmHg'. Candidate should state they would continue fluid resuscitation.*	0 1 –
Diability			
Pupils	• Check that pupils are equal and reactive to light.	**'PEARL'**	0 1 –
GCS / AVPU	• Score the patient on the GCS or AVPU scale.	**'GCS 15/15'**	0 1 –
Capillary BM	• Ask for BM.	**'BM 4.1'**	0 1 –
Pain	• Ask if patient is in pain.	**'Patient is pain free'.**	0 1 –
Treat	Nil required		0 1 –
Exposure			
	• State 'I would fully expose the patient and examine them from head to toe'.	*'Right renal angle tenderness* *Cloudy urine* *Dip - 4+++ leuc 4+++ blood pos nitrites'.*	
	• STATE 'I WOULD SEEK SENIOR HELP AT APPROPRIATE TIME'.		0 1 –

STAGE	KEY POINTS AND ACTIONS	SCORE

AMPLE HISTORY

When able, use the mnemonic—AMPLE.
Allergies: *Penicillin allergy*
Medications: *Nil regular*
Past medical history: *Previously well*
Last meal: *Had lunch*
Events: *Fevers started 1 day ago, right flank pain and dysuria persisting for 2 days.*

MANAGEMENT

Sepsis

This patient is exhibiting the whole gamut of the systemic inflammatory response syndrome with a likely infectious source; this is the definition of sepsis (*see* below). Treatment should be immediate and appropriate, and is often bundled in A&E following the Surviving Sepsis campaign. The mnemonic [FLOCCA] is useful here.

Fluids: IV crystalloids in all resuscitation scenarios; if the patient responds continue aggressive fluids if no contraindications.
Lactate: ABG shows a lactate of 3.9, this is a marker of end-organ dysfunction and severe sepsis.
Oxygen: If appropriate.
Catheter: For oliguric patients, as in this case, but be careful in patients with already suspected urinary tract infections; discuss with a senior if just for fluid monitoring.
Cultures: As soon as possible, ideally > 2 sets at least 8-10mL of blood in each bottle. Underfilled blood culture bottles are the number one cause of blood culture negative sepsis. (Repeating the cultures again at 30-60 minutes will greatly increase the likelihood of making a culture diagnosis.)
Antibiotics: Mortality increases exponentially with every hour before initial antibiotic administration. Which antibiotic will depend on local policy and the patient's allergy status, but do not wait for the nurse to administer it; if there will be any delay give it yourself.

EXAMINER'S EVALUATION

Overall assessment of sepsis management	0 1 2 3 4 5

Total mark out of 26

EXEMPLAR PRESENTATION

'Mr B is a 62-year-old hydroelectric engineer presenting with a two-day history of fevers, right flank pain, and dysuria. He is awake and alert, but looks unwell. The airway is patent. The lungs are clear, the respiratory rate is 26 and the saturation is maintained in air. An ABG showed a lactic acidosis. The heart rate was 119 and the blood pressure is 90 systolic, with a cap refill of 5 seconds and a temperature of 38.6 C. Blood pressure improved to 101 systolic with 500mL crystalloid fluid challenge and I have started the patient on a fluid resuscitation regimen. GCS is 15, blood glucose is borderline low at 4.1, and I would like to repeat this measurement in due course. I have sent bloods for FBC, U&E, LFT, and CRP and taken a full septic screen including 2 sets of blood cultures with 10mL blood in each bottle, urine dip and MCS, and chest x-ray. He is previously well and has some right flank pain and dysuria. The diagnosis here is sepsis, most likely from a urinary source but my differential would include the chest as well. There were no skin rashes, boils, or visible abscesses, no meningism or photophobia to suggest another source. My initial management would be empirical antibiotic administration following local policy in a penicillin allergic patient as soon as possible, fluid resuscitation, oxygen as required, and catheterization if appropriate. Further investigations might include renal tract imaging. I would like to notify the registrar on-call to review, handover the patient using an SBAR technique, and not leave the patient until a senior arrived'. ■

SURVIVING SEPSIS

Definition

Systemic Inflammatory Response Syndrome (SIRS) Criteria (adapted from the Surviving Sepsis Guidelines)

Respiratory rate- >25 OR a PaCO2 <4.3kPa
Heart rate- >90
Temperature- >37.5 degrees or <36 C ('cool' sepsis)
WCC >10 or <4

Sepsis

SIRS + the suspected or proven presence of infection

Severe sepsis

The above + presence of end-organ dysfunction (abnormal clotting, thrombocytopenia, oliguria, hypoxemia, lactic acidosis)

Septic shock

The above + hypoperfusion of major organs persistent despite adequate fluid resuscitation

Mortality

Retrospective study data shows an estimated increase of approximately 8% for every hour delay in administration of antibiotics from the time of first presentation. To put that simply; a patient waiting for 1 hour has a 92% chance of survival, while someone waiting for 6 hours has only a 52% chance.

Treatment

Measure lactate, take cultures and administer antibiotics as soon as humanly possible.

Persistent hypotension requires vasopressors and CVP monitoring- this patient will require ITU input.

Further reading
www.survivingsepsis.org

04.5
HYPOGLYCAEMIA

INSTRUCTIONS You are a foundation year House Officer in A&E when the nursing staff ask you to see Ms Y next, a 22-year-old who has presented confused and agitated. Please examine and manage this acutely unwell patient in a structured manner.

STAGE	KEY POINTS AND ACTIONS		SCORE
	CANDIDATE	**EXAMINER RESPONSE**	
Danger	• Check around the bedside for potential hazards; e.g. spills, wires, blood.	'Safe to approach'.	0 1 –
Response	• Introduce yourself. Ask a simple question.	*'"Groaning and confused" Follow-up information – patient will not communicate further'.*	0 1 –
Airway	Recognise airway patency as patient is speaking.		0 1 –
Look	• Look for signs of airway obstruction. • Be able to state them.	'No abnormality'.	0 1 –
Listen	• Listen for gargling or snoring obstructive sounds. • Look in the mouth.	*'Speaking in complete sentences No upper airway noises Responds to voice'.*	0 1 –
Treat	*Nil required*		0 1 –
Breathing			
Look	• Look for signs of respiratory distress. • Be able to state signs (*see* table above).	*'Looks unwell, pale, clammy'.*	0 1 –
Feel	• Check chest expansion. • Percuss chest.	*'Chest expansion – equal, bilateral Percussion – resonant throughout No chest tenderness'.*	0 1 –
Listen	• Auscultate front and back.	*'No crackles, rubs or wheezes, good breath sounds throughout, bases clear'.*	0 1 –

STAGE	KEY POINTS AND ACTIONS		SCORE
Measure	• Respiratory rate • Saturations • Consider arterial blood gases • Chest x-ray	'Respiratory rate – 12 Saturations – 98% in air ABG results (if asked for) – pH 7.39 pCO2 4.5kPa PO2 16.8kPa Lac 0.1 Glu 1.9 BE 2 Bicarbonate 28 **(Correct interpretation**; normal acid-base, hypoglycaemia CXR: NAD)'.	0 1 –
Treat	• Mention oral glucose.		0 1 –
Re-assess	• State 'I would re-assess patient'.	**'BM 4.0 after oral sugar and biscuit'.**	0 1 –
Circulation			
Look	• Peripherally: cap refill, cyanosis; Centrally: conjunctival pallor, hydration status • JVP	'Peripherally: cap refill < 2 seconds, warm peripheries Centrally: looks unwell, JVP not raised'.	0 1 –
Feel	• Peripheral pulses, apex beat	'Peripheral pulses: Heart rate is 83 and regular, good volume Apex: non-displaced'.	0 1 –
Listen	• Auscultate heart.	**'Normal auscultation'.**	0 1 –
Measure	• Urine output • Temperature • Capillary refill • Heart rate and rhythm • Blood pressure	'Urine output – 30ml/hr (patient weighs 48kg) Temperature – 35.6 C Capillary refill – as above Heart rate and rhythm – as above Blood pressure – 109/54 mmHg'.	0 1 –
Treat	Insert two wide-bore cannula in each anterior cubital fossa and send bloods – FBC, U&E, LFTs, CRP and two sets of blood cultures. • Fluid challenge – not indicated • Mention IV glucose bolus +/- IM glucagon.	'ECG – normal sinus rhythm'.	0 1 –
Reassess	• State 'I would re-assess patient'.	'BM increases to 4.0 with 20% glucose bolus (if not given oral glucose already)'.	0 1 –
Diability			
Pupils	• Check that pupils are equal and reactive to light.	'PEARL'	0 1 –
GCS / AVPU	• Score the patient on the GCS or AVPU scale.	'GCS 14/15 -Motor – obeys commands -Voice – confused speech -Eyes – open and alert'.	0 1 –
Capillary BM	• Ask for BM.	'Glucose 2.0'.	0 1 –
Pain	• Ask if patient is in pain.	'Mild pain in chest'.	0 1 –

STAGE	KEY POINTS AND ACTIONS		SCORE
Treat	Correct hypoglycaemia – 1. Oral glucose (e.g. Hypostop). 2. Mention sugary drink and biscuit. 3. If IV access in-100mL bolus of 20% glucose (give thiamine IV first if any suspicion of alcoholism or malnutrition). Glucagon can also be given.	'BM improves to 4.2 after further administration of oral glucose'.	0 1 –
Exposure	Fully expose the patient and examine them from head to toe.		
	• State 'I would fully expose the patient and examine them from head to toe'.	*'Multiple injection sites at single area above the right iliac fossa* *Low BMI'.*	
	STATE 'I WOULD SEEK SENIOR HELP AT APPROPRIATE TIME.		0 1 –

AMPLE HISTORY

Not available from patient

MANAGEMENT

Hypoglycaemia

The protocol will vary where you are and on the individual patient but the overriding message is to recognise hypoglycaemia in any unwell patient early and promptly get glucose into them, by whatever means possible.

If patient is awake and able to take oral medications:

1. Oral glucose load; e.g. sugar lumps, biscuits, or sugary drinks/fruit juice
2. Oral glucose gel; e.g. Hypostop or GlucoGel

If obtunded, seizing, or unconscious:

1. Consider airway at all times.
2. IV access – 80-100mL of 20% glucose stat.
3. IM Glucagon 1mg.
4. Repeat IV glucose if no improvement; set up a glucose infusion if persistent hypoglycaemia.
5. Get expert help; ITU may be required for central line treatment, reversal of overdoses and treatment of cerebral oedema (mannitol and dexamethasone).

Useful points

-Diabetic patients with frequent hypoglycaemia episodes get increasingly acclimatized to low blood sugars; whenever you see a patient with any history of hypoglycaemia ask them at what blood glucose level do they begin to get symptomatic. Frequent hypos will result in patients being asymptomatic at blood glucose levels of < 2; these are the patients at highest risk of fatal complications such as seizures and cerebral injury as they will have no pre-warning the blood glucose is already low before it is too late.
-Always check the injection site and technique of insulin-dependant patients. Accidental overdose can occur if injecting in a site of lipohypertrophy or into a very low fat area especially in very thin patients; insulin is absorbed too rapidly and hypoglycaemia can occur as a result.

STAGE	KEY POINTS AND ACTIONS	SCORE

-Hypoglycaemia occurs in other contexts; alcoholism is an important one. Any patient at risk of thiamine deficiency—conditions including alcoholism, malnutrition, anorexia nervosa and bulimia—should be given thiamine prior to correcting the blood glucose. Acute treatment with glucose can precipitate or worsen Wernicke's encephalopathy; pre-treat with thiamine to prevent this.

-In patients presenting with hypoglycaemia who are not on insulin, testing the C-Peptide level in the blood can be useful. This will be raised in patients with endogenous insulin overproduction (very rare; e.g. insulinoma) but will be absent in factitious hypoglycaemia; e.g. deliberate overdose of insulin.

Further reading
http://pathways.nice.org.uk/pathways/diabetes#path=view%3A/pathways/diabetes/managing-type-1-diabetes-in-adults.xml&content=view-node%3Anodes-managing-hypoglycaemia

---

EXAMINER'S EVALUATION

Overall assessment of hypoglycaemia management

0 1 2 3 4 5

Total mark out of 29

EXEMPLAR PRESENTATION

'Ms Y is a 22-year-old lighting technician presenting to A&E with confusion and agitation. We were unable to get any other history from the patient. She looked unwell, alert but confused with a GCS of 14/15. The airway was not compromised. The lungs were clear, respiratory rate was 12, and saturations were 98% in air. The heart rate was 83 and blood pressure 109 systolic. Urine output was in the normal range for her weight, which was 48kg. Her blood sugar on capillary testing was 2.0; this was confirmed on the ABG at 1.9. On examination of the abdomen there were multiple injection sites and an area of lipohypertrophy consistent with long-term insulin use, with poor rotation of injection sites. Her BMI was also notably low. As she was co-operative oral glucose was administered with 100mL of fruit juice and three sugar cubes. Repeat blood glucose was 4.2. The diagnosis here is hypoglycaemia, most likely secondary to accidental insulin overdose, although the differential must include deliberate overdose. I would like to monitor her blood glucose over the next four hours. Should she require further treatment, a glucose infusion would be useful, 100mL/hr of 10% glucose with 30-60 minute BMs would be appropriate. I would also like to take a full history, discuss injection site and medication use technique, and explore any risk factors for deliberate overdose. I would like to notify the registrar on-call to review, handover the patient using an SBAR technique, and not leave the patient until a senior arrived. Should the patient deteriorate I would discuss her urgently with ITU'. ∎

04.6 DKA

INSTRUCTIONS You are a foundation year House Officer in A&E when the nursing staff ask you to see Mr Y next, a 23-year-old who has presented confused and drowsy. Please examine and manage this acutely unwell patient in a structured manner.

STAGE	KEY POINTS AND ACTIONS		SCORE
	CANDIDATE	**EXAMINER RESPONSE**	
Danger	• Check around the bedside for potential hazards; e.g. spills, wires, blood.	'Safe to approach'.	0 1 –
Response	• Introduce yourself. Ask a simple question.	*'"Groaning and confused" Follow-up information – patient will not communicate further'.*	0 1 –
Airway	Recognise airway patency as patient is speaking.		0 1 –
Look	• Look for signs of airway obstruction. • Be able to state them.	*'No obvious abnormality Responding to voice Nothing obvious in the mouth'.*	0 1 –
Listen	• Listen for gargling or snoring obstructive sounds. • Look in the mouth.	*'Some upper airway noises, occasional snores'.*	0 1 –
Treat	*Get help.* *Head-tilt chin-lift.* *Attempt airway adjunct; e.g. nasopharyngeal airway.* *Place in recovery position.*	*'Patient comfortable Airway now secured with nasopharyngeal airway'.*	0 1 –
Breathing			
Look	• Look for signs of respiratory distress. • Be able to state signs (*see* table above).	*'Looks drowsy and unwell'.*	0 1 –
Feel	• Check chest expansion. • Percuss chest.	*'Decreased chest expansion right sided – deep inspiratory efforts Dull to percussion at the right base'.*	0 1 –
Listen	• Auscultate front and back.	*'Auscultate – decreased breath sounds with bronchial breathing and crackles at the right base'.*	0 1 –

STAGE	KEY POINTS AND ACTIONS		SCORE
Measure	• Respiratory rate • Saturations • Consider arterial blood gases • Chest x-ray	*'Respiratory rate – 32 – very deep Saturations – 100% in air ABG results (if asked for) – pH 7.21 pCO2 2.0kPa PO2 18.8kPa Lac 1.2 Glu 48 BE -16 Bicarbonate 11 **(Correct interpretation**; severe metabolic acidosis, hyperglycaemia CXR: Right lower lobe consolidation)'.*	0 1 –
Treat	*Administer oxygen* • *Treat as DKA if diagnosed at this stage (see below) and ensure senior help.*		0 1 –
Re-assess	• State 'I would re-assess patient'.	*'Re-assess patient – no change with oxygen'.*	0 1 –
Circulation			
Look	• Peripherally: cap refill, cyanosis Centrally: conjunctival pallor, hydration status • JVP	*'Peripherally: cap refill 2-3 seconds, cool peripheries Centrally: looks unwell, JVP absent, dry mucous membranes'.*	0 1 –
Feel	• Peripheral temperatures, apex beat	*'Peripheral pulses: Heart rate is 122 and regular, thready volumes Apex: non-displaced'.*	0 1 –
Listen	• Auscultate heart	***'Normal auscultation'.***	0 1 –
Measure	• Urine output • Temperature • Capillary refill • Heart rate and rhythm • Blood pressure	*'Urine output – 2mL/hr (patient weighs 88kg) Temperature – 38.6 C Capillary refill – as above Heart rate and rhythm – as above Blood pressure – 92/54 mmHg'.*	0 1 –
Treat	*Insert two wide-bore cannula in each anterior cubital fossa and send bloods – FBC, U&E, LFTs, CRP, glucose, and two sets of blood cultures. Fluid challenge - give stat 1000mL of normal saline over 20 minutes. Then follow DKA protocol (if diagnosis made at this point) see below.* • *Community acquired pneumonia antibiotics regimen following allergy status and local guidelines.*	*'ECG – normal sinus rhythm'.*	0 1 –
Reassess	• State 'I would re-assess patient'.	*'BP increases to 109 systolic after fluid challenge, HR to 100; should state would continue IV fluid therapy'.*	0 1 –
Diability			
Pupils	• Check that pupils are equal and reactive to light.	'PEARL'	0 1 –

STAGE	KEY POINTS AND ACTIONS		SCORE
GCS / AVPU	• Score the patient on the GCS or AVPU scale.	'GCS 11/15 - Motor – localizes to pain - 5 -Voice – inappropriate speech - 3 -Eyes – responds to voice - 3'.	0 1 –
Capillary BM	• Ask for BM.	'Glucose - +++ unreadable on BM ABG- 49 Ketones 5.1mmol/L (if asked for) or ++++ on urine dip'.	0 1 –
Pain	• Ask if patient is in pain.	'Pain free'.	0 1 –
Treat	*See below*		0 1 –
Re-assess	• State 'I would re-assess patient'.	'Repeat ABG at 2 hours after fluids and insulin infusion shows *pH 7.26 pCO2 3.1kPa PO2 18.8kPa Lac 0.5 Glu 41 BE -10.3 Bicarbonate 16'.	0 1 –
Exposure	Fully expose the patient and examine them from head to toe.		
	• State 'I would fully expose the patient and examine them from head to toe'.	'Multiple injection sites around abdomen'.	
	STATE 'I WOULD SEEK SENIOR HELP AT APPROPRIATE TIME'.		0 1 –

AMPLE HISTORY

Not available from patient

MANAGEMENT

Diabetic Ketoacidosis
The situation is complex as there are two required treatments here. The first is a right basal pneumonia which will require antibiotic therapy in line with local guidelines; in this context IV antibiotics are indicated.
The second is the diagnosis of diabetic ketoacidosis based on the triad of raised ketones, acidosis, and hyperglycaemia. This can be present in previously undiagnosed diabetics, known insulin-dependant diabetes mellitus and, uncommonly, in non-insulin dependant diabetes mellitus. There is usually a precipitant—in this case a community acquired pneumonia.

Acute treatment is three-fold in the following order of priority:

1. Rehydration – Aggressive fluid resuscitation following local protocol, –usually a bolus of 500mL-1000mL of normal saline and then a progressively spaced regime; e.g. 1L over 1 hours, 2 hours, then 4 hours, then 8 hours, etc. This will vary with individual departments.

2. Hyperglycaemia – Treat with a fixed rate insulin infusion depending on the patient's weight and their subsequent response. Again, the rate and administration will vary with individual departments; check the local protocol. Aim to reduce blood glucose no more than 3mmol/hour – this is to avoid precipitating cerebral oedema.

3. Hypokalaemia – The patient will be total body potassium deplete, despite initial potassium being intravascularly normal or even high. Once insulin is administered this will rapidly fall as potassium is driven back into cells with co-transport of glucose. Potassium should begin to be replaced early on in treatment.

STAGE	KEY POINTS AND ACTIONS	SCORE

These patients are also particularly susceptible to venous thromboembolism and require prophylactic low-molecular weight heparin and anti-thromboembolic stockings.

In severe disease an HDU/ITU based setting may be appropriate; early senior review and ITU involvement is essential.

Once they are recovered (normal bicarbonate, ketones < 0.1) they will require regular insulin and education. They can switch to subcutaneous insulin once background insulin has been established (e.g. Lantus) and they are eating and drinking with biochemical recovery. Make sure they know about 'sick day' rules for taking insulin, have a good injection technique, and understand how to monitor their BMs during illness. They might need a regime change; make sure their GP is involved in the discharge. This is an entirely treatable but potentially fatal condition; handle these patients with care, and get senior help ASAP.

Further reading
http://guidance.nice.org.uk/CG15/Guidance

EXAMINER'S EVALUATION

Overall assessment of diabetic ketoacidosis management

0   1   2   3   4   5

Total mark out of 30

EXEMPLAR PRESENTATION

'Mr Y is a 23-year-old kite-surfing instructor presenting to A&E with confusion and drowsiness. We were unable to get any other further history from the patient. He looked unwell, responding to voice only. He was making some upper airway obstructive noises, so was placed in the recovery position and a nasopharyngeal airway placed that was tolerated. There were crackles and bronchial breathing with reduced breath sounds and expansion at the right base; saturations were maintained at 100% in air but the respiratory rate was 35 with deep inspirations in a Kussmaul breathing pattern. Oxygen was applied and an ABG showed a pH of 7.2 with a PCO2 of 2.1 and PAO2 of 18, glucose of 49 and BE -10 with a bicarbonate of 11. A CXR showed a right basal pneumonia. The diagnosis is diabetic ketoacidosis, likely secondary to a right lower lobe pneumonia. Capillary refill was 2-3 seconds and BP was 90 systolic with a heart of 123, urine output was only 2mL/hour and he was febrile. I have taken bloods for FBC, U&E, VBG for glucose, CRP, and two sets of blood cultures. After a 1000mL fluid challenge of 0.9% normal saline, blood pressure improved to 109 systolic and heart rate to 100. BM was unreadable at the bedside and ketonuria was 4+ with bedside capillary ketones measured at 5.1. GCS is currently 11 – localizing to pain, inappropriate speech, and eyes opening to voice. I have started this patient on the DKA protocol – set up a fixed rate insulin infusion based on the patient's weight and continuing aggressive fluid resuscitation with potassium replacement. I have also started IV antibiotics for severe community acquired pneumonia; this will need review at 48 hours. I would like to notify the registrar on-call to review urgently, handover the patient using an SBAR technique, and not leave the patient until a senior arrived. I would also like to discuss the patient with HDU'. ∎

04.7
UPPER GI BLEED

INSTRUCTIONS You are a foundation year House Officer on the ward when the ward staff ask you to see Mr C, a 72-year-old, who has been having coffee-ground vomits for the past 2 hours.

STAGE	KEY POINTS AND ACTIONS		SCORE
	CANDIDATE	**EXAMINER RESPONSE**	
Danger	• Check around the bedside for potential hazards; e.g. spills, wires, blood.	'Safe to approach'.	0 1 –
Response	• Introduce yourself. Ask a simple question.	*'I feel terrible doctor'.* *Follow-up information: vomited 6x in the last 2 hours, some fresh blood on first vomit and coffee-grounds since, epigastric pain, admitted for elective knee replacement, takes 1200mg Ibuprofen a day and drinks heavily.*	0 1 –
Airway	Recognise airway patency as patient is speaking.		0 1 –
Breathing			
Look	• Look for signs of respiratory distress. • Be able to state signs (*see* table above).	*'Looks unwell and pale Slightly tachypneoic'.*	0 1 –
Feel	• Check chest expansion. • Percuss chest.	*'Normal chest expansion Resonant to percussion'.*	0 1 –
Listen	• Auscultate front and back.	*'Auscultate – normal breath sounds, no crackles, rubs or wheeze'.*	0 1 –
Measure	• Respiratory rate • Saturations • Consider arterial blood gases • Chest x-ray	*'Respiratory rate – 40 Saturations – 100% in air ABG results (if asked for) – pH 7.36 pCO2 2.0 kPa PO2 18.8kPa Lac 0.2 Glu 5 BE 4 Bicarbonate 27 Hb 7.4* **(Correct interpretation**; *normal ABG, anaemic)* *erect CXR: (if asked for) free air under both diaphragms'.*	0 1 –
Treat	*Administer oxygen.*		0 1

STAGE	KEY POINTS AND ACTIONS		SCORE		
Re-assess	• State 'I would re-assess patient'.	'Re-assess patient – no change with oxygen'.	0	1	–
Circulation					
Look	• Peripherally: cap refill, cyanosis Centrally: conjunctival pallor, hydration status • JVP	'Peripherally: cap refill 4 seconds, cool peripheries Centrally: looks unwell, JVP absent, dry mucous membranes'.	0	1	–
Feel	• Peripheral pulses, apex beat	'Peripheral pulses: Heart rate is 135 and regular, thready volume Apex: non-displaced'.	0	1	–
Listen	• Auscultate heart.	**'Normal auscultation'.**	0	1	–
Measure	• Urine output • Temperature • Capillary refill • Heart rate and rhythm • Blood pressure	'Urine output – 10mL/hr (patient weighs 78kg) Temperature – 37.4 C Capillary refill – as above Heart rate and rhythm – as above Blood pressure – 89/54 mmHg'.	0	1	–
Treat	*Insert two wide-bore cannula in each anterior cubital fossa and send bloods – FBC, U&E, LFTs, CRP, glucose, and cross match 4 units.* *Fluid challenge: give 500mL of 0.9% normal saline STAT.* • *Upper GI bleed management; see below.*	ECG: sinus tachycardia	0	1	–
Reassess	• State 'I would re-assess patient'.	'BP increases to 112 systolic after fluid challenge, HR to 123; continue IV fluids'.	0	1	–
Diability					
Pupils	• Check that pupils are equal and reactive to light.	'PEARL'.	0	1	–
GCS / AVPU	• Score the patient on the GCS or AVPU scale.	'GCS 15/15'.	0	1	–
Capillary BM	• Ask for BM.	'5'.	0	1	–
Pain	• Ask if patient is in pain.	'Pain free'.	0	1	–
Treat	*See below*		0	1	–
Exposure	Fully expose the patient and examine them from head to toe.				
	• State 'I would fully expose the patient and examine them from head to toe'.	'Very tender epigastrically Rigid abdomen with guarding above umbilicus'.			

STAGE	KEY POINTS AND ACTIONS	SCOR
	STATE 'I WOULD SEEK SENIOR HELP AT APPROPRIATE TIME'.	0 1

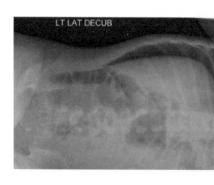

Fig 4.1 Left lateral decubitus film

Source: Tristan Barrett, Nadeem Shaida, and Ashley Shaw. *Radiology for Undergraduate Finals and Foundation Years.* London: Radcliffe Publishing; 2010.

AMPLE HISTORY

Allergies: No allergies
Medications: 400mg ibuprofen TDS, heavy alcohol intake
Past medical history: ETOH excess, knee osteoarthritis
Last meal: Ate breakfast 4 hours ago
Events: Vomiting began for 2 hours, pre-operative admission for elective knee replacement, fresh blood then coffee-ground vomiting, epigastric pain, bowels not open today

MANAGEMENT

There are three elements of the history to pick up on: 1) the epigastric pain and coffee ground vomiting suggests a UGI bleed; 2) the ABG shows an Hb of 7.4—this is a severe haemorrhage requiring transfusion; 3) the erect chest x-ray showed free-air under the diaphragm—this is evidence of a perforated abdominal viscus.

The differential for pneumoperitoneum is:
-Perforated diverticulae
-Perforated small or large bowel (unusual, unless related to malignancy)
-Perforated gallbladder
-Abdominal trauma or recent surgery (including laparoscopic)

Additionally, the patient is on ibuprofen 1200mg a day, which is a significant risk factor for duodenal or gastric ulceration and subsequent perforation.

Treatment for non-variceal upper GI bleeding
-Fluid resuscitate the patient, apply oxygen, monitor their blood pressure closely.
-Consider the airway if the patient becomes obtunded.
-Think about possible causes of the bleed—duodenal or gastric ulcers, gastritis, Mallory-Weiss tear, oesophageal or gastric variceal bleeding.
-Reverse any reversible coagulopathy; e.g. patients on warfarin.
-Involve gastroenterology early for urgent endoscopy.

-For perforation get an immediate surgical opinion and senior help.
-Crossmatch 4-6 units of blood and make the patient nil-by-mouth.

STAGE	KEY POINTS AND ACTIONS	SCORE

NB: Treatment for variceal UGI bleeds
-Fluid resuscitate, apply oxygen and monitor blood pressure.
-IV terlipressin in the acute setting.
-Prophylactic antibiotics are shown to reduce mortality from variceal bleeding and are recommended by NICE.
-Reverse any reversible coagulopathy; e.g. Vitamin K in liver cirrhosis—if patient is thrombocytopenic (< 50) consider transfusing platelets. This patient may need clotting factor replacement as well. Many hospitals have a Massive Transfusion Protocol; check locally the best way to sort this out quickly.
-Get urgent gastroenterology input for immediate endoscopy.
-IV PPIs are not recommended pre-endoscopy although this is controversial—consult your local hospital policy.

Further reading;
http://www.nice.org.uk/nicemedia/live/13762/59549/59549.pdf

EXAMINER'S EVALUATION

Overall assessment of upper GI bleed management	0 1 2 3 4 5

Total mark out of 26

EXEMPLAR PRESENTATION

'Mr C is a 73-year-old retired paratrooper admitted for an elective knee replacement, now presenting with a two-hour history of coffee-ground vomiting. He takes 1200mg ibuprofen daily and is a heavy drinker. He looked unwell, pale, and tachypnoeic. Airway was patent and GCS was 15/15. Lungs were clear, and saturations were maintained at 98% in room air with a respiratory rate of 38. Oxygen was applied. The capillary refill was 5 seconds and the patient was cool peripherally. The blood pressure was 89 systolic with a heart rate of 133. An ECG showed a sinus tachycardia. There was no active bleeding at the time. Two wide-bore cannulae were inserted into both anterior cubital fossae and blood was taken for FBC, U&E, CRP, and X-Match for 4 units. An ABG showed an Hb of 7.6 and an erect chest x-ray showed free-air under the diaphragm. A fluid challenge of 500mL crystalloid STAT was administered and blood pressure improved to 112 systolic. IV fluids are on-going. BM was 5 and GCS remained 15. On examining the patient from head-to-toe I found a tender epigastrium, with guarding and rigidity. In the context of the x-ray findings and clinical findings the leading diagnosis is a perforated duodenal or gastric ulcer, with a differential of other perforated viscus and variceal bleeding. I would like to transfuse the patient 2-4 units of packed red cells, continue IV resuscitation, and keep them nil-by-mouth. I would like to notify the surgical registrar on-call to review immediately, handover the patient using an SBAR technique, and not leave the patient until a senior arrived. I would also discuss the patient with my senior and involve HDU should this become appropriate'. ∎

UPPER GI BLEEDING

Rockall scoring system

Pre-endoscopy (Blatchford score)	Score
Age	< 60 – 0 points
	60-79 – 1 point
	> 80 – 2 points
Blood pressure/pulse	Systolic BP > 100, pulse < 100 – 0 points
	Systolic BP > 100, pulse > 100 – 1 point
	Systolic BP < 100 – 2 points
Co-morbidities	No major co-morbidity – 0 points
	Cardiac failure, IHD, or any major co-morbidity – 2 points
	Renal or liver failure, disseminated malignancy – 3 points
	Any score > 1 should be for endoscopy, > 4 to HDU
Post-endoscopy (Full Rockall)	
Diagnosis	Mallory-Weiss tear or no lesion – 0 points
	All other diagnoses – 1 point
	Malignancy of upper GI tract – 2 points
Evidence of bleed	None or dark spot only – 0 points
	Visible blood or active bleeding – 2 points

NICE Guideline: Acute UGI Bleed June 2012

section **05**

PRESCRIBING

05.1 GENERAL TIPS

NOTE: Medical pharmacology is constantly being updated and treatment protocols differ from hospital to hospital. The information provided here is only a guide. You should make every effort to check the local guidance for your medical school.

GENERAL TIPS

Prescribing is a vital skill. In many ways the entire medical school curriculum and qualification is designed to ensure you have the ability to safely prescribe medications.

General Rules for Prescribing

1. **ALWAYS** fill out the patient's name, date of birth, and hospital number. The patient's weight, where known, is often very useful.
2. **ALWAYS** document **ALLERGIES** – record what the drug is, what the reaction was, the source of this information (e.g. patient, notes) and sign and date this recording. Specifically document Anaphylaxis like this.

*PENICILLIN ALLERGY ** ANAPHYLAXIS** FROM PATIENT Signed 6/6/14*

3. Different drug charts have different areas for particular drug types or situations; this varies slightly from hospital to hospital but generally they are laid out similarly to the Sample Drug Chart at the end of the chapter.
   a. The 'ONCE ONLY & PREMEDICATION DRUGS' or 'STAT' side is usually on the front and is for drugs to be given as a one-off, usually immediately. This is for prescribing in emergencies; e.g. morphine and aspirin in acute myocardial infarction.
   b. The 'REGULAR PRESCRIPTIONS' area is for medications to be given at regular intervals; this can be weekly, daily, twice daily, etc.
   c. The 'AS REQUIRED PRESCRIPTIONS' or 'PRN' side is for any medication you wish the patient to have only when needed; e.g. analgesia, anti-emetics. Nursing staff can administer these when indicated as long as they are prescribed. Always document the indication; e.g. cyclizine, 50mg TDS, IV/IM/PO, *For Nausea.*
   d. The 'INTRAVENOUS & SUBCUTANEOUS INFUSIONS' section is usually on the back and is for prescribing fluids and other infusion medication; e.g. insulin sliding scale.
   e. Other sections – some drug charts may have extra areas for the following:
      i. Oxygen – this is a drug and should be prescribed for any patient on oxygen, indicating the target saturations and method for oxygen delivery.
      ii. Drug history – this is usually filled out by the pharmacist after consolidating the medications with GP and patient on admission.
      iii. Nebuliser therapy.
      iv. Sliding scales – sometimes these are pre-written and just require your signature and circling the appropriate regimen.
      v. Infusions – sometimes these are separate from the IV side.

. **ALWAYS** write the following for every prescription:

   a. The drug name.

   b. The drug dose.

   c. The route of administration.

   d. The time interval – e.g. STAT, once a day (OD), weekly and the time of day to be given; e.g. TDS 0800, 1400, 2200.

   e. The start date.

   f. Your signature.

   g. Your full name (PRINTED).

   h. Your bleep or other contact number.

   i. For antibiotics or any medication where it is not clear you should document the Indication as well.

. **ALWAYS** write legibly.

. **ALWAYS** check any dose you are not certain of with local policy or the BNF (most hospitals offer free smartphone access for the BNF nowadays). This includes when a senior tells you the dose; if it's your signature it's your responsibility that the dose is correct, no one else's. If you aren't comfortable **DON'T PRESCRIBE IT.**

. When stopping a drug cross through the entire box including the administration record clearly and sign and date the line and reason for stopping. Like so:

Amoxicillin 500mg TDS PO
Signed   `End of course`
~~*Dr A Bu̶p 4309*~~   *1/6/14*   /   /   /   `Signed 6/6/14`

. Use standard acronyms only (*see* chart).

. Use generic drug names where possible.

0. For complicated prescriptions; e.g. weight-based prescribing, it is good practice to write out the calculations as well as the dose; e.g. Gentamicin 5mg/kg – 300mg OD IV.

1. The drug chart is not a legal document; if you think it would be clearer to write additional instructions anywhere on the chart then that is perfectly admissible.

2. It is also permissible to write a range of doses where appropriate for nursing staff to decide; e.g. codeine 30-60mg QDS PO.

3. Document on the front of the drug chart any useful information for prescribing; e.g. renal failure, liver failure, heart failure, etc.

4. **DO NOT** write 'U' instead of UNITS. This is to avoid misinterpretation of U as an additional 0 and the dose being read as x10 the required; e.g. 12U can be read as *120*

5. **DO NOT** write '.5' instead of '0.5'. This is to avoid misinterpretation of .5 as 5. Better yet, write 0.5g as 500mg to avoid confusion entirely.

Accepted prescribing acronyms

ACRONYM	MEANING
PO	Per oral – oral medication
IM	Intramuscular
IV	Intravenous
NEB	Nebulised
INH	Inhaled
TOP	Topical
2°	2 hourly (It is clearer to write hourly however)
OD	Once daily
BD	Twice daily
TDS	Three times a day
QDS	Four times a day
MICROG	Micrograms
MG	Milligrams
G	Grams
PRN	'Pro re nata' (for what is born) – as required

05.2
GI BLEED

INSTRUCTIONS You are a foundation year House Officer on the ward when the ward staff ask you to see Mr C, a 72-year-old man who has been having coffee-ground vomits for the past 2 hours. He looks unwell, pale, and tachypnoeic. His BP is 89/50 and his heart rate is 133. He is tender over the epigastrium and melaena is noted PR. His repeat prescription is provided. He is allergic to penicillin. Complete his inpatient drug chart using information from the repeat prescription provided, and administer appropriate acute treatment. There is no patient in this scenario.

NOTE: Medical pharmacology is constantly being updated and treatment protocols differ from hospital to hospital. The information provided here is only a guide. You should make every effort to contact a specialist at your medical school or further guidance to treatments and dosages.

Mr C, DOB 11/5/42, Hospital no. 758473
Ibuprofen 400mg TDS
Ramipril 5mg OD

STAGE	KEY POINTS AND ACTIONS	SCORE		
	DRUG CHART LABEL			
Name	Complete forename and surname clearly.	0	1	–
DoB	Fill out patient's date of birth.	0	1	–
Hospital No.	Complete patient's hospital number.	0	1	–
Allergy	Circle appropriate – YES – box for allergy and record correct allergy.	0	1	2
	ACUTE MEDICAL MANAGEMENT			
STAT Fluids	Correctly prescribe a stat dose of IV 0.9% normal saline 500mL.	0	1	2
Anti-emetic	Prescribe an appropriate stat dose of IV anti-emetic; i.e. cyclizine 50mg IV/IM.	0	1	2

STAGE	KEY POINTS AND ACTIONS	SCORE

CONTINUING MEDICAL MANAGEMENT

Ibuprofen	Stop ibuprofen.	0	1	–
Ramipril	Hold ramipril (as low BP).	0	1	–
Fluids	Write up one bag of 0.9% normal saline 1000mL with 20mmol/L potassium chloride over 4 hours.	0	1	2
5% Dextrose	Write up two successive bags of 5% dextrose 1000mL with KCL 20mmol/L over 6 hours (or any equivalent regime). (Allow leeway for not knowing the response to the fluid challenge; any combination of bolus plus ongoing fluids is acceptable.)	0	1	2

AS REQUIRED MEDICINES

Anti-Emetic	Correctly prescribe IV/IM cyclizine TDS.	0	1	–
Analgesia	Prescribe alternative analgesia PRN; i.e. IV morphine 2.5mg, PO codeine 30mg.	0	1	–

GENERAL PRESCRIBING

Writing	Complete all sections clearly, legibly, and in black ink.	0	1	–
Admission	Record all the patient's drugs on admission in relevant section.	0	1	–
Generic	Prescribe generic drugs and avoid the use of brand names. Avoid any of the DO NOTs listed in 5.1 General Tips. Avoid giving PPIs pre-endoscopy as per NICE guidance; consult local policy.	0	1	–

EXAMINER'S EVALUATION

Overall assessment of prescribing in acute GI bleed	0	1	2	3	4	5

Total mark out of 25

St. Somewhere or Another Hospital Trust
Drug Prescription and Administration

WARD – *RADCLIFFE WARD*
HOSPITAL NO. - *758473*
SURNAME - *C*
FIRST NAME- *MR*
DOB – *11/5/42*

CONSULTANT – *MR SO AND SO*
HOUSE OFFICER – *DR PIMENTA*
BLEEP- *1202*
DATE OF ADMISSION- *1/6/14*

DRUG ALLERGIES

YES/~~NO~~/~~NOT KNOWN~~
DRUGS:*PENICILLIN*   REACTION: *RASH*

DATED: *1/6/14*
SIGNED: DP

Once only & Premedication drugs								
DATE	DRUG	DOSE	TIME	ROUTE	DRS SIGNATURE	TIME GIVEN	GIVEN BY	PHARMACY
1/6/14	*CYCLIZINE*	*50MG*	*15:00*	*IV/IM*	DP			

REGULAR PRESCRIPTIONS

ADMINISTRATION RECORD

DRUG Ibuprofen	DOSE 400mg	ROUTE PO
DATE 1/6/14	BLP 1001	SIGNATURE DP

	1/6	2/6	3/6	4/6	5/6	6/6	7/6	8/6
0800	DO							
1200								
1800								
0000								

DRUG Ramipril	DOSE 5mg	ROUTE PO
DATE 1/6/14	BLP 1001	SIGNATURE DP

	1/6	2/6	3/6	4/6	5/6	6/6	7/6	8/6
0800	X	X	X	X				
1200								
1800								
0000								

DRUG	DOSE	ROUTE
DATE	BLP	SIGNATURE

	1/6	2/6	3/6	4/6	5/6	6/6	7/6	8/6
0800								
1200								
1800								
0000								

DRUG	DOSE	ROUTE
DATE	BLP	SIGNATURE

	1/6	2/6	3/6	4/6	5/6	6/6	7/6	8/6
0800								
1200								
1800								
0000								

DRUG	DOSE	ROUTE
DATE	BLP	SIGNATURE

	1/6	2/6	3/6	4/6	5/6	6/6	7/6	8/6
0800								
1200								
1800								
0000								

AS REQUIRED PRESCRIPTIONS

DRUG *Cyclizine*			Date	DO								
DOSE *50mg*	Route *IV/IM*	Start date *1/6/14*	Time									
Signature DP		Max Freq. *TDS*	Dose									
Additional information- *for nausea*			Given									

DRUG *Morphine*			Date	DO								
DOSE 2.5mg	Route *IV*	Start date *1/6/14*	Time									
Signature DP		Max Freq. *4 hourly*	Dose									
Additional information			Given									

DRUG *CODEINE*			Date	DO								
DOSE 30-60mg	Route *IM*	Start date *1/6/14*	Time									
Signature DP		Max Freq. *qds*	Dose									
DRUG			Given									

INTRAVENOUS & SUBCUTANEOUS INFUSIONS

USE OF CHART

Prescribe only those drugs to be given by infusion on the IV chart.

State clearly the line through which the infusion fluid is to be administered, e.g. intravenous, central venous pressure (CVP) line, subcutaneous

Date	Additions to infusion		Infusion fluid		IV or SC	Time to run or mL/hr	Signatures	
	Drug	Dose	Type/strength	Volume			Prescriber	Given
1/6/14	*Nil*		0.9% NaCl	500mL	*IV*	*STAT*	DP	
1/6/14	KCl	20mmol	0.9% NaCl	1000mL	*IV*	4 hrs	DP	
1/6/14	KCl	20mmol	5% dextrose	1000mL	*IV*	6 hrs	DP	
1/6/14	KCl	20mmol	5% dextrose	1000mL	*IV*	6 hrs	DP	

05.3 ACUTE ASTHMA ATTACK

INSTRUCTIONS Mr Banbury has been brought into hospital by ambulance complaining of shortness of breath. He is a known asthmatic with three previous hospital admissions and one admission to ITU. He is having difficulty in completing sentences when speaking. His oxygen saturation is 94% in air and pulse rate is 120 regular. A polyphonic wheeze is apparent throughout the chest. He is allergic to eggs. Complete the inpatient drug chart using information from the repeat prescription provided and administer appropriate acute treatment. There is no patient in this scenario.

NOTE: Medical pharmacology is constantly being updated and treatment protocols differ from hospital to hospital. The information provided here is only a guide. You should make every effort to check the local guidance for your medical school.

Mr B, DOB 22/3/52, Hosp no. 123498
Paracetamol 1g QDS
Seretide 250 Evohaler (fluticasone 250 microg+ salmeterol 25 microg) – two puffs BD

STAGE	KEY POINTS AND ACTIONS	SCORE		
Name	Complete forename and surname clearly.	0	1	–
DoB	Fill out patient's date of birth.	0	1	–
Hospital No.	Complete patient's hospital number.	0	1	–
Allergy	Circle appropriate – YES – box for allergy and record correct allergy.	0	1	2

Score			Drug	Dose	Route	Freq	Duration	Notes
			Acute medical management (STAT side)					
0	1	2	Oxygen	Titrate to sats 94–98%	Controlled; e.g. Venturi 24%	STAT and regular medications	As required	
0	1	2	Salbutamol	5mg	Nebulized	STAT	–	Specify the driving gas as oxygen.
0	1	2	Hydrocortisone	200mg	IV	STAT	–	
			Continuing medical management (Regular side)					
0	1	2	Salbutamol	5mg	Nebulized	2–4 hourly	Review daily	Stretch to 4 hourly and then switch to inhalers once stable; specify driving gas.
0	1		Prednisolone	40mg	Oral	OD	5 days	Wean dose after 5 days if multiple courses during the year.
0	1		Paracetamol	1g	Oral	QDS	Ongoing	
			As required medication (PRN side)					
0	1		Salbutamol	5mg	Nebulized	2 hourly	As required	Specify driving gas.
			Infusion therapy (IVI side)					
0	1		Nil					

STAGE	KEY POINTS AND ACTIONS	SCORE		
General Prescribing	Recognise the need to prescribe oxygen.	0	1	2
Writing	Complete all sections clearly, legibly, and in black ink.	0	1	–
Admission	Record all the patient's drugs on admission in relevant section.	0	1	–
Generic	Prescribe generic drugs and avoid the use of brand names. Avoid any of the DO NOTs listed in 5.1 General Tips.	0	1	–

EXAMINER'S EVALUATION

Overall assessment of prescribing in acute asthma	0	1	2	3	4	5

Total mark out of 27

05.4 COPD EXACERBATION

INSTRUCTIONS Mr Collins has been brought into hospital by ambulance complaining of shortness of breath. He is a known COPD sufferer with five previous hospital admissions and two admissions to ITU. He mentions that he has been coughing up green phlegm for the past three days. His temperature is 38.1 C, oxygen saturation is 91% in air and pulse is 120. There is poor air entry throughout the chest and right basal crepitations. A polyphonic wheeze is apparent throughout the chest. He is allergic to penicillin. Complete the inpatient drug chart using information from the repeat prescription provided and administer appropriate acute treatment. There is no patient in this scenario.

NOTE: Medical pharmacology is constantly being updated and treatment protocols differ from hospital to hospital. The information provided here is only a guide. You should make every effort to contact a specialist at your medical school for further guidance to treatments and dosages.

Mr P Colins, DOB 14/8/32, Hosp no. 7249298
Salbutamol 2 PUFFS QDS
Tiotropium bromide 5 microg 2 PUFFS OD

STAGE	KEY POINTS AND ACTIONS	SCORE		
Name	Complete forename and surname clearly.	0	1	–
DoB	Fill out patient's date of birth.	0	1	–
Hospital No.	Complete patient's hospital number.	0	1	–
Allergy	Circle appropriate – YES – box for allergy and record correct allergy.	0	1	2

Score			Drug	Dose	Route	Freq	Duration	Notes
			Acute medical management (STAT side)					
0	1	2	Oxygen	Titrate to sats 88–92%	Controlled; e.g. Venturi 24%	STAT and regular medications	As required	Represcribe after ABG results available.
0	1	2	Salbutamol	5mg	Nebulized	STAT	–	Specify the driving gas; oxygen if very hypoxic or air if not.
0	1	2	Ipratropium	500 microg	Nebulized	STAT	–	
0	1	2	Prednisolone	30mg	Oral	STAT	–	Continue on regular side.
0	1	2	Antibiotics; e.g. Clarithromycin	500mg	Oral	STAT	–	Follow local policy for penicillin allergy.
			Continuing medical management (Regular side)					
0	1	2	Salbutamol	5mg	Nebulized	2–4 hourly	Review daily	Stretch to 4 hourly and then switch to inhalers once stable; specify driving gas as air.
0	1	2	Ipratropium	500 microg	Nebulized	QDS	Review daily	Switch to inhalers once stable; specify driving gas as air.
0	1		Clarithromycin	500mg	Oral	BD	5–7 days	Follow local policy.
0	1		Prednisolone	30mg	Oral	OD	7 days	Wean dose after 7 days if multiple courses during the year.
			As required medication (PRN side)					
0	1		Salbutamol	5mg	Nebulized	2 hourly	As required	Specify driving gas as air.
			Infusion therapy (IVI side)					
0	1		Nil					

STAGE	KEY POINTS AND ACTIONS	SCORE
	GENERAL PRESCRIBING	
Writing	Complete all sections clearly, legibly, and in black ink.	0 1 –
Admission	Record all the patient's drugs on admission in relevant section.	0 1 –
Generic	Prescribe generic drugs and avoid the use of brand names. Avoid any of the DO NOTs listed in 5.1 General Tips.	0 1 –
	EXAMINER'S EVALUATION	
	Overall assessment of prescribing in exacerbation of COPD	0 1 2 3 4 5
	Total mark out of 31	

05.5 ACUTE CORONARY SYNDROME

INSTRUCTIONS Mr F is a 65-year-old recruitment consultant presenting with acute onset, left sided, crushing central chest pain. His ECG shows > 4mm ST elevation in leads V1-V4 with reciprocal inferior depression. Observations are stable and examination is normal. Complete the inpatient drug chart using information from the repeat prescription provided and administer appropriate acute treatment. There is no patient in this scenario.

NOTE: Medical pharmacology is constantly being updated and treatment protocols differ from hospital to hospital. The information provided here is only a guide. You should make every effort to check the local guidance for your medical school.

Mr F, DOB 14/8/49, Hosp no. 7249298
Ibuprofen 200mg TDS

STAGE	KEY POINTS AND ACTIONS	SCORE		
Name	Complete forename and surname clearly.	0	1	–
DoB	Fill out patient's date of birth.	0	1	–
Hospital No.	Complete patient's hospital number.	0	1	–
Allergy	Circle appropriate – NO – box for allergy.	0	1	2

Score			Drug	Dose	Route	Freq	Duration	Notes
			Acute medical management (STAT side)					
0	1	2	Oxygen	Titrate to sats > 94%	Controlled; e.g. Venturi 24%	STAT and regular medications	As required	
0	1	2	Aspirin	300mg	PO	STAT		
0	1	2	GTN Spray	2 puffs	Sublingual	STAT		
0	1	2	Morphine	2.5mg	IV	STAT		
			Continuing medical management (Regular side)					
0	1	–	Aspirin **	75mg	PO	OD	From day of MI	
			As required medication (PRN side)					
0	1	–	GTN spray	2 puffs	Sublingual	PRN	As required	
0	1	–	Metoclopramide	10mg	PO	TDS	As required	
			Infusion therapy (IVI side)					
0	1	-	Nil					

http://www.nice.org.uk/guidance/CG167
**Local guidance will vary on antiplatelet therapies.
For ST-Elevated Myocardial Infarction with intention for PCI;
Ticagrelor: 180mg STAT PO and then 90mg BD PO for 12 months with aspirin
Bivalirudin (in combination with clopidogrel and aspirin) Given when undergoing PCI as body-weight infusion

STAGE	KEY POINTS AND ACTIONS	SCORE					
	GENERAL PRESCRIBING						
Writing	Complete all sections clearly, legibly, and in black ink.	0	1	–			
Admission	Record all the patient's drugs on admission in relevant section.	0	1	–			
Generic	Prescribe generic drugs and avoid the use of brand names. Avoid any of the DO NOTs listed in 5.1 General Tips.	0	1	–			
	EXAMINER'S EVALUATION						
	Overall assessment of prescribing in acute coronary syndrome	0	1	2	3	4	5
	Total mark out of 25						

05.6 ACUTE LEFT VENTRICULAR FAILURE

INSTRUCTIONS Mrs Beatty has been brought into hospital by ambulance complaining of shortness of breath. She suffers from hypertension and back pain. On examination she has a raised JVP and widespread bilateral crackles in her chest. Her blood pressure is 130/80mmHg. She is allergic to codeine. Her repeat prescription is provided. Complete her inpatient drug chart and administer appropriate acute treatment. There is no patient in this scenario.

NOTE: Medical pharmacology is constantly being updated and treatment protocols differ from hospital to hospital. The information provided here is only a guide. You should make every effort to check the local guidance for your medical school.

Mrs Eve Beatty, DOB: 12/5/45
Hosp. No. 343556
Aspirin 75mg
Atenolol 50mg BD
Ramipril 5mg OD
Simvastatin 20mg
Ibuprofen 400mg prn

STAGE	KEY POINTS AND ACTIONS	SCORE		
Name	Complete forename and surname clearly.	0	1	–
DoB	Fill out patient's date of birth.	0	1	–
Hospital No.	Complete patient's hospital number.	0	1	–
Allergy	Circle appropriate – YES – box for allergy and record correct allergy.	0	1	2

Score	Drug	Dose	Route	Freq	Duration	Notes
	Acute medical management (STAT side)					
0 1 2	Oxygen	Titrate to sats > 94%	Controlled; e.g. Venturi 24%	STAT and regular medications	As required	
0 1 2	Furosemide	40-80mg	IV	STAT		
	Continuing medical management (Regular side)					
0 1 2	Aspirin	75mg	PO	OD		
0 1 2	Atenolol*	50mg	PO	BD		See * comment.
0 1 2	Ramipril	5mg	PO	OD		
0 1 2	Simvastatin	20mg	PO	NOCTE		
0 1 2	Furosemide	40mg	IV	0800 and 1200		
	As required medication (PRN side)					
0 1 –	Cyclizine	50mg	IV/IM/PO	TDS	As required	
	Infusion therapy (IVI side)					
0 1 –	GTN infusion	50mg in 50mL NaCl 0.9%	IV	Titrate rate starting at 1ml/hr to 10ml/hr		Titrate to breathlessness, keep BP > 110mmHg.

In stable patients without hypotension continued beta-blocker therapy is safe if maintained previously > 3 months. If hypotensive, beta-blockers should be omitted but restarted once stabilized.

Further reading:
http://www.escardio.org/guidelines-surveys/esc-guidelines/guidelinesdocuments/guidelines-acute%20and%20chronic-hf-ft.pdf

STAGE	KEY POINTS AND ACTIONS	SCORE
	GENERAL PRESCRIBING	
Writing	Complete all sections clearly, legibly, and in black ink.	0 1 –
Admission	Record all the patient's drugs on admission in relevant section.	0 1 –
Generic	Prescribe generic drugs and avoid the use of brand names. Avoid any of the DO NOTs listed in 5.1 General Tips.	0 1 –
	EXAMINER'S EVALUATION	
	Overall assessment of prescribing in acute left ventricular failure	0 1 2 3 4 5
	Total mark out of 29	

05.7
HYPERKALAEMIA

INSTRUCTIONS Miss G is an 80-year-old woman with a history of renal failure. She has come in to hospital with pneumonia, for which she is on co-amoxiclav at a reduced dose. Her latest potassium result comes back at 6.8mmol/L. Prescribe appropriate management therapy.

NOTE: Medical pharmacology is constantly being updated and treatment protocols differ from hospital to hospital. The information provided here is only a guide. You should make every effort to check the local guidance for your medical school.

Miss G, DOB: 9/6/34
Hosp. No. 1029394
Aspirin 75mg
Co-amoxiclav 1.2g IV TDS

STAGE	KEY POINTS AND ACTIONS	SCORE		
Name	Complete forename and surname clearly.	0	1	–
DoB	Fill out patient's date of birth.	0	1	–
Hospital No.	Complete patient's hospital number.	0	1	–
Allergy	Circle appropriate – NO – box for allergy.	0	1	2

Score			Drug	Dose	Route	Freq	Duration	Notes
			Acute medical management (STAT side)					
0	1	2	Oxygen	Titrate to sats > 94%	Controlled; e.g. Venturi 24%	STAT and regular medications	As required	
0	1	2	Calcium Gluconate 10%	10mL	IV	STAT		
			Continuing medical management (Regular side)					
0	1	2	Aspirin	75mg	PO	OD		
0	1	2	Co-amoxiclav	1.2g	IV	TDS		
			As required medication (PRN side)					
			Infusion therapy (IVI side)					
0	1	2	Actrapid in 100mL of 20% glucose	15 units	IV	STAT	Over 20 minutes	

STAGE	KEY POINTS AND ACTIONS	SCORE
	GENERAL PRESCRIBING	
Writing	Complete all sections clearly, legibly, and in black ink.	0 1 –
Admission	Record all the patient's drugs on admission in relevant section.	0 1 –
Generic	Prescribe generic drugs and avoid the use of brand names. Avoid any of the DO NOTs listed in 5.1 General Tips.	0 1 –

EXAMINER'S EVALUATION

Overall assessment of prescribing in hyperkalaemia	0 1 2 3 4 5

Total mark out of 23

PRACTICE DRUG CHARTS

Sample Chart 1 of 3

St. Somewhere or Another Hospital Trust

Drug Prescription and Administration

WARD –	CONSULTANT –
HOSPITAL NO. -	HOUSE OFFICER
SURNAME -	BLEEP-
FIRST NAME-	DATE OF ADMISSION-
DOB –	

DRUG ALLERGIES

YES/NO/NOT KNOWN   DATE:

DRUGS: REACTION: SIGNED:

Once only & Premedication drugs

DATE	DRUG	DOSE	TIME	ROUTE	DRS SIGNATURE	TIME GIVEN	GIVEN BY	PHARMACY

REGULAR PRESCRIPTIONS

ADMINISTRATION RECORD

DRUG		DOSE	ROUTE
DATE	BLP	SIGNATURE	

	1/6	2/6	3/6	4/6	5/6	6/6	7/6	8/6
0800								
1200								
1800								
0000								

DRUG		DOSE	ROUTE
DATE	BLP	SIGNATURE	

	1/6	2/6	3/6	4/6	5/6	6/6	7/6	8/6
0800								
1200								
1800								
0000								

DRUG		DOSE	ROUTE
DATE	BLP	SIGNATURE	

	1/6	2/6	3/6	4/6	5/6	6/6	7/6	8/6
0800								
1200								
1800								
0000								

DRUG		DOSE	ROUTE
DATE	BLP	SIGNATURE	

	1/6	2/6	3/6	4/6	5/6	6/6	7/6	8/6
0800								
1200								
1800								
0000								

DRUG		DOSE	ROUTE
DATE	BLP	SIGNATURE	

	1/6	2/6	3/6	4/6	5/6	6/6	7/6	8/6
0800								
1200								
1800								
0000								

AS REQUIRED PRESCRIPTIONS

DRUG				Date									
DOSE	Route		Start date	Time									
Signature			Max Freq.	Dose									
Additional information				Given									

DRUG				Date									
DOSE	Route		Start date	Time									
				Dose									
Signature				Given									
Additional information													

DRUG				Date									
DOSE	Route		Start date	Time									
				Dose									
Signature				Given									
Additional information													

INTRAVENOUS & SUBCUTANEOUS INFUSIONS

USE OF CHART

Prescribe only those drugs to be given by infusion on the IV chart.

State clearly the line through which the infusion fluid is to be administered, e.g. intravenous, central venous pressure (CVP) line, subcutaneous

Date	Additions to infusion		Infusion fluid		IV or SC	Time to run or	Signatures	
	Drug	Dose	Type/strength	Volume		mL/hr	Prescriber	Given

section 06

COMMUNICATION SKILLS

06.1 HIV TEST COUNSELLING

INSTRUCTIONS Mr D has recently returned from a trip to Thailand. He has presented to you complaining of a urethral discharge and is requesting an HIV test. Take a brief sexual history and give him the appropriate advice.

STAGE	KEY POINTS AND ACTIONS	SCORE		
	INTRODUCTION			
Introduction	Introduce yourself. Elicit name, age, and occupation. Establish rapport.	0	1	–
Patient Agenda	Establish why the patient has booked the appointment. Elicit patient's ideas, concerns, and expectations.	0	1	2
	'I am going to ask you a few personal questions to find out more about your problem. Although the questions may be embarrassing, you do not have to answer them if you do not wish to. We ask these questions of all our patients and everything that you say will remain strictly confidential'.			
	SEXUAL HISTORY			
Symptoms	Do you have any discharge? Any fevers? Any urinary symptoms?	0	1	–
Contacts	Do you have a regular partner? Male or female? Any casual partners?	0	1	–
	HIV RISK SPECIFIC QUESTIONS: Have you ever had a partner: -with known HIV? -from Sub-Saharan Africa or East Asia? -who was a sex worker? -who was bisexual? -who injected drugs?			
Types of SI	When was the last time you had sexual intercourse (SI)? What type of intercourse did you have? Was it anal or vaginal?	0	1	–
Contraception	Did you use any form of contraception; e.g. condoms?	0	1	–
Other Activity	Have you ever used intravenous drugs? Have you ever shared needles? Have you ever had a blood transfusion?	0	1	–
Past History	Do you suffer from any STDs? Have you ever had an HIV test before?			

STAGE	KEY POINTS AND ACTIONS	SCORE
Drug History	Are you using any medicines? Do you have any allergies?	
	HIV TESTING	
Understanding	Elicit patient's understanding of HIV and testing.	0 1 –
	'Have you ever had an HIV test before? Can you please tell me what you understand by HIV'?	
HIV & AIDS	Explain in clear and simple terms the difference between HIV and AIDS.	0 1 2
	'HIV is a virus that invades the body and weakens its defences against other infections. It can be passed in different ways, the most common being through unprotected sexual intercourse (between male and female or male and male); or by sharing infected needles. AIDS is a condition which is caused by HIV and is characterised by specific infections which infect the body as a result of the weakened immune system. The time period between HIV and developing AIDS varies from person to person and can often be many years'.	
HIV Test	Explain how the HIV test works.	0 1 –
	'We will take some blood from your arm and send this to the laboratory for analysis. When a person has HIV, the body produces antibodies that we can test for. If these antibodies are present it means HIV has been detected; if not, it means you do not have HIV'.	
Window Period	Give appropriate advice regarding a possible negative test.	0 1 2
	'It is important to appreciate that it can take up to three months after being infected with HIV for these antibodies to be produced. In essence we are assessing your HIV status three months ago. If you were recently infected because of unprotected sex, then the antibodies may not necessarily be present and we may get a negative result. This is known as the "window period" and we may need to repeat the test in a few months to be sure of your status'.	
	TEST RESULTS	
Results	Explain how he will be informed of results.	0 1 –
	'As I mentioned previously, everything that we have discussed remains confidential. The same applies for your blood results. We will not ring you or write to you with your results. Rather we will send you an appointment to attend the clinic. Some clinics have the facility to text a negative result to your mobile phone. Would this be of benefit to you'?	
Implications	Explain the possible advantages and disadvantages of having the test.	0 1 2
	'Before taking the HIV test you may wish to consider what implications the results may have for you. One of the advantages of doing the test includes knowing whether you have HIV or not. If positive then we can commence treatment immediately. Although treatment is not curative, it can delay progression to AIDS. Also by knowing your status you can take precautions from spreading the virus to your partner. However, by knowing your status, this may have a negative impact on your relationship with your partner and you may also have to inform your insurance company'.	

STAGE	KEY POINTS AND ACTIONS	SCORE
Support Group	Enquire about a support network and whether he would like more counselling.	0 1 –
	'If the results are positive is there anyone from your friends or family you think you can talk to? We have specially trained professionals who can counsel you if the test is positive. I can put them in touch with you if you think that may help'.	
	FINISHING OFF	
Understanding	Confirm patient understands what has been discussed.	0 1 –
	Encourage questions and deal with concerns accordingly.	
Follow-Up	Mention the need for an out-patient follow-up to review symptoms.	0 1 –
Offer Leaflet	Close the interview and offer HIV information leaflet.	0 1 –

EXAMINER'S EVALUATION

Overall assessment of explaining pre-assessment HIV testing	0 1 2 3 4 5

Total mark out of 26

06.2
PEAK FLOW

You are in general practice. Mr F has presented to you with symptoms of nocturnal cough and a wheeze on examination. You suspect that he may be asthmatic and wish to carry out a Peak Flow to confirm this. Explain to the patient what you are going to do.

STAGE	KEY POINTS AND ACTIONS	SCORE
	INTRODUCTION	
Introduction	Introduce yourself. Elicit name, age, and occupation. Establish rapport.	0 1 –
Understanding	Elicit patient's understanding of asthma and peak flow measurement.	0 1 –
	'I understand that you have had symptoms of a night cough and wheeze for a while now. I wish to carry out a peak flow test to rule out the possibility of asthma. Have you ever had one of these tests before? Could you please tell me what you understand by the term asthma'?	
Explain	Explain in clear and simple terms what the peak flow is measuring.	0 1 –
	'The peak flow meter is a simple device which measures how air flows out of your lungs and tells us how good your ability to push air out is. In asthma, due to the airway constriction, this reading is usually lower than normal. I will now show you how to use the peak flow meter'.	
	THE PROCEDURE	
Position	Ensure that the patient is standing for the test.	0 1 –
Preparation	Take the peak flow device and reset the pointer to zero. Place a fresh mouthpiece into the peak flow meter.	0 1 –
Inhale	Advise the patient to inhale fully, filling their lungs with air.	0 1 –
Holding	Hold the meter correctly with fingers not interfering with the pointer. Make a tight seal around the mouthpiece.	0 1 –
Exhale	Demonstrate to the patient how to blow as hard and as fast as possible through the peak flow meter.	0 1 –
Repeat	Advise the patient to repeat the test three times taking the highest reading.	0 1 –
Reading	Instruct the patient how to take a correct reading and record this in a diary.	0 1 –

STAGE	KEY POINTS AND ACTIONS	SCORE
Comprehension	Check whether the patient understood the process and ask him to demonstrate.	0 1 –
Compare	Check the patient's reading against a standardised chart taking into account the age, sex, and height of the patient.	0 1 –
	'This tubelike device is the peak flow meter. These graduations are used to check the flow of air. This end is for you to place your mouth over via a mouthpiece. Before you take a reading, stand up and take a few breaths. Take one final deep breath and place the mouthpiece in your mouth ensuring that you make a tight seal around it with your lips. Hold the peak flow meter with your dominant hand and make sure your fingers do not interfere with the pointer. Ensure the pointer is placed to zero. Blow as hard and fast as you can, as if you are blowing through the meter. Repeat this three times and record the highest reading in the peak flow diary provided. The best times to take a peak flow are first thing in the morning and just before you go to sleep. Also take readings when you experience symptoms such as coughing or wheeze. Record all these readings in this peak flow diary'.	

EXPLANATION

STAGE	KEY POINTS AND ACTIONS	SCORE
Interpret	Interpret the results against the chart accordingly and confirm or negate possibility of asthma.	0 1 –
Advice	Provide appropriate medical advice regarding cause of the symptoms and suggest appropriate investigation or management strategies.	0 1 –
Understanding	Confirm that the patient has understood what has been explained to them. Elicit any questions or concerns.	0 1 –
Follow-up	Mention the need for follow-up to review symptoms.	0 1 –

EXAMINER'S EVALUATION

Overall assessment of demonstration of peak flow meter use	0 1 2 3 4 5

Total mark out of 21

06.3
CT HEAD SCAN

INSTRUCTIONS Mrs G, a 38-year-old woman, has been admitted with sudden onset right hemiparesis. Your Consultant has requested a CT head scan to investigate the cause of the weakness. You have been instructed to explain the procedure to the patient.

STAGE	KEY POINTS AND ACTIONS	SCORE
	INTRODUCTION	
Introduction	Introduce yourself. Elicit name, age, and occupation. Establish rapport.	0 1 –
Understanding	Elicit patient's understanding of a CT scan.	0 1 –
	'I understand that you have noticed weakness of the right side of your body. In order to try and establish what exactly is going on we need to carry out a CT head scan. Do you know what this is? What do you understand by a CT'?	
Concerns	Elicit patient's concerns of CT and stroke.	0 1 –
	'Do you have any particular concerns about having the CT scan? What do you think is the cause of your weakness'?	
	EXPLAINING	
CT Scan	Clarify to the patient what a CT scan is.	0 1 –
	'CT stands for computerised tomography. A CT scan uses x-rays to produce images of the body. The images are produced from data which the scanner acquires which are then turned into cross-sectional images of the body, like slices in a loaf of bread'.	
Procedure	Explain to the patient the procedure in simple terms.	0 1 –
	'You will be taken tomorrow for the CT head scan. You should stop eating and drinking around 2 hours before the scan. The CT scanner looks much like a giant washing machine and you will be placed inside it. You may feel a little claustrophobic. The scanning is a painless procedure and should take around 10 minutes. When you are in the room you will be left alone with the scanner. However, in the next adjacent room will be the operator and another assistant with whom you will be able to speak through an intercom system'.	
Safety	Explain to the patient issues of safety regarding the CT.	0 1 –
	'Generally speaking, the CT scan is a safe procedure. Although CT scanners use x-rays at the lowest practical dose, you still are having exposure to radiation. The benefits of having a CT scan outweigh the risk of exposure to radiation, as the information obtained from the scan is vital for diagnosis and treatment'.	

STAGE	KEY POINTS AND ACTIONS	SCORE
Risks	Check for any contraindications to the CT scan.	0 1 –
	'The CT scan is not recommended for some people such as those who are pregnant. Is there a possibility that you are pregnant'?	
Injection	Warn the patient that she may have an IV contrast injection.	0 1 –
	'In order to make the images as beneficial as possible, you may have an injection of a harmless dye into a vein in your arm. The injection should leave no after-effects. Have you ever had any allergies before'?	

FINISHING OFF

Understanding	Check whether patient has understood what has been explained.	0 1 –
Questions	Encourage patient to ask questions and deal with them appropriately.	0 1 –
Consent	Provide appropriate summary to patient and take consent.	0 1 –
Respond	Acknowledge patient's feelings and react positively to them.	0 1 –

EXAMINER'S EVALUATION

Overall assessment of explaining CT head scan	0 1 2 3 4 5

Total mark out of 17

06.4
MRI SCAN

INSTRUCTIONS Mr G has been admitted for further investigation for severe back pain and right foot weakness. Your registrar has booked an MRI scan for him and has requested you to explain the procedure to the patient.

STAGE	KEY POINTS AND ACTIONS	SCORE		
	INTRODUCTION			
Introduction	Introduce yourself. Elicit name, age, and occupation. Establish rapport.	0	1	–
Understanding	Elicit patient's understanding of an MRI scan.	0	1	–
	'I understand that you have had quite severe back pain and problems with your right foot. In order to try and establish what exactly is going on we need to carry out an MRI scan. Do you know what an MRI scan is? What do you understand by it'?			
Concerns	Elicit patient's concerns of MRI and disability secondary to back pain.	0	1	–
	'Do you have any particular concerns about having the MRI scan? What do you think is causing your problems'?			
	EXPLAINING			
MRI Scan	Clarify to the patient what an MRI scan is.	0	1	–
	'MRI stands for magnetic resonance imaging and is a non-invasive way of getting pictures of the human body. The process uses a magnetic field to obtain accurate pictures of the area in question and does not involve x-rays'.			
Procedure	Explain to the patient the procedure in simple terms.	0	1	2
	'You will be taken tomorrow for the MRI scan. You will be allowed to eat and drink freely before it. The MRI scanner is a large tube like machine in which you will be placed. You may feel a little claustrophobic. MRI is a painless procedure and should take around 30 minutes. When you are in the room you will be left alone. In the adjacent room will be the operator and an assistant with whom you will be able to speak through an intercom system'.			
Noisy	Warn the patient about the noise and need to wear ear protection.	0	1	–
	'Because of the way the MRI scan works, the procedure may be a little noisy and may hurt your ears. Consequently, we advise all patients to wear the earplugs which will be provided to you'.			
Safety	Explain to the patient issues of safety regarding the MRI.	0	1	–
	'The MRI scan is an extremely safe procedure which as yet has no proven risks or side effects. Consequently you can have repeated scans without the risks associated with repeated x-ray exposure'.			

STAGE	KEY POINTS AND ACTIONS	SCORE
Risks	Check for any contraindications to the MRI scan.	0　1　2
	'Although the MRI scan is extremely safe, it is not recommended for some people such as those who have a pacemaker, surgical clips in their body, or metallic heart valves. In addition, anyone who has the possibility of metal fragments in their eyes should be x-rayed prior to MRI scanning. Does any of what I said apply to you'?	
Injection	Warn the patient that he may have an IV contrast injection.	0　1　–
	'Although this is unlikely in your case, I must still warn you that you may have an injection of a harmless dye into a vein in your arm. This will help to make the images as beneficial as possible. The injection should leave no after-effects. Have you ever had any allergies before'?	

FINISHING OFF

Understanding	Check whether the patient has understood what has been explained.	0　1　–
Questions	Encourage the patient to ask questions and deal with them appropriately.	0　1　–
Consent	Provide appropriate summary to patient and take consent.	0　1　–
Respond	Acknowledge patient's feelings and react positively to them.	0　1　–

EXAMINER'S EVALUATION

Overall assessment of explaining MRI scan	0　1　2　3　4　5
Total mark out of 20	

06.5 OGD ENDOSCOPY

INSTRUCTIONS Mr D, a 35-year-old man with a history of alcohol abuse, has been having worsening dyspnoea on exertion. He also reports the passing of black stools. He has been admitted for a day case upper gastro-intestinal endoscopy. Your SHO has requested you to explain the procedure to the patient.

STAGE	KEY POINTS AND ACTIONS	SCORE		
	INTRODUCTION			
Introduction	Introduce yourself. Elicit name, age, and occupation. Establish rapport.	0	1	–
Understanding	Elicit patient's understanding of the endoscopic procedure.	0	1	–
	'I understand that you have had episodes of passing black stools. In order to establish what exactly is going on we need to carry out an endoscopy. Do you know what an endoscopy is? What do you understand by it'?			
Concerns	Elicit patient's concerns of GI bleed; i.e. cancer and procedure.	0	1	–
	'Do you have any particular concerns about the endoscope test? What do you think is causing your black motions'?			
	EXPLAINING			
Endoscope	Clarify to the patient what the endoscope is.	0	1	–
	'The upper endoscopy test is a procedure that allows the doctor to look directly at the lining of the oesophagus (food pipe), the stomach, and the first part of the intestine. The endoscope is a long thin flexible tube with a bright light on its tip. The doctor may take a small sample of tissue or a biopsy from inside which will be taken painlessly using tiny forceps'.			
Pre-procedure	Explain to the patient the pre-procedure preparation.	0	1	2
	'You will be taken for the endoscopy tomorrow. To allow a clear view inside, you will not be allowed to eat and drink at least six hours prior to the procedure. A spray may be applied into your nose or an injection given to make you feel relaxed and not feel any discomfort during the procedure'.			
Procedure	Explain to the patient the procedure.	0	1	2
	'The doctor will place a mouth-guard to keep your mouth open. The thin endoscope will be passed painlessly into your stomach. During the procedure air may be placed into your stomach to allow a clearer view. The whole procedure may take between fifteen minutes and half an hour'.			

STAGE	KEY POINTS AND ACTIONS	SCORE		
Post-procedure	Explain to the patient post-operative procedure.	0	1	–
	'Because of the medication you would have taken you may feel a little weak and uneasy and you should not drive. It is important that you have someone with you to take you home. You should be feeling much better tomorrow and can go back to work'.			

FINISHING OFF

Understanding	Check whether patient has understood what has been explained.	0	1	–
Questions	Encourage patient to ask questions and deal with them appropriately.	0	1	–
Summary	Provide appropriate summary to the patient of the procedure.	0	1	–
Follow-up	Mention the need for out-patient follow-up for results.	0	1	–
Respond	Acknowledge patient's feelings and react positively to them.	0	1	–

EXAMINER'S EVALUATION

Overall assessment of explaining endoscopy	0	1	2	3	4	5

Total mark out of 19

06.6 BARIUM ENEMA

INSTRUCTIONS Ms E, a 45-year-old woman, has been having bloody diarrhoea for the past three months. She has been booked for a barium enema by her GP, who has not yet explained the procedure. She has requested you to explain the procedure to her today.

STAGE	KEY POINTS AND ACTIONS	SCORE
	INTRODUCTION	
Introduction	Introduce yourself. Elicit name, age and occupation. Establish rapport.	0 1 –
Understanding	Elicit patient's understanding of a barium enema.	0 1 –
	'I understand that you have had bouts of bloody diarrhoea. In order to try and establish what exactly is going on we need to carry out a barium enema. Do you know what this is? What do you understand by the test'?	
Concerns	Elicit patient's concerns of bowel cancer and procedure.	0 1 –
	'Do you have any particular concerns about the test? What do you think is causing your symptoms'?	
	EXPLAINING	
Barium Enema	Clarify to the patient what a barium enema is.	0 1 –
	'A barium enema is used to look for problems in your lower bowel. The gut does not show up very well on ordinary x-ray pictures. However, if barium liquid is placed in the gut, the outline of the gut (intestines) shows up more clearly. Barium is a soft white metal which can be placed in the lower bowel through an enema'.	
Preparation	Explain to the patient how to prepare for the test.	0 1 2
	'You will be given some strong laxatives to take the day before the test. This will help wash out your lower bowel and allow for better x-ray pictures. These laxatives are quite strong and may make you feel weak. We usually advise not to go to work on this day. You will be given an advice leaflet on what you may and may not eat prior to the test. However, you should generally eat a light diet. If the test is in the morning you are advised not to eat anything the night before'.	
Procedure	Explain to the patient the procedure.	0 1 –
	'When you come in for the test you will be changed into a gown and asked to lie on your side. A small tube will be inserted into your back passage and the barium will be passed through this. Some air will also be passed into the lower bowel and this can feel a little uncomfortable. The whole test may take up to twenty minutes'.	

STAGE	KEY POINTS AND ACTIONS	SCORE
Positioning	Explain that the patient, during the procedure, may have to move around.	0 1 –
	'In order for us to obtain clear pictures of different parts of the bowel you will be asked to move into different positions during the procedure. The bed you will be lying on may be tilted and there will be hand rails which you will be able to steady yourself with'.	
Side Effects	Explain the side effects of barium.	0 1 2
	'Although barium is not absorbed into the body, it still can cause a few unpleasant side effects. The most usual being mild stomach cramps and constipation, which occur for a few hours after the procedure. You may also find that your stools become white; this is quite normal'.	

FINISHING OFF

Understanding	Check whether patient has understood what has been explained.	0 1 –
Questions	Encourage patient to ask questions and deal with them appropriately.	0 1 –
Summary	Provide appropriate summary to patient of the procedure.	0 1 –
Follow-up	Mention need for out-patient follow-up for results.	0 1 –
Respond	Acknowledge patient's feelings and react positively to them.	0 1 –

EXAMINER'S EVALUATION

Overall assessment of explaining barium enema	0 1 2 3 4 5

Total mark out of 20

06.7 TRANSURETHRAL RESECTION OF PROSTATE

INSTRUCTIONS Mr O'Shea has been referred for a transurethral resection of the prostate under spinal anaesthesia. Elicit his concerns and explain the procedure to him including possible post-operative complications.

STAGE	KEY POINTS AND ACTIONS	SCORE		
	INTRODUCTION			
Introduction	Introduce yourself. Elicit name, age, and occupation. Establish rapport.	0	1	–
Understanding	Elicit patient's understanding of transurethral resection of the prostate.	0	1	–
	'I understand that you are here today for a transurethral resection of the prostate. Can you tell me what you understand by this procedure'?			
Concerns	Elicit patient's concerns of the operation; i.e. post-op pain and impotence.	0	1	–
	'Do you have any particular concerns about the operation? Are there any matters you wish me to clarify'?			
	EXPLAINING			
Operation	Explain to the patient what the operation is.	0	1	2
	'The transurethral resection of the prostate is a procedure performed to remove part of your prostate gland. A small telescope will be passed through the urethra of your penis and the area of blockage will be cut away. You will be required to come into the hospital the night before the operation and may be kept in hospital for up to four days after it'.			
Fasting	Explain to the patient the need to fast before the operation.	0	1	–
	'If you are having the operation in the morning we advise that you do not eat or drink anything after midnight. Otherwise you should not eat anything six hours prior to the operation and avoid any fluids four hours before'.			
Anaesthetic	Explain to the patient about the spinal anaesthetic and pre-med.	0	1	2
	'When you first come to theatre, you will meet a nurse who will take your details and provide a gown for you to change into. You will be taken into the anaesthetic room where the anaesthetist will prepare you for surgery by giving you medicines through a line in your arm. As you are having a spinal block, a small tube will be inserted between the bones of your back and the anaesthetist will inject pain relief there. This will cause your body to become numb from the waist downward ensuring that you do not feel anything during the operation'.			

STAGE	KEY POINTS AND ACTIONS	SCORE
Recovery	Explain that the patient will be transferred to recovery.	0 1 2
	'Once the operation is complete, you will be transferred into a recovery room where you will awake. Don't be startled by the change in surroundings! You may feel ill or groggy once you are awake and will be given medicines to reduce any pain or sickness you may feel'.	
Catheter	Explain to the patient regarding catheter and bladder wash out.	0 1 –
	'You will find a catheter in your urethra (water pipe) so you won't need to go to the toilet to pass urine. There will be some bags of fluid attached to the catheter which will help wash out any debris and blood from your bladder. This will remain in place for two days after the operation'.	

COMPLICATIONS

STAGE	KEY POINTS AND ACTIONS	SCORE
Haematuria	Explain to the patient the possibility of post-op bleeding.	0 1 –
	'For up to two weeks after the operation you may notice blood in your urine. A small amount of blood in the urine can often make the urine look bright red. Do not be alarmed by this as it is entirely normal'.	
Impotence	Explain to the patient the possibility of impotence.	0 1 –
	'A small percentage of people report problems sustaining an erection after the operation. Do not be disheartened as there are a number of medications (Viagra, etc.) available that can be used to help achieve erections'.	
Infertility	Explain to the patient the possibility of infertility due to retrograde ejaculation.	0 1 –
	'A number of patients note when they ejaculate after the operation, the amount of semen is less than before. This is because the semen passes into the bladder and can make your urine look cloudy. Although this is quite harmless, it may lead to problems later on with conceiving children'.	
Infection	Explain to the patient the possibility of infection.	0 1 –
	'As with any operation, there is a small risk that you may develop an infection. If you feel feverish, pain on passing urine, or notice a penile discharge, you should seek medical help from your GP'.	
Frequency	Explain to the patient the possibility of change in urine stream.	0 1 –
	'After the operation you may feel the need to go to the toilet more often than before. This unpleasant sensation may last up to six weeks after the operation. However, it should settle down. If it has not resolved by this time, I would recommend speaking with your GP'.	
Pain	Explain to the patient the possibility of continuing pain.	0 1 –
	'There is a possibility that you may still experience pain a few weeks after the operation. You should take the painkillers which we will prescribe you on discharge. If you are concerned about the pain you should contact your GP'.	

POST-OP ADVICE

STAGE	KEY POINTS AND ACTIONS	SCORE
Fluid	Explain the need to drink up to three litres of fluid per day.	0 1 –
	'Once you are discharged home it is important that you continue to drink plenty of fluids to help reduce the amount of blood you pass in your urine. We suggest drinking between two and three litres a day'.	
Intercourse	Explain to the patient regarding sexual intercourse.	0 1 –
	'Due to the nature of your operation, you will be feeling quite sore down below. We advise all patients not to engage in sexual intercourse until at least two weeks after the operation'.	

STAGE	KEY POINTS AND ACTIONS	SCORE
Work	Explain to the patient issues regarding work.	0 1 –
	'Generally speaking, we advise people to return to work two weeks after the operation. By that time the wound should have healed well and the pain should be minimal if present'.	

FINISHING OFF

Understanding	Check whether patient has understood what has been explained.	0 1 –
Questions	Encourage patient to ask questions and deal with them appropriately.	0 1 –
Summary	Provide appropriate summary to the patient about the procedure.	0 1 –
Follow-up	Mention need to be seen in out-patient clinic in three months' time.	0 1 –
Respond	Acknowledge patient's feelings and react positively to them.	0 1 –

EXAMINER'S EVALUATION

Overall assessment of explaining transurethral resection of the prostate	0 1 2 3 4 5

Total mark out of 30

06.8 HERNIA REPAIR

INSTRUCTIONS Mr B, a 60-year-old man, has had a reducible inguinal hernia for six months and has been sent for a hernia repair. He has attended day surgery today for the operation under a local anaesthetic. Elicit his concerns and explain to him the procedure.

STAGE	KEY POINTS AND ACTIONS	SCORE		
	INTRODUCTION			
Introduction	Introduce yourself. Elicit name, age, and occupation. Establish rapport.	0	1	–
Understanding	Elicit patient's understanding of hernia procedure.	0	1	–
	'I understand that you are here today for a hernia operation. What do you understand by the procedure and what it entails'?			
Concerns	Elicit patient's concerns of the operation; i.e. being awake during operation, post-op pain, and when he can return to work.	0	1	–
	'Do you have any particular concerns about the operation? Are there any matters you wish me to clarify'?			
	EXPLAINING			
Operation	Clarify to the patient what the operation is.	0	1	2
	'The hernia repair is a procedure that involves returning the swelling which you have, back into its normal position within the abdomen. The weakness in the wall will then be repaired and covered with a mesh to prevent the lump appearing again. This operation is usually carried out as a day-case with no overnight stay in hospital'.			
Anaesthetic	Explain to the patient the anaesthetic procedure.	0	1	2
	'You will be having a local anaesthetic which will be delivered by injection in and around the hernia area in your groin as well as higher up. This will completely block any feeling in your groin region for the duration of the operation and will make you feel numb for a number of hours afterward. As you are having a local anaesthetic procedure, you will be awake during the operation'.			
Screen	Explain to the patient about the screen.	0	1	–
	'Many patients do not wish to see the operation and for this reason a screen will be put up to prevent you from seeing what is going on. The whole procedure should be over within half an hour'.			

STAGE	KEY POINTS AND ACTIONS	SCORE
Recovery	Explain to the patient that he will be transferred to recovery.	0 1 –
	'Because the local anaesthetic can make you feel weak and uneasy, we will transfer you to a recovery room where you will be monitored by a nurse for a short period. It is unlikely that you will experience any pain at this time; however if you do, you may ask the nurse for more pain relief'.	

POST-OP ADVICE

Complications	Explain to the patient complications of the procedure.	0 1 2
	'The hernia repair is a very common operation with more than 95,000 of these operations taking place in the UK each year. There are very few complications as a result of the operation, but these may include mild discomfort in the area, an adverse reaction to the local anaesthetic, post-operation bleeding, wound infection, and possible hernia recurrence'.	
Going Home	Explain to the patient issues regarding driving.	0 1 –
	'It is important that you organise someone to take you home after the operation as you should not drive. You should only resume driving once you are confident that you are able to perform an emergency stop; this is usually two weeks after the operation'.	
Stitches	Explain to the patient issues regarding wound and stitches.	0 1 –
	'The surgeon would usually insert dissolvable stitches into the operation site which disappear themselves after a few days and do not need removing. Once the wound is dry it should be left uncovered. We advise patients to get the wound checked by their practice nurse within four to five days of the operation'.	
Exercise	Explain to the patient issues regarding exercise and lifting.	0 1 –
	'In general you should rest two to three days after the operation. Although you should be able to perform your normal activities after this, you should avoid performing any strenuous exercise or undertaking any heavy lifting for up to six weeks after the operation'.	
Work	Explain to the patient issues regarding work.	0 1 –
	'The surgeon may advise you differently depending on the exact nature of your work; however, generally speaking we advise people to return to work two weeks after the operation. By that time the wound should have healed well and the pain should be minimal, if present. You can obtain a sickness certificate from your GP to allow you the time off'.	

FINISHING OFF

Understanding	Check whether patient has understood what has been explained.	0 1 –
Questions	Encourage patient to ask questions and deal with them appropriately.	0 1 –
Summary	Provide appropriate summary to the patient of the procedure.	0 1 –
Respond	Acknowledge patient's feelings and react positively.	0 1 –

EXAMINER'S EVALUATION

Overall assessment of explaining hernia repair		0 1 2 3 4 5
Total mark out of 24		

06.9 LAPAROSCOPIC CHOLECYSTECTOMY

INSTRUCTIONS Mr G has been admitted for a laparoscopic cholecystectomy procedure under general anaesthetic booked for tomorrow. Elicit his concerns and explain the procedure to him including possible post-operative complications.

STAGE	KEY POINTS AND ACTIONS	SCORE
	INTRODUCTION	
Introduction	Introduce yourself. Elicit name, age, and occupation. Establish rapport.	0 1 –
Understanding	Elicit patient's understanding of laparoscopic cholecystectomy.	0 1 –
	'I understand that you are here today for a laparoscopic cholecystectomy. What do you understand by this procedure and what it entails'?	
Concerns	Elicit patient's concerns of the operation; i.e. post-op pain and open surgery.	0 1 –
	'Do you have any particular concerns about the operation? Are there any matters you wish me to clarify'?	
	EXPLAINING	
Operation	Explain to the patient what the operation is.	0 1 –
	'The laparoscopic cholecystectomy is a procedure performed to remove your gallbladder. A small camera and two prongs will be inserted into your tummy so that the surgeon can cut out and remove your gallbladder. The operation will leave only three small scars once completed'.	
Fasting	Explain to the patient the need to fast before the operation.	0 1 –
	'If you are having the operation in the morning we advise that you do not eat or drink anything after midnight. Otherwise you should not eat or drink anything six hours prior to the operation'.	
Anaesthetic	Explain to the patient the general anaesthetic and pre-med.	0 1 2
	'When you first come to theatre, you will meet a nurse who will take your details and provide a gown for you to change into. You will be taken into the anaesthetic room where the anaesthetist will prepare you for surgery by giving you medicines through a line in your arm. You will be given injections to relax you and the general anaesthetic, which will make you sleep and not feel any pain during the procedure. The anaesthetist will monitor you continuously throughout the procedure to make sure you are well'.	

STAGE	KEY POINTS AND ACTIONS	SCORE
Recovery	Explain that the patient will be transferred to recovery.	0 1 –
	'Once the operation is complete, you will be transferred into a recovery room where you will awake. Don't be startled by the change in surroundings! You may feel ill or groggy once you are awake and will be given medicines to reduce any pain or sickness you may feel'.	

COMPLICATIONS

Open Surgery	Explain to the patient the possibility of having open surgery.	0 1 –
	'During the operation, the surgeon may decide that it is safer for you to have open surgery rather than continuing with the camera. Although this is a rare occurrence, you should be aware of its possibility'.	
Bile Duct	Explain to the patient the possibility of damage to the bile duct.	0 1 –
	'Although this procedure is performed routinely, there is a small possibility of complications. During gallbladder removal, the bile duct may be damaged or injured and this may lead you to develop jaundice'.	
Infection	Explain to the patient the possibility of infection.	0 1 –
	'There is also a small possibility of the skin around the operation site becoming infected, or more rarely an infection inside the abdomen. If you notice continuing pain, discharge, or fevers you should seek medical help'.	
Pain	Explain to the patient the possibility of continuing pain.	
	'As with any operation, there is a possibility that you may still experience pain a few weeks after the operation. You should take the painkillers which we will prescribe you when you are discharged home. If you are ever concerned about the pain you should contact your GP'.	
Bleeding	Explain to the patient the possibility of post-op bleeding.	0 1 –
	'For a few days after the operation you may notice a discharge from the operation site. This is entirely normal and we will send you home when this has stopped. However, if you notice blood coming out of the wound, although this may be normal, we recommend that you contact your GP'.	

POST-OP ADVICE

Clips	Explain to the patient the use of surgical clips.	0 1 –
	'The surgeon may insert some metal clips into the operation site which will need removing. This should normally be performed seven to ten days after the procedure by your GP's practice nurse'.	
Work	Explain to the patient issues regarding work.	0 1 –
	'Generally speaking, we advise people to return to work two weeks after the operation. By that time the wound should have healed well and the pain should be minimal if present'.	

FINISHING OFF

Understanding	Check whether the patient has understood what has been explained.	0 1 –
Questions	Encourage patient to ask questions and deal with them appropriately.	0 1 –
Summary	Provide appropriate summary to the patient about the procedure.	0 1 –

STAGE	KEY POINTS AND ACTIONS	SCORE
Respond	Acknowledge patient's feelings and react positively to them.	0 1 –

EXAMINER'S EVALUATION

Overall assessment of explaining laparoscopic cholecystectomy	0 1 2 3 4 5

Total mark out of 23

06.10 INHALER TECHNIQUE

INSTRUCTIONS You are in General Practice. Mr F has attended your clinic on several occasions with breathlessness and a wheeze. Following a markedly reduced peak flow you postulate that he may be asthmatic. Explain to the patient his diagnosis and show him how to use his salbutamol inhaler.

STAGE	KEY POINTS AND ACTIONS	SCORE
	INTRODUCTION	
Introduction	Introduce yourself. Elicit name, age, and occupation. Establish rapport.	0 1 –
Understanding	Elicit patient's understanding of asthma.	0 1 –
	'I understand that you have had symptoms of breathlessness and wheezing for a while. Following the peak flow test, I suspect that you may be asthmatic. Could you please tell me what you understand by the term asthma'?	
Explain	Clarify to the patient how salbutamol relieves symptoms of asthma.	0 1 2
	'Asthma is a lung condition which is characterised by difficulty in breathing. People who have asthma may have sensitive airways which react by narrowing when they become irritated, making it difficult for air to move in or out. This narrowing causes the symptoms you have been experiencing. In order for us to relieve this, we use the drug salbutamol, which is delivered from an inhaler that allows us to deliver the medicine exactly where it is needed. Salbutamol works by opening up the air passages in the lungs so that air can flow into the lungs more freely. Today I wish to demonstrate how to use an asthma inhaler with the correct technique. Do you have any questions about what I have said'?	
Position	Ensure that the patient is sitting up in the chair.	0 1 –
	THE PROCEDURE	
Inhaler	Choose the correct (blue) inhaler and show patient how to shake the inhaler before use.	0 1 –
Exhale	Advise the patient to fully exhale air from their lungs, removing the cap from the inhaler in the process.	0 1 –
Inhalation	Demonstrate to the patient how to co-ordinate inhaler whilst taking a deep breath in.	0 1 –
Hold Breath	Advise the patient to hold their breath for ten seconds after taking the inhaler.	0 1 –

STAGE	KEY POINTS AND ACTIONS	SCORE
Comprehension	Check whether the patient has understood the process and ask to demonstrate.	0 1
Repeat	Advise the patient that he has to wait at least a minute before repeating the process and taking another puff of the inhaler.	0 1

'This blue inhaler is the salbutamol inhaler. The medicine is held in the metal canister and is released when it is pressed. Before you take the inhaler, it is important to shake it well so that the medicine is mixed with the gas propellant. Exhale fully before using the inhaler, and remove the cap. Hold the inhaler between your thumb and index finger with your index finger on the canister. Make a seal with your lips around the mouth of the inhaler. As you press down on the inhaler, it is important to simultaneously start taking a deep breath in. Close your mouth and hold your breath for at least ten seconds. If you feel that you need another dose of the medicine, it is important that you wait at least a minute. This will allow the medicine to mix properly again with the propellant. Repeat the whole process again exactly as I mentioned the first time, beginning with shaking it. Are you happy with what I have just explained? Please show me how to use this inhaler'.

EXPLANATION

Side Effects	Explain to the patient the possible side effects of using salbutamol such as fast heart rate, shakiness, or headaches.	0 1
Regularity	Explain to the patient how often the salbutamol inhaler should be taken; i.e. two puffs PRN (as required) up to four times a day.	0 1
Seek Help	Explain to the patient when they should seek help or medical advice.	0 1 2

'The blue inhaler can be used as and when you have your symptoms of wheeze or breathlessness. However, we would initially recommend using a maximum of two puffs four times a day. If you are finding that you need more than this, you may benefit from other medications and it is important that you consult your doctor. Although salbutamol is extremely safe in this form, some patients often experience some unwanted side effects. These may include mild headaches, a fast heartbeat, or feeling shaky. If you are concerned about these please seek medical advice'.

Understanding	Confirm that the patient has understood what you have explained to them. Ask if they have any questions or concerns.	0 1
Follow-up	Mention the need for follow-up to review symptoms.	0 1

EXAMINER'S EVALUATION

Overall assessment of demonstrating inhaler use	0 1 2 3 4 5

Total mark out of 22

06.11 SPACER DEVICE

INSTRUCTIONS You are in General Practice. Mrs G, a 75-year-old woman with a history of rheumatoid arthritis, has recently been diagnosed with asthma. Despite prescribing her a salbutamol inhaler her symptoms of wheeze and breathlessness remain. She attends today complaining of difficulty in using the inhaler.

STAGE	KEY POINTS AND ACTIONS	SCORE		
	INTRODUCTION			
Introduction	Introduce yourself. Elicit name, age, and occupation. Establish rapport.	0	1	–
Understanding	Elicit patient's understanding of asthma and inhalers.	0	1	–
	'I understand that you have been recently diagnosed with asthma and given an inhaler to use. Could you please tell me what you understand by asthma and how you think the inhaler may help you'?			
Concerns	Elicit patient's fears, concerns, and expectations.	0	1	–
	Correctly identify the patient's poor technique due to RA.			
	'Despite taking the inhaler I understand that you are still experiencing symptoms. Can I ask how comfortable you feel with using the inhaler device? Have you had any problems with it'?			
Explain	Explain the need for a spacer device.	0	1	2
	'As you suffer from asthma it is important that you take the salbutamol inhaler to relieve your symptoms. However, I feel you are having some difficulty in using the inhaler correctly due to your rheumatoid arthritis and therefore I would recommend using a spacer device. The spacer gives you greater ease in delivering the medicine to your lungs and eliminates the need to co-ordinate the small inhaler with your breathing. I will now demonstrate how to use this device'.			
	THE PROCEDURE			
Spacer	Choose the two correct opposing ends of the spacer device, assembling it easily and skilfully.	0	1	–
Inhaler	Shake the inhaler and connect to the correct side, releasing two puffs into the spacer device.	0	1	–
Inhalation	Attach mouth with a good seal onto the mouthpiece and inhale and exhale deeply and slowly.	0	1	–

STAGE	KEY POINTS AND ACTIONS	SCORE
Comprehension	Check whether patient has understood the process and ask to demonstrate.	0 1 2
	'This device is known as a volumatic spacer. It consists of these two pieces which slot together easily. On one end is the mouthpiece (sticking out) which also has a release valve and the other end is where the inhaler is to be attached. Once the device is assembled, shake your inhaler well and connect it to the far end. Release two puffs into the spacer. As the spacer has a valve, the medicine will remain inside. Attach your mouth to the nearside, which has the mouthpiece, ensuring you make a tight seal. Breathe in and out deeply and at a slow pace with your mouth still attached. Do this around three to four times. This will ensure that your lungs have taken enough of the medication. Have you understood what I have said? Please could you show me how you would use this spacer device'?	

EXPLANATION

Cleaning	Explain to the patient how to care for and clean the device.	0 1 -
Storage	Explain to the patient how to store the device and how to prevent scratches.	0 1 -
Replacement	Explain to the patient when to replace the spacer device; i.e. between six and twelve months of use.	0 1 -
	'The spacer device should be washed with warm water at least once a week and left to drip dry. You should not use any detergents or materials to dry it since they may create static and reduce the effectiveness of the device. It is also important to store the device in its box in a cool area to prevent scratching. I would recommend changing the device after between six and twelve months regular usage to ensure optimum functioning'.	
Understanding	Confirm that the patient has understood what you have explained to them. Ask if they have any questions or concerns.	0 1 -
Follow-up	Mention the need for follow-up to review symptoms.	0 1 -

EXAMINER'S EVALUATION

Overall assessment of explanation of volumatic spacer usage	0 1 2 3 4 5

Total mark out of 20

06.12 GTN SPRAY

INSTRUCTIONS You are a foundation year House Officer in Cardiology. Mr S, a 45-year-old man, has been diagnosed as having angina brought on by exercise. Today he is going to be discharged from the ward and it is your job to explain to him how and when to use his GTN spray.

STAGE	KEY POINTS AND ACTIONS	SCORE		
	INTRODUCTION			
Introduction	Introduce yourself. Elicit name, age, and occupation. Establish rapport.	0	1	–
Understanding	Elicit patient's understanding of angina and when to use GTN spray.	0	1	–
	'I understand that you were admitted to hospital due to chest pains when exercising. We have found that this is due to stable angina. Have you heard this term before? Could you please tell me what you understand by angina? I am also aware that you have been given a spray to treat the pain. Can you please tell me what you know about the spray'?			
Explain	Explain in clear and simple terms what angina is and how the GTN spray works.	0	1	2
	'Angina is chest pain or discomfort that occurs when your heart is not getting sufficient blood supply. Angina occurs when a small plaque builds up in the arteries supplying the heart, reducing blood flow and oxygen supply to the heart muscle and causing pain. The type of angina you have is known as stable angina because the pain comes only when you are exercising as the heart muscle requires more oxygen'.			
	'The GTN spray works by relaxing the vessels in the body making it easier for the heart to pump blood around the body and as well allows more blood to flow to the heart muscle reducing by-product formation. I will now show you how to use the spray. Do you have any questions before I start'?			
	THE PROCEDURE			
Position	Explain to the patient the need to cease activities and sit down before using the spray.	0	1	–
Shake	Explain to the patient the need to shake the spray well and remove the cap.	0	1	–
Spray	Advise the patient to raise their tongue and deliver two puffs underneath it.	0	1	–
Repeat	Advise the patient to repeat procedure in ten minutes if pain persists.	0	1	–

STAGE	KEY POINTS AND ACTIONS	SCORE
When to Use	Explain to the patient when to use the GTN spray; i.e. when he has chest pain or prophylactically before carrying out any strenuous exercise.	0 1 –
Side Effects	Explain to the patient common side effects of the spray; i.e. lightheadedness, flushing, or dizziness.	0 1 2
Seeking Help	Advise the patient to seek urgent medical help if pain is not resolving fifteen minutes from onset.	0 1 –
	'You should use the spray whenever you experience chest pain or before you carry out any activity that brings on the pain. Before you take the spray you should stop what you are doing and sit down. Shake the spray well and remove the cap. Lift up your tongue and deliver two sharp bursts of the spray, one after the other, underneath the tongue. If the pain is not resolving then you may take another two puffs after ten minutes. If after fifteen minutes the pain is still present, I would call an ambulance or seek medical help urgently. Although the spray is not harmful if used in this way, some people may feel lightheaded, dizzy, or flushed when taking it. That is why we recommend you sit down before using the spray'.	

EVALUATION

Understanding	Confirm that the patient has understood what you have explained to them. Ask if they have any questions or concerns.	0 1 –
Follow-up	Mention the need for follow-up to review symptoms.	0 1 –
Summarise	Provide a brief and appropriate summary of salient points. Thank the patient.	0 1 –

EXAMINER'S EVALUATION

Overall assessment of explaining use of GTN spray	0 1 2 3 4 5

Total mark out of 20

06.13 INSTILLING EYE DROPS

INSTRUCTIONS You are in General Practice. Mr E has attended your clinic with an itchy, gritty, red eye which he has had for two weeks. Give him the appropriate advice and show him how to instil eye drops.

STAGE	KEY POINTS AND ACTIONS	SCORE		
	INTRODUCTION			
Introduction	Introduce yourself. Elicit name, age, and occupation. Establish rapport.	0	1	–
History	Take a brief history eliciting red, sticky, and itchy right eye. No change in vision nor trauma. No allergies.	0	1	–
Diagnosis	Clarify to the patient likelihood of viral infection but possibility of bacterial conjunctivitis.	0	1	–
Transmission	Explain likely infection routes through direct touch or droplets. Elicit young son had similar symptoms one week ago.	0	1	–
Advice	Give appropriate advice to avoid spread by regularly washing hands and by using own towels and pillowcases. Warn that infection may still spread to the other eye despite these precautions.	0	1	2
Treatment	Appropriately recommend chloramphenicol eye drops for affected eye.	0	1	–
	'I understand that you have had symptoms of an itchy and sticky right eye. The likely cause of this is an infection causing conjunctivitis, which explains why your eye is also red. Although the most common cause is viral, often bacteria can cause symptoms as well. Therefore, I wish to start some antibiotic eye drops to help relieve your symptoms. It is important that you take simple precautions to prevent your other eye from becoming infected as well as protecting other members of your family, since this type of conjunctivitis is quite easily spread through touch. Each time you touch your affected eye you should wash your hands thoroughly. You should only dry your hands and face with a towel that should not be used by others and when you sleep you should use a pillowcase which is personal to you'.			
	THE PROCEDURE			
Wash Hands	Advise patient to wash hands thoroughly before instilling eye drops.	0	1	–
Position	Advise patient to stand and look upward with head tilted backwards.	0	1	–

STAGE	KEY POINTS AND ACTIONS	SCORE
Instil	Pull down the eyelid and drop one or two drops into lower lid.	0 1 –
Close	Close eye tightly and seal the medication bottle.	0 1 –
Understanding	Check whether patient understood the process and ask to demonstrate.	0 1 –
Follow-up	Mention the need for medical follow-up if the symptoms are not relieved by two weeks or if there is any change in vision.	0 1 –

'I will now explain how to put the eye drops in your affected eye. Firstly, wash your hands thoroughly. Get the eye drops and check that they are not out of date. Stand up and tilt your head backward. Look up and pull down the bottom eyelid. Take off the cap from the eye drop bottle. Hold the bottle a few centimetres away from your eye, ensuring that the bottle does not touch it. Drop one or two drops into the eyelid and shut your eye; this will help spread the antibiotic all over. Do this four times a day. If your symptoms continue for more than two weeks, or you notice any change in vision, it is important that you seek advice from your medical doctor'.

EXAMINER'S EVALUATION

Overall assessment of explaining how to instil eye drops   0 1 2 3 4 5

Total mark out of 18

06.14 BLOOD PRESSURE MANAGEMENT

INSTRUCTIONS Ms H, a 50-year-old woman, has been recently diagnosed with hypertension. She has booked an appointment with you, her GP, as she wants to know what can be done to control her pressure. Offer her the appropriate advice regarding her blood pressure and suggest possible treatment options.

STAGE	KEY POINTS AND ACTIONS	SCORE
	THE HISTORY	
Introduction	Introduce yourself. Elicit name, age, and occupation. Establish rapport.	0 1 –
Explain	'I understand that you have been recently diagnosed with high blood pressure, is that correct? I would like to ask a few brief questions before I discuss how we can go about reducing your blood pressure'.	0 1 –
Ideas	What do you understand by high blood pressure? Do you have any idea as to what may be causing it?	0 1 –
Concerns	Do you have any issues or concerns you would like to raise regarding your blood pressure?	0 1 –
	ASSOCIATED HISTORY	
Symptoms	Establish whether patient has experienced any symptoms of hypertension such as headaches, vomiting, visual disturbances, or fits.	0 1 –
Duration	How long has the patient been diagnosed with hypertension? Establish whether they have had more than two raised blood pressure readings on two separate occasions.	0 1 –
Risk Factors	Establish the presence of any risk factors which could explain the recent rise in the patient's blood pressure.	0 1 –

Risk Factors for Hypertension

- Smoking
- Alcohol
- Stress
- Weight
- Exercise (lack of)
- Diet (high cholesterol and salt)

STAGE	KEY POINTS AND ACTIONS	SCORE
Medical History	Establish past medical history of the following: angina, MI, CVA, TIA.	0 1
Family History	Establish any family history of hypertension or ischaemic heart disease.	
Drug History	Is patient on any medication for their hypertension? Are they taking those medications (concordance)? If not, why not?	0 1

THE MEDICAL ADVICE

Discussion

Reason	Discuss the possible reasons why the patient's blood pressure may be elevated outlining the presence of contributing risk factors.	0 1
Lifestyle	Stress the importance of reducing associated risk factors of hypertension by performing a number of lifestyle changes. Tailor the advice based upon the risk factors present in the patient.	0 1 2
Smoking	Reduce or stop smoking.	
Diet	Eat a more healthy diet, low in fat and salt.	
Alcohol	Reduce alcohol consumption.	
Exercise	Take regular exercise such as a daily brisk 30 minute walk.	
Weight	Consider weight reduction to BMI 20–25kg/m^2.	
Stress	Advise to alter environment to relieve stress or consult a counsellor or engage in relaxation techniques.	
Investigations	Request to perform a number of investigations in order to identify end-organ damage and those patients with secondary causes of hypertension.	0 1 2
	Urine: Diabetes (glucose), renal disease (haematuria, proteinuria). U&Es: Renal impairment, hyperaldosteronism. ECG: Myocardial ischaemia, left ventricular hypertrophy, angina. CXR: Cardiac failure, coarctation of aorta (in young hypertensives).	
Treatment	Take into account the class and dose of the medication the patient is already on. Consider either increasing the dose, changing the class or adding another drug of a different class if appropriate.	0 1

British Hypertensive Society Guidelines

It is important to take into account the NICE Hypertension guidelines. NICE defines hypertension as Stage I or Stage II

- Stage I – clinic blood pressure 140/90mmHg or ambulatory blood pressure monitoring > 135/65mmHg
- Stage II – clinic blood pressure 160/100mmHg and ambulatory blood pressure monitoring 150/95mmHg

Medication is needed if:

1. Stage 1 hypertension in any under 80 plus any of: target organ damage, established cardiovascular disease, renal disease, diabetes, 10-year cardiovascular risk equivalent to 20% or more.
2. Stage II hypertension in age group.

Aims of treatment

1. People aged under 80 years, clinic blood pressure lower than 140/90mmHg, ambulatory blood pressure lower than 135/85mmHg

2. People aged over 80 years, clinic blood pressure lower than 150/90mmHg, ambulatory blood pressure lower than 145/85mmHg

Medication algorithm

1. Step 1 –
   a. Under 55 – ACE inhibitor
   b. Over 55 or Afro-Caribbean background- Calcium channel antagonist

2. Step 2 –
   a. Ace inhibitor + Calcium channel antagonist

3. Step 3 –
   a. Ace inhibitor + Calcium channel antagonist + thiazide-like diuretic

4. Step 4 –
   a. ACE inhibitor + Calcium channel antagonist + thiazide-like diuretic + Spironolactone

Medications   0   1   2

Medications	Contraindications	Side effects
ACE inhibitors	Renal artery stenosis	First dose hypotension, dry cough, hyperkalaemia
Beta blockers	(Mnemonic: AB) Asthma*, Block (heart block), COPD*, Diabetes mellitus, (*these are only relative contraindications and can be tolerated quite well in practice)	Bradycardia, bronchospasm, hypotension
Calcium antagonists		Bradycardia, headaches, ankle oedema
Diuretics (thiazide-like diuretic), loop diuretics in renal disease		Hyponatraemia, hypokalaemia
Spironolactone	Hyperkalaemia	

http://pathways.nice.org.uk/pathways/hypertension#path=view%3A/pathways/hypertension/antihypertensive-drug-treatment.xml&content=view-node%3Anodes-step-3-ace-inhibitor-or-angiotensin-ii-receptor-blocker-calcium-channel-blocker-thiazide-like-diuretic

STAGE	KEY POINTS AND ACTIONS	SCORE
Interactions	Advise to avoid NSAIDs, steroids, OCP (or other oestrogen containing drug) which can be responsible for elevating blood pressure levels.	0 1
Understanding	Check for patient's understanding of diagnosis and management.	0 1
Questions	Respond appropriately to any patient's questions.	0 1
Follow-up	Arrange an appropriate follow-up by organising another appointment in several weeks' time.	0 1
Leaflet	Offer to provide more information in the form of a handout. Give contact details for other sources of advice such as a dietician or hypertensive support groups.	0 1
Finishing Off	Thank the patient and answer any possible questions.	

EXAMINER'S EVALUATION

Overall assessment of blood pressure management advice	0 1 2 3 4

Total mark out of 27

06.15 DIABETIC MANAGEMENT

INSTRUCTIONS Mr B has been recently diagnosed with diabetes. He has booked an appointment with you, his GP, as he wants to know what can be done to control his high BMs. Offer him the appropriate advice regarding diabetic management and suggest possible treatment options.

STAGE	KEY POINTS AND ACTIONS	SCORE
	THE HISTORY	
Introduction	Introduce yourself. Elicit name, age, and occupation. Establish rapport.	0 1 –
Explain	'I understand that you have been diagnosed with diabetes; is that correct? Before I discuss with you how we can bring your diabetes under control, I would like to ask you some questions. Is that ok with you'?	0 1 –
Ideas	'What do you understand by the term diabetes'?	0 1 –
Concerns	'Do you have any issues or concerns you would like to raise regarding diabetes'?	0 1 –
	ASSOCIATED HISTORY	
Symptoms	Establish whether the patient has noticed any symptoms of diabetes such as polyuria (urinary frequency), polydipsia (thirst), weight loss, and lethargy. Also elicit evidence of diabetic complications.	0 1 2
	Complications of Diabetes	
	• Abdominal pain & vomiting	
	• Diabetic ketoacidosis	
	• Visual disturbances	
	• Retinopathy	
	• Numbness or pins and needles	
	• Neuropathy	
	• Nocturia, polyuria	
	• Nephropathy	
	• Foot ulcers	
	• Vascular disease	
Duration	How long has the patient been diagnosed with diabetes? Establish what type (1 or 2 or insulin/non-insulin dependent) diabetes the patient has.	0 1 –

STAGE	KEY POINTS AND ACTIONS	SCORE
Risk Factors	Establish the presence of any risk factors which could explain the lack of control of the patient's diabetes.	0　1　2
	Risk Factors for Diabetes	
	• Smoking	
	• Alcohol	
	• Weight (obesity)	
	• Diet (high cholesterol and salt)	
Medical History	Establish past medical history of the following: IHD, MI, CVA, TIA.	
Family History	Establish any family history of diabetes.	
Drug History	How is their diabetes managed: diet only/diet and medication/insulin? If they are on medication establish which type of medication. If they are on insulin establish which type of insulin, when they take it and what the dosage is. Are they taking their medications as directed (concordance)? If not, why not (e.g. side effects)?	0　1　–

THE MEDICAL ADVICE

Discussion

STAGE	KEY POINTS AND ACTIONS	SCORE
Reason	Discuss the possible reasons why the patient's diabetic control may be poor outlining the presence of contributing risk factors.	0　1　–
Lifestyle	Stress the importance of reducing any associated risk factors of diabetes by performing a number of lifestyle changes. Tailor the advice based upon the risk factors present in the patient.	0　1　2
Smoking	Reduce or stop smoking.	
Alcohol	Reduce alcohol consumption.	
Weight	Consider weight reduction to BMI 20–25kg/m^2.	
Exercise	Engage in regular aerobic physical activity, such as brisk walking for at least 30 minutes on most days.	
Diet	Eat a more healthy diet low in fat and sugar. Complex carbohydrates, such as bread, pasta, and rice, are good as they release energy slowly. However, saturated fats, such as pastries and fast food, are bad. Reserve cakes and sweets for special occasions.	
Concordance	Emphasise the importance of concordance with medications in order to control their diabetes and avoid future complications.	0　1　2
	Short & Long Term Complications of Diabetes	
	Short term	
	• Life threatening complications:	
	Ketoacidosis and hyperosmolar non-ketotic acidosis	
	Long term	
	• Irreversible long-term damage to the body:	
	Damage to your eyes, kidneys, and nerves; increased risk of strokes, heart attacks	

STAGE	KEY POINTS AND ACTIONS	SCORE
	Monitoring	
BM Testing	Emphasise the need to keep a diary of blood glucose measurements. Perform self-tests on two days per week, four times per day. Take this diary to all your doctor's appointments.	0 1 –
	Emergencies	
Hypoglycaemia	'If you become increasingly hungry or sweaty and notice your heart beat, this could be because your blood sugar levels are low. Start sipping a glass of sugary water until you feel better. It may be a good idea for you to keep a sugary drink with you at all times. If these feelings persist, or if you start to feel drowsy, take yourself immediately to A&E'.	0 1 2
	Additional Points	
Medication	Remind the patient to always take their medication even if they miss a meal or are feeling ill as missing a dose often results in diabetic ketoacidosis.	0 1 –
Understanding	Check for patient's understanding of diagnosis and management.	0 1 –
Questions	Respond appropriately to patient's questions.	0 1 –
Follow-up	Arrange an appropriate follow-up; i.e. with the diabetic nurse/dietician.	0 1 –
Leaflet	Offer to provide them with more information in the form of a handout. Give contact details for other sources of advice such as a dietician or diabetic support groups.	0 1 –
Finishing Off	Thank the patient and answer any questions.	

EXAMINER'S EVALUATION

Overall assessment of diabetic management advice	0 1 2 3 4 5

Total mark out of 28

06.16 WARFARIN THERAPY

INSTRUCTIONS Ms K has been admitted to the hospital following experiencing shortness of breath and an irregular heartbeat. She has been recommended to commence warfarin by the cardiologist. As the foundation year House Officer in Medicine, you have been asked to explain this to Ms K and deal with her ensuing questions.

STAGE	KEY POINTS AND ACTIONS	SCORE
	THE HISTORY	
Introduction	Introduce yourself. Elicit name, age, and occupation. Establish rapport.	0 1 –
Explain	'I understand that because of the symptoms you presented with, the cardiologist has recommended you should be started on warfarin, is that correct? Before I begin explaining a bit more about warfarin, I would like to ask you some questions. Is that ok'?	0 1 –
Ideas	'What do you understand by warfarin and what it is used for? Are you aware of any of the side effects of warfarin'?	0 1 –
Concerns	'Do you have any issues or concerns you would like to raise regarding your treatment with warfarin'?	0 1 –
	ASSOCIATED HISTORY	
Reason	'Do you know why you are being treated with warfarin'? Establish if the patient has atrial fibrillation, DVT, PE, TIAs, rheumatic heart disease or a prosthetic (metallic) heart valve.	0 1 –
Suitability	'In order to assess your suitability for warfarin, I would like to ask you some questions about your general health'.	0 1 2
	Checking Warfarin Suitability	
	'Are you on any medication? Are you pregnant or breastfeeding? Have you ever had a stroke? Or undertaken a recent operation? Do you have stomach ulcers? Do you suffer from hypertension? Do you have any heart infections (SBE)'?	

STAGE	KEY POINTS AND ACTIONS	SCORE

THE MEDICAL ADVICE

Taking Warfarin

Explanation	'Warfarin is a drug that thins your blood and makes it less likely to clot. The reason you are taking it is because you are suffering from a condition that makes you more likely to form clots'.	0	1	–
Side Effects	'The possible side effects of warfarin treatment include jaundice, skin rashes, hair thinning (alopecia), diarrhoea, bleeding, nausea, and vomiting'.	0	1	–
Toxicity	Warn about symptoms of over-anticoagulation; i.e. bleeding.	0	1	–
	'If you notice any prolonged bleeding or blood in the urine, do not take another dose of warfarin; inform your doctor immediately'.			
Precautions	'When you are on warfarin it is important to take a number of precautions'.			
Trauma	Take precautions at work and during hobbies. It is important to avoid contact sports.	0	1	–
Alcohol Intake	Excessive alcohol may increase the effect of anticoagulants and increase the risk of bleeding. You should not take more than two drinks each day.	0	1	–
Diet	Avoid large changes to your diet especially foods containing vitamin K, such as liver and green vegetables, without first discussing these with your doctor.			
Pregnancy	Warfarin is dangerous during pregnancy especially in the first trimester. If you think that you are at risk of being pregnant, stop taking the warfarin and see your GP immediately.			

Drugs	**Analgesia** NSAIDs are not safe (e.g. Ibuprofen, Diclofenac). Paracetamol is safe.	0	1	2
	Interactions Explain that many drugs may interact with warfarin leading to side effects including bleeding.			
	OTC drugs You should always check with the pharmacist to see if it is safe to take over-the-counter medications along with warfarin.			

Regular Blood Tests

Reason	'We need to tailor the dose of warfarin to be the right level for you. This means that we need to check how well your blood clots at regular intervals. A number of blood tests may be needed at first; but the number of checks will reduce as the warfarin level in the blood stabilises'.	0	1	–

Warfarin Blood Test Intervals

1 Every day for 1 week
2 Every week for 3 weeks
3 Every month for 3 months
4 Every 8 weeks beyond that

Warfarin Book

INR Book	Check that the patient has a warfarin book and if they do not, give them one.	0	1	–

STAGE	KEY POINTS AND ACTIONS	SCOR
Explain	'In this book we record your dose and the results of your blood clotting test and the INR values, which tell us how thin your blood is. This helps us to keep track of your treatment and modify it as necessary. Your warfarin dose may be altered often until you reach a steady level. You should show this book to any health professional that is treating you'.	0 1
	Additional Points	
Bracelet	'Wear a bracelet if undergoing long-term treatment in case of an emergency or accident so that the doctors are aware of your condition and can treat you accordingly'.	0 1
Dentist	'Also warn the dentist that you are taking warfarin before undertaking any dental procedures'.	0 1
Dose	'Take your dose at the same time each day. Anticoagulants may be taken with or without food. Make a mark on your calendar when you have taken today's dose. If you miss a daily dose, do not take double the next day. Just take your normal dose and inform your doctor for further advice'.	0 1
Concordance	'It is important that you do not suddenly stop taking warfarin without seeking advice first from your GP or doctor'.	0 1
Understanding	Check for patient's understanding of diagnosis and management.	0 1
Questions	Respond appropriately to patient's questions.	0 1
Leaflet	Offer to give them more information in the form of a handout. Advise that the warfarin book contains much of the information you have mentioned.	0 1
Finishing Off	Thank the patient and answer any possible questions.	

EXAMINER'S EVALUATION	
Overall assessment of warfarin therapy advice	0 1 2 3 4
Total mark out of 31	

06.17 STEROID THERAPY

INSTRUCTIONS Mrs N has had pain, stiffness, and problems using her arms for many months. A recent ESR was raised at 100. The consultant rheumatologist has written to you suggesting that she should commence long-term steroids. You have arranged for Mrs N to visit you today to explain this and deal with her questions.

STAGE	KEY POINTS AND ACTIONS	SCORE		
	THE HISTORY			
Introduction	Introduce yourself. Elicit name, age, and occupation. Establish rapport.	0	1	–
Explain	'I understand that you recently saw a specialist doctor regarding the problems with your arms. The doctor has written to me advising that you should be started on steroid therapy. Before I begin explaining what it entails, I would like to ask a few brief questions'.	0	1	–
Ideas	'What do you understand by steroid therapy and what it does? Are you aware of any of the side effects of steroids'?	0	1	–
Concerns	'Do you have any issues or concerns you would like to raise regarding steroid treatment'?	0	1	–
	ASSOCIATED HISTORY			
Reason	'Do you know why you have been prescribed steroids'?	0	1	–
	Establish if the patient has asthma, rheumatoid arthritis, inflammatory bowel disease, systemic lupus erythematosus, or polymyalgia rheumatica.			
Dose	'Do you know the dose of steroid treatment you are on'?	0	1	–
Medical History	'Do you suffer from epilepsy, osteoporosis, diabetes, or hypertension? Do you have any problems with bleeding excessively? Have you ever had tuberculosis or chickenpox? Have you ever suffered from stomach ulcers'?	0	1	2
Drug History	'Are you taking any painkillers such as ibuprofen (increases risk of peptic ulceration)? Are you on any other medication? Do you have any drug allergies'?	0	1	–
Social History	'Do you smoke or drink alcohol'?	0	1	–

STAGE	KEY POINTS AND ACTIONS	SCORE

THE MEDICAL ADVICE

Taking Steroids

Explanation	'Steroids are substances that are naturally produced in the body (joints, lung, and bowel) and help to reduce inflammation and swelling. They can also be made artificially and used as drugs. Many people take and use steroid tablets for a health problem they have. It is important to understand that these steroids are different to the ones that athletes and body builders take which are known as anabolic steroids and act differently on the body'.	0 1 2
Side Effects	'As with all medications there are side effects which I would like to discuss with you. Such side effects are more likely to occur in people taking higher doses over a longer period of time; i.e. between 2 and 3 months. Some of these may include . . .'	
Infection	'Due to the immunosuppressive properties of steroids, avoid contact with people with chickenpox or shingles'.	0 1 –
Increased BP	'Taking steroids causes your blood pressure to rise. Have your blood pressure monitored regularly'.	0 1 –
Diabetes	'You may notice that you feel thirsty or are passing urine more frequently. If this happens consult your GP'.	
Osteoporosis	'Steroids may cause thinning of bones. We can offer calcium and Vitamin D supplements to build bone strength or bisphosphonate therapy to counter this effect. In females, HRT may be recommended to those at risk'.	0 1 –
Weight Gain	'You may notice fullness around the face and an increase in your appetite'.	0 1 –
Skin Thinning	'You may bruise more easily than normal'.	0 1 –
Mood Change	'Steroids may make you feel irritable and depressed'.	
Dyspepsia	'Steroids may make you experience indigestion or stomach upsets'.	

Steroid Card

Blue Card	Check that the patient has a blue steroid card and if not, provide one.	0 1 –
	'To inform doctors what steroids you are on and give guidance so they can keep side effects to a minimum, you must show this card to any doctor or nurse who is involved in your treatment'.	

Additional Points

Bracelet	'Wear a steroid bracelet if undergoing long-term treatment in case of any emergency or accident so that the doctors are aware of your condition and can treat you accordingly'.	0 1 –
Avoid	If the patient smokes or drinks they should cut down when on steroids. Patients should avoid ibuprofen analgesics.	0 1 2
	'It is important not to take any analgesics like ibuprofen without discussing with doctors first, since they increase the risk of stomach ulceration. You should also reduce the amount you smoke or drink whilst you are taking the steroid medication'.	
Concordance	Explain that it is extremely dangerous to suddenly stop taking steroids for periods at a time (can lead to Addisonian crisis). This risk exists if the patient is taking steroids for more than three weeks or taking a dose of more than 40mg.	0 1 2

STAGE	KEY POINTS AND ACTIONS	SCORE
Understanding	Check for patient's understanding of diagnosis and management.	0 1 –
Questions	Respond appropriately to patient's questions.	0 1 –
Leaflet	Offer to give the patient more information in the form of a handout. Advise that the steroid card contains much of the information you have mentioned.	0 1 –
Finishing Off	Thank the patient and answer any possible questions.	

EXAMINER'S EVALUATION

Overall assessment of long-term steroid treatment advice	0 1 2 3 4 5

Total mark out of 31

06.18 EPILEPTIC STARTING A FAMILY

INSTRUCTIONS Mrs Michaels, a long-term epileptic, has recently married and wishes to start a family. She has booked in to your GP clinic to speak with you. Offer the patient appropriate advice and deal with any relevant concerns.

STAGE	KEY POINTS AND ACTIONS	SCORE
	THE HISTORY	
Introduction	Introduce yourself. Confirm name, age, and occupation. Establish rapport.	0 1 -
Purpose	Establish why the patient has attended the practice.	0 1 -
	Elicit Patient's Understanding	
Ideas	'What do you understand of the difficulties of having a child whilst on anti-epileptic medication? Has anything already been explained to you'?	0 1 -
Concerns	'Do you have any particular worries or concerns regarding having a child as an epileptic'?	0 1 -
Expectations	'Is there anything in particular you would like to know from me? How would you like me to help you today'?	0 1 -
	Brief History	
Epilepsy	Elicit when patient was diagnosed with epilepsy and what type; e.g. grand mal.	0 1 -
Fits	Elicit how often patient fits, for how long, and when the last fit was.	0 1 -
Medication	Elicit what anti-epileptic medication the patient is taking.	0 1 -
	Explanation of Problem	
Pregnancy	Explain the issues relating to having a child in an epileptic in terms the patient understands and avoid using jargon.	0 1 -
	'Your epilepsy seems to be under reasonable control with the medication you are currently on. For this reason we recommend you carry on taking medicine during the pregnancy to minimise the risk of fitting. The frequency of your fits may change during your pregnancy; however most commonly they remain the same'.	

STAGE	KEY POINTS AND ACTIONS	SCORE
Off Medication	Explain in simple terms what effect stopping medicines may have.	0 1 2
	'If you decide to stop taking your medications whilst you are pregnant you have an increased chance of fitting. Having a fit during pregnancy can be extremely harmful to the baby and may even cause you to miscarry. You also risk falling, hitting your head, or injuring yourself'.	
On Medication	Explain in simple terms and accurately the risks to the foetus associated with anti-epileptic medication.	0 1 2
	'I must warn you that taking epileptic medications during pregnancy carries a small but significant risk of causing defects to the unborn child. Using the anti-epileptic drug carbamazepine carries a 1% risk of the child having spina bifida or other associated anomalies. In addition to this, because of how the medication works, some babies are prone to bleed more than normal later in pregnancy. Although you may feel that this is a risk you do not wish to take for your unborn child, I must stress once again that the risk to your baby from not taking your medicines is far greater than from taking the medications'.	
Reassurance	Pace the information appropriately. Reassure the patient when explaining complications.	0 1 –
	'Although I have told you some of the problems that taking anti-epileptic drugs may cause to your child, we have a number of ways that help prevent their complications'.	
	Management	
Complications	Advise patient of ways that can reduce complication rates; i.e. use of carbamazepine, reduce multiple agents to a single drug, give prophylactic folate, and intramuscular Vitamin K.	0 1 2
	'The first way to reduce the risk of complications is to try and reduce the number of your anti-epileptic medications to a single agent. We normally use carbamazepine, because it is the safest to take during pregnancy and is less likely to induce changes in the unborn child. You will be referred to a consultant neurologist who will alter your medications as required'.	
	'Secondly, we will try and minimise any deformities in the child by offering you folate 5mg. You should take this daily, three months before trying to get pregnant and three months into the pregnancy. This is a higher dose than that which non-epileptic women take and helps prevent spina bifida (problems associated with failure of the spine to close properly)'.	
	'Lastly, in the remaining four weeks of your pregnancy, you will be given Vitamin K tablets which will help prevent any bleeding that the epilepsy tablets may cause. In addition, as is usual practice for the majority of babies born in the UK, the child will receive a Vitamin K injection, which too will help against any bleeding'.	
Neurologist	Mention referring the patient to a neurologist for follow-up and alteration of medication.	
Understanding	Check patient's understanding before moving on.	0 1 –
	'I know that I have spoken a lot already. Are you happy that you understand all of what I have told you? Do you have any questions'?	

STAGE	KEY POINTS AND ACTIONS	SCORE

What Happens Next?

Medical Team Mention the multidisciplinary team who will be involved in patient care. `0  1`

'Your care will involve a number of different health professionals including a neurologist, midwife, and GP and will be headed by a consultant obstetrician. You will be seen more frequently in antenatal clinics to ensure that all things are progressing smoothly'.

US Scans Explain that serial ultrasounds may be performed. `0  1`

'In addition to this, we will be performing regular ultrasounds to ensure that the baby is growing well and that no abnormalities are present'.

Delivery Explain the need for the delivery to take place in hospital. `0  1`

'Provided all things go well, we expect the delivery to take place in the hospital under the supervision of the obstetrician. The baby may need to be taken to the Special Care Baby Unit for routine tests and checks but this will be discussed with you nearer the time'.

Post Birth Mention that there is a 10% chance the child will develop epilepsy later in life. `0  1`

Breastfeeding Mention that it is safe to breastfeed the child whilst taking anti-epileptics. `0  1`

Questions Encourage patient to ask questions and deal with them appropriately. `0  1`

Summarise Summarise the problem appropriately. Thank the patient and offer patient advice leaflet. Offer follow-up appointment. `0  1`

'I understand that you have had a lot to take in today. A lot of what I have said will be explained to you again by the other health professionals involved in your care. I have with me a leaflet detailing all that we have discussed today which may be of interest to you. Perhaps you wish to discuss this with your partner before making a concrete decision as to when you wish to start a family. You can always come back and see me when you both have come to a final decision'.

EXAMINER'S EVALUATION

Overall assessment of explaining epilepsy and pregnancy `0  1  2  3  4  5`

Total mark out of 29

06.19 BREAKING BAD NEWS

INSTRUCTIONS You are a foundation year House Officer in Rheumatology. Mr B, a 36-year-old man, has had pain and swelling in his joints for a few months. He has attended today seeking the results of a blood test, which confirms rheumatoid arthritis. Explain to the patient what the results mean.

STAGE	KEY POINTS AND ACTIONS	SCORE		
	THE HISTORY			
Introduction	Introduce yourself. Confirm name, age, and occupation. Establish rapport.	0	1	–
Purpose	'What symptoms have you been having recently? Is there anything today I could help you with'?	0	1	–
	Elicit Patient's Understanding			
Understanding	'What have you been told so far? Has anything been explained to you'?	0	1	–
Ideas	'Do you have any idea as to what may be causing your symptoms'?	0	1	–
Concerns	'Do you have any particular worries and concerns about your symptoms'?	0	1	–
Expectations	'Is there anything in particular you would like to know? How would you like me to help you'?	0	1	–
	Breaking Bad News			
Blood Results	Break the bad news empathically, using pauses where appropriate. Information is paced with good use of body language.	0	1	–
	'The results of the blood tests that you had recently are back. Unfortunately, I am afraid it is more serious than we hoped. Your symptoms have been going on for a while now and you were particularly concerned how this would affect your work. I am sorry to have to tell you that your test indicates that you have rheumatoid arthritis (RA)'.			

STAGE	KEY POINTS AND ACTIONS	SCOR
Explain RA	Explain the diagnosis in simple terms the patient understands.	0 1
	'Would you like me to explain what the disease means? RA is a condition that affects your joints. For an unknown reason, your body begins to attack the linings in the joint causing destruction which results in pain and swelling. Although at present we cannot cure the disease we can delay its progress and control the symptoms'.	
Management	Explain the management options in simple terms.	0 1
	'There are a number of treatment options available. We can give you medication to slow the disease down. Other treatments can reduce the symptoms. We will make a follow-up appointment to monitor you and address any further questions you have'.	
Questions	'Do you have any questions about what I have told you? Is there anything that still concerns you? Would you like any more information'?	0 1
Understanding	'I know you have had a lot to take in today. Please could you tell me what you understand by your condition'?	0 1
Summarise	'I am sorry to have had to break the news to you. It must have been quite a shock to you. I suggest you think about what I said and we can discuss things further when you come back in a month's time'.	0 1
	COMMUNICATION SKILLS	
Rapport	Establish and maintain rapport throughout interview.	0 1
Listening	Demonstrate interest and concern in what the patient says. Listen to the patient empathically.	0 1
Pauses	Demonstrate the use of pacing of information and use appropriate pauses. Allow the patient to speak his feelings freely and without interruption.	0 1
Verbal Cues	Use non-verbal and verbal cues; i.e. tone and pace of voice, nodding head aptly where appropriate.	0 1

EXAMINER'S EVALUATION		
Overall assessment of breaking bad news	0 1 2 3 4	
Role player's assessment	0 1 2 3 4	
Total mark out of 28		

CLINICAL CASES

You are a foundation year House Officer in Medicine. Ms T, a 25-year-old woman, has had bouts of poor vision and tingling in the lower limbs for the past few months. She had a diagnosed optic neuritis two months ago. She has attended today seeking the results of an MRI, which confirms multiple sclerosis. Explain to the patient what the diagnosis means.

You are a foundation year House Officer in Medicine of the Elderly. You have been asked to see Mrs Beakers who is a heavy smoker. Her notes tell you that she was admitted two days ago for weight loss and shortness of breath. Her C shows a probable lung primary. Explain to the patient what the results mean.

06.20 ANGRY PATIENT

INSTRUCTIONS You are a foundation year House Officer in Accident & Emergency. Mr James has been in the waiting area for two hours and is becoming aggressive and demanding to see a doctor. There are still three patients waiting before him. The Charge Nurse has given you the task of speaking to the patient and dealing with his issues.

STAGE	KEY POINTS AND ACTIONS	SCORE
	THE HISTORY	
Introduction	Introduce yourself. Obtain patient's name.	0 1 –
Rapport	Attempt to establish rapport with the patient through the use of appropriate eye contact. Maintain appropriate body language and open posture throughout interview.	0 1 –
	THE PROBLEM	
Problem	Elicit the main problems and concerns of the patient.	0 1 –
	'I am one of the doctors here. I understand that you have been waiting to see a doctor for a while. What seems to be the problem'?	
Ideas	'Do you have any idea as to why you have had to wait so long'?	0 1 –
Concerns	'Do you have any particular concerns regarding your wait'?	0 1 –
Expectations	'Is there anything in particular you would like to know'?	
	THE SOLUTION	
Respond	Recognise that the patient is angry and respond appropriately. Remain non-confrontational, calm, and non-dismissive at all times.	0 1 2
	'I am sorry that you have been waiting so long and that you feel the way you do. We assess patients according to their medical need. Although there are three patients in front of you, we are working as best as we can in the circumstances. You will be seen as quickly as possible'.	
Reflection	Reflect back to the patient checking understanding.	0 1 –
Questions	Encourage and respond to patient's questions.	0 1 –

STAGE	KEY POINTS AND ACTIONS	SCORE
Management	Come to an agreed negotiated conclusion.	0 1 2
	'I must reiterate once again that we are sorry that you have had to wait so long. I understand that you are in pain and as we have agreed I will ensure that we give you some pain relief before a doctor comes to fully assess you. You will be seen as soon as your turn arrives. Are you happy with this'?	

COMMUNICATION SKILLS

STAGE	KEY POINTS AND ACTIONS	SCORE
Rapport	Establish and maintain rapport throughout the interview.	0 1 –
Listening	Demonstrate interest and concern in what the patient says. Listen empathically.	0 1 –
Pauses	Demonstrate the use of pacing of information and use appropriate pauses. Allow the patient to speak his feelings freely and without interruption.	0 1 –
Verbal Cues	Use non-verbal and verbal cues; i.e. tone and pace of voice, nodding head aptly where appropriate.	0 1 –

EXAMINER'S EVALUATION

Overall assessment of managing angry patient	0 1 2 3 4 5
Role player's assessment	0 1 2 3 4 5
Total mark out of 25	

CLINICAL CASES

You are a foundation year House Officer in General Practice. Ms M, a 35-year-old woman, attends the surgery for an appointment she believes she had booked, and has taken time off work to attend today. The receptionist can find no record of the appointment and fails to reassure Ms M, who is getting increasingly angry. You are called to deal with the situation.

You are a foundation year House Officer in Medicine of the Elderly. You have been looking after Mrs B, an elderly woman who was admitted 4 days previously with lower lobe pneumonia. She has moved wards three times and now is being transferred into a side-room because gentamicin-resistant E. coli was grown from sputum cultures. You have been asked to see Mrs B's relatives, who wish to complain about her treatment.

06.21
NEGOTIATION

INSTRUCTIONS You are in General Practice. Ms B, an Egyptologist, has made an appointment to see you. Interview the patient, eliciting the reason for attendance and negotiate a management plan.

STAGE	KEY POINTS AND ACTIONS	SCORE
	THE HISTORY	
Introduction	Introduce yourself. Confirm name, age, and occupation.	0 1 –
Rapport	Attempt to establish rapport with the patient through the use of appropriate eye contact. Maintain appropriate body language and open posture throughout interview.	0 1 –
Purpose	Elicit purpose of consultation.	0 1 –
	'I am one of the GPs here. How can I be of help to you today'?	
	NEGOTIATING SKILLS	
Patient's Agenda	Elicit patient's ideas, concerns, and expectations.	0 1 –
	'I understand that things are very difficult for you; you have done the right thing in seeking help regarding your drug habit. I am here to listen and help you. Is there anything specific you wish to discuss with me'?	
Own Agenda	Explain that you do not wish to prescribe more methadone.	0 1 –
	'I am sorry, but as you may know it is normally a specified doctor who prescribes this medication for you. Have you tried contacting them for more medication'?	
Compromise	Negotiate an agreed compromise. Offer alternative medications that may reduce withdrawal symptoms; i.e. benzodiazepines/beta-blockers.	0 1 –
	'Let us think about what you have said and see what I can do for you. There are a number of medications I can offer you that can also work to reduce the symptoms of drug withdrawal which you are experiencing and make you feel better than you are currently. For example, for your shaky feeling and palpitations we can offer beta-blockers to reduce this. For the problems you are having with sleeping or with the excessive feelings of fear we can offer benzodiazepines. Do you think that these options may be of use to you'?	
	RELEVANT HISTORY	
Drug Usage	Elicit current and previous drug usage. What different drugs have they used and their types? Is their drug usage increasing or decreasing?	0 1 –

STAGE	KEY POINTS AND ACTIONS	SCORE		
Treatments	Elicit details of any drug rehabilitation courses they have been on and for how long they have been with them.	0	1	–
Symptoms	Are they experiencing symptoms of withdrawal; i.e. sweating, tremors, fits, agitation, anger, fear, or personality change?	0	1	2
Effect on Life	Elicit any negative social, psychological and financial effects on the patient's life. Enquire about criminality, forensic history and alcohol use.	0	1	–
Questions	Encourage and respond to patient's questions.	0	1	–
Summarise	Summarise what has been agreed and come up with an action plan.	0	1	–

COMMUNICATION SKILLS

Rapport	Establish and maintain rapport throughout interview.	0	1	–
Listening	Demonstrate interest and concern in what the patient says. Show active listening and listen empathically.	0	1	–
Pauses	Demonstrate the use of pacing of information and use appropriate pauses. Allow the patient to speak her feelings freely and without interruption.	0	1	–
Verbal Cues	Use non-verbal and verbal cues; i.e. tone and pace of voice, nodding head aptly where appropriate.	0	1	–

EXAMINER'S EVALUATION

Overall assessment of negotiating request for methadone	0	1	2	3	4	5
Role player's assessment	0	1	2	3	4	5
Total mark out of 27						

CLINICAL CASE

You are a foundation year House Officer in Orthopaedics. Ms B has had lower back pain for the past two weeks since a fall. She has already had an x-ray and blood tests, which were normal. The back pain is still present despite taking neurofen. Ms B attends today demanding an MRI.

06.22

INTERPROFESSIONAL

INSTRUCTIONS You are a newly qualified foundation year House Officer in General Medicine. You have just returned from lunch when the Nurse in Charge hands you the SHO's bleep stating that he is leaving early to study for his MRCP exams in a few weeks. Your SHO has not discussed this with anyone senior. The Consultant is busy in outpatients' and the Registrar is off sick. You notice your SHO emerging from the staff room about to leave.

STAGE	KEY POINTS AND ACTIONS	SCORE
	THE HISTORY	
Introduction	Use an appropriate introduction. Establish rapport.	0 1 –
	'How are your studies going for the MRCP? You seem quite concerned with the exam'.	
Purpose	Explain the reason for the meeting.	0 1 –
	'There is something troubling me and I need to talk to you about it. Could we go somewhere private and discuss this matter'?	
	MENTION PROBLEM	
Explain	Explain in an objective way what the issues and problems are relating to the SHO leaving early.	0 1 –
	Highlight the lack of any further senior support, i.e. Registrar away.	
Concerns	Explain personal concerns and worries of taking responsibility.	0 1 –
	'As you know, I have just recently qualified as a doctor. I do not feel I have sufficient experience in medicine to deal with an emergency without senior support and supervision'.	
Response	Deal with senior's reassurances appropriately and empathically.	0 1 –
	'I understand that these examinations are important for you and require much study. However, I feel that my workload is increasing and I am finding it difficult to cope myself'.	
Offer Advice	Demonstrate understanding of the situation and offer possible solutions.	0 1 –
	'I appreciate that you do need some time off to study for your exams. Perhaps you could speak with the Registrar or the Consultant and arrange some study leave or senior cover'.	

STAGE	KEY POINTS AND ACTIONS	SCORE
Summarise	Give a brief summary to the SHO about what has been discussed. Jointly agree upon a plan of action. Do not collude with the SHO.	0 1 2
	'I am happy that we have had the opportunity to discuss this. As we have agreed, we will go to see the Consultant together tomorrow regarding your educational needs and the need for me to have senior support present. I am sorry I am unable to carry your bleep on this occasion'.	

COMMUNICATION SKILLS

STAGE	KEY POINTS AND ACTIONS	SCORE
Rapport	Establish and maintain rapport throughout interview.	0 1 –
Listening	Demonstrate interest and concern in what the SHO says. Show active listening and listen empathically.	0 1 –
Pauses	Demonstrate the use of pacing of information and use appropriate pauses. Allow the SHO to speak his feelings freely and without interruption.	0 1 –
Verbal Cues	Use non-verbal and verbal cues; i.e. tone and pace of voice, nodding head aptly where appropriate.	0 1 –

EXAMINER'S EVALUATION

Overall assessment of interprofessional negotiation	0 1 2 3 4 5
Role player's assessment	0 1 2 3 4 5
Total mark out of 22	

CLINICAL CASES

You are a foundation year House Officer in Medicine. You have concluded the Consultant ward round and have been told that Mrs S, who was admitted and treated for pyelonephritis, needs another 24 hours of IV antibiotics. The nurse in charge has returned from her break and says due to the bed shortage, the patient should be discharged home with oral antibiotics.

You are providing ward cover as a foundation year House Officer in Surgery. You have written up IV fluids for a dehydrated patient post-op and handed this to the nurse to give them. When you return to the ward five hours later you notice the fluids have not yet been given. The nurse is seated by the nurses' station.

06.23 CROSS CULTURAL

INSTRUCTIONS You have been asked to see Mr H, a 57-year-old toymaker, in outpatients' clinic. He is a newly diagnosed insulin diabetic with a urine infection diagnosed two days ago, for which he is taking antibiotics. The month of Ramadan begins tomorrow and due to his medical illnesses, he is to be advised not to observe the fast.

STAGE	KEY POINTS AND ACTIONS	SCORE
	THE HISTORY	
Introduction	Introduce yourself. Confirm name, age, and occupation.	0 1 –
Rapport	Attempt to establish rapport including appropriate eye contact. Maintain appropriate body language and open posture throughout consultation.	0 1 –
Purpose	Elicit purpose of consultation.	0 1 –
	Elicit Patient's Understanding	
Understanding	'What have you been advised so far? Has anything been explained to you'?	0 1 –
Ideas	'Do you have any idea as to what may be causing your symptoms'?	0 1 –
Concerns	'Do you have any particular concerns or issues with your illness'?	0 1 –
Expectations	'Is there anything in particular you would like to know'?	0 1 –
	Cultural Consideration	
Religion	Correctly identify religion and upcoming month of fasting.	0 1 –
	'You must be quite excited and full of anticipation for the upcoming month of Ramadan'.	
Understanding	Elicit patient's own understanding of his illness and fasting.	0 1 –
	'Do you think there are any issues with your health and the upcoming fast'?	

STAGE	KEY POINTS AND ACTIONS	SCOR

Medical Advice

Explore Issues — Establish the key points of issue. Explain situation in simple terms; i.e. weigh up apparent religious duty versus health problems.   0 1

'Ramadan must be a very difficult time for you especially with an illness that requires regular treatment. How do you think you will manage to control your diabetes during this month? Have you thought about the implications of not taking your medications'?

Correct Advice — Give accurate medical advice.   0 1

'I understand how important this month is for you. However, I must advise you that your medical health may deteriorate if you fail to take your required medication as a result of the fast. This may have serious repercussions for your health not only in the short term, but in the long term as well. As you may well know, diabetes can affect all of your body. In particular it can damage your kidneys, heart, vision, and sense of feeling if not controlled well. From a medical point of view, I must strongly advise you of the necessity of taking your medications in spite of the fast. Would you like to speak with a minister of religion such as an Imam regarding this as I understand there may be some flexibility on medical grounds in not partaking in the fast'?

Understanding — Check patient's understanding of the information provided.   0 1

'I know you have had a lot to take in today. However, I wish to check that you have understood everything we have spoken about today. Please can you tell me now what you understand by your condition and the upcoming fast'?

Questions — Encourage and respond to patient's questions.   0 1

'Do you have any questions about what I have told you? Is there anything that still concerns you'?

Summarise — Give a brief summary to the patient about what has been discussed. Jointly agree on an action plan and conclude the interview.   0 1

'You are a Muslim who has a chronic illness that needs regular treatment. With Ramadan coming up, you will be in a difficult situation and you may not get the treatment your body needs to improve your health. You may wish to consult your religious leader for advice as to whether it is acceptable in these circumstances to compromise your religious duties'.

COMMUNICATION SKILLS

Rapport — Establish and maintain rapport throughout interview.   0 1

Listening — Demonstrate interest and concern in what the patient says. Show active listening and listen empathically.   0 1

Pauses — Demonstrate the use of pacing of information and use appropriate pauses. Allow the patient to speak his feelings freely and without interruption.   0 1

Verbal Cues — Use non-verbal and verbal cues; i.e. tone and pace of voice, nodding head aptly where appropriate.   0 1

STAGE	KEY POINTS AND ACTIONS	SCORE
Respect	Do not be condescending toward the patient's beliefs. Afford appropriate respect and understanding to the subject matter.	0 1 –

EXAMINER'S EVALUATION

Overall assessment of explaining Ramadan and diabetes		0 1 2 3 4 5
Role player's assessment		0 1 2 3 4 5
Total mark out of 32		

CLINICAL CASES

You are a foundation year House Officer in Medicine. Your patient, Mr C, passed away within 24 hours of being admitted with the cause of death still undetermined. He is likely to go for an autopsy which will delay his burial. His mother wishes to speak with you.

You are a foundation year House Officer in Accident & Emergency. Mr Dogan has recently arrived from Turkey and speaks little English. He has had coryzal symptoms for a couple of days and is demanding antibiotics. You have been given the task of dealing with his request. [Hint: you may wish to use a pen and paper.]

06.24 RADIOLOGY REQUEST

INSTRUCTIONS Ms Fitzgerald, 19/6/94, is an obese 20-year-old who has presented with a two-day history of acute pleuritic sounding chest pain. The pain is located on the right side of her chest, worse on deep inspiration and sharp in nature. In addition to the pain, she has experienced breathlessness on exertion and feels that she is breathing faster than usual. She denies any cough, fever, sputum production, or haemoptysis. She is currently on the COC pill and only two days prior returned from Turkey.

STAGE	KEY POINTS AND ACTIONS	SCORE		
	Examiner asks candidate what their working diagnosis is	0	1	2
	The history is consistent with a presentation of acute pulmonary embolism. However, I wish to exclude other diagnoses such as pneumonia, muscle strain, and costochondritis.			
	Examiner asks candidate what radiological investigations they would like to do			
Tests	Candidate mentions full inspiratory CXR followed by CTPA if CXR is normal.	0	1	–
Fills Out Form	Candidate chooses the correct request form (chest x-ray) and fills it out appropriately including:			
Name	Record patient's forename and surname.	0	1	–
DOB	Record patient's date of birth.	0	1	–
Date	Write down today's date.	0	1	–
Status	Write clearly your own name and status; i.e. PRHO.			
Request	Request inspiratory chest film/CTPA.	0	1	–
Details	Provide sufficient clinical details as per findings.	0	1	–

EXAMINER'S EVALUATION							
Overall assessment of preparation of radiology request form	0	1	2	3	4	5
Total mark out of 13							

SAMPLE FORM

St. Somewhere Hospital Trust – RADIOLOGY REQUEST FORM

NHS No: *345498x*

Surname: *Fatima*

Forename: *Osgul*

Title: *Ms*

DOB: *12.01.85*　　Sex: M / F
　　　　　　　　　　　　　　Female

Address:

Tel no:　　　　　　　X-ray no:

Ref Con:

Specialty:

Ward:

Report Dest:

Status NHS / CAT II / Private / Contract / Trial

DEPT USE ONLY

Number of films taken:　　Radiographer:
Radiologist:
Date:　　　　　　　　　　Comments:

ALL PREVIOUS SCANS MUST ACCOMPANY PATIENT

Clinical Details and Previous Surgery:
　2 day history of acute right pleuritic chest pain. Recently returned from Turkey. On the contraceptive pill and obese.

What Questions do you want answered?
　Exclude acute Pulmonary Embolus

Signature: *Dr Anybody*　　　Bleep number:

Print name: *Dr Anybody*　　Date: *110505*

MRI SCAN CRITERIA

Has the patient any of the following:
Pacemaker or artificial valve?　☐
Aneurysm clips?　☐
Metal clips in eyes?　☐
Metal implants?　☐

If you have ticked any of the above, please contact the MRI unit.

I certify I am not pregnant:
Signature:
LMP:

EXAMINATION REQUIRED
Full Inspiratory Chest X Ray

Appointment Date:

Time:　　　　　　　　　Room:

INADEQUATELY FILLED IN FORMS WILL BE RETURNED

06.25 BLOOD REQUEST

INSTRUCTIONS Mr Hugo, 28/9/1984, a 30-year-old businessman, has presented with a three-day history of fevers and severe headaches. The fevers are accompanied with sweating, a feeling of general malaise, and rigors. He has experienced these symptoms since returning from a holiday in East Africa five days ago. He denies any diarrhoea or urinary symptoms. He began taking his chloroquine tablets since returning to the UK and did not use any nets or mosquito repellents whilst on holiday. He has no other medical problems and denies any drug allergies.

STAGE	KEY POINTS AND ACTIONS	SCORE		
	Examiner asks candidate what their working diagnosis is	0	1	2
	The findings are consistent with a possible presentation of malaria infection. But I wish to exclude other possible sources of infection including chest, urine, and GI. I also would wish to exclude acute hepatitis.			
	Examiner asks candidate what investigation they would like to perform			
Tests	Candidate mentions malaria blood test (thick and thin blood films) and chooses appropriate form.	0	1	–
Fills Out Form	Candidate chooses the correct request form (haematology) and fills it out appropriately including:			
Name	Record patient's forename and surname.	0	1	–
DOB	Record patient's date of birth.	0	1	–
Date	Write down today's date.	0	1	–
Request	Tick Malaria box or in additional tests write malarial parasites, thick and thin blood films.	0	1	–
Details	Provide sufficient clinical details including places visited and mention poor prophylactic malarial compliance.	0	1	–
	Examiner informs results are positive for falciparum malaria and asks what they will do			
Consultant	Mention that you will contact the consultant microbiologist or communicable disease specialist.	0	1	–

STAGE	KEY POINTS AND ACTIONS	SCORE

Summary Mention possible need for anti-malarial medication and oral rehydration solution.

EXAMINER'S EVALUATION

Overall assessment of preparation of blood request form   0 1 2 3 4 5

Total mark out of 14

SAMPLE FORM

St. Somewhere or Another Hospital Trust
Clinical Laboratory Services - ROUTINE REQUEST FORM

Surname .... Franks
Forename .... Keith
DOB .... 02.12.75 .... Gender: M / F ...... Male
Hosp No. 344690x

Report Destination ....
Consultant / GP ...... Dr. Anybody
Specialty ...... Accident and Emergency

CLINICAL DETAILS – What questions do you have answered?
3 day history of fevers and headaches
Recently returned from East Africa
ETHNIC ORIGIN ....

TREATMENT   *Poor Chloroquine compliance*
Date of Onset ....
Pregnancy: Y / N ....   Immunocompromised: Y / N ....
EDD   Month   Year   Danger of infection: Y / N ....

CHEMISTRY
Renal profile ☒
Bone profile ☐
Lipid profile ☐
Thyroid profile ☐
Glucose ☐
HbA1C ☐
Uric Acid ☐
Magnesium ☐
Amylase ☐
CRP ☒
CK ☐

HAEMATOLOGY
Malaria Studies ☒
FBC (+ WBC) ☒
ESR ☐
Reticulocytes ☐
Paul Bunnell ☐
Sickle Test ☐
Thalassaemia Screen ☐
G6PD Screen ☐

BLOOD TRANSFUSION
Group & Antibody Screen ☐
Coombs Test ☐
Cross Match
No. of units ....
Date required ....
Time required ....

HAEMATINICS
Vitamin B12 ☐
Folate ☐
Ferritin ☐
Erythropoietin ☐

VIROLOGY
Pre Hep B Vaccine ☐
Post Hep B Vaccine ☐
Rubella Screen (non preg) ☐
ANC Screen ☐
Dialysis Screen ☐
CMV IgG screen ☐
VZV ab screen ☐
Toxoplasma ☐
Syphilis ☐
HIV (+ consent) ☐
IgE ☐
Hep A IgM ☐
Hep B Surface Ag ☐
Hep C IgG ☐
Atypical Pneumonia ☐
Glandular fever ☐
EBV ☐
Tx Screen – Renal ☐
      – Corneal ☐
      – BM ☐

IMMUNOLOGY
Antinuclear antibodies ☐
Rheumatoid Factor ☐
DNA ☐
ENA ☐
ANCA ☐
C3 + C4 ☐
Immune Complex ☐
Thyroid antibodies ☐
Gastric Parietal Cell Abs. ☐
IgE ☐
Liver Disease Profile ☐
Complement activity ☐
CSF Immunochemistry ☐

ENDOCRINE
LH / FSH ☐
Prolactin ☐
Progesterone ☐
Testosterone ☐

HAEMOSTASIS
Clotting Screen ☐
Anticoagulant Therapy ☐
Heparin ☐
Streptokinase ☐

OTHER

THIS REQUEST HAS A 'ROUTINE' PRIORITY
DOCTOR'S NAME (PRINT) ...... Dr Anybody
BLEEP No .... DATE 110505
SIGNATURE ...... Dr Anybody

MALARIA INFECTION

Malaria is a disease mostly of tropical and subtropical areas caused by five genera of Plasmodium—ovale, vivax, malariae, knowlesi and falciparum. Plasmodium protozoa, injected by female anopheles mosquitoes, multiply in red blood cells causing haemolysis, sequestration, and cytokine release. Malaria is one of the most common causes of fever and illness in the tropics with an estimated two million deaths each year. Falciparum malaria, which is the most morbid of the types of the disease, usually presents within the first month of infection. Classically, flu like prodrome is experienced followed by fever and chills with a recurring periodicity of three days. Signs such as anaemia, tachycardia, jaundice, and hepatosplenomegaly can often also be found.

Complications [Mnemonic—CHAPLIN] include **C**erebral manifestations, **H**ypoglycaemia, **A**naemia, **P**ulmonary oedema, **L**actic acidosis, **I**nfection, and **N**ecrosis of renal tubules. Investigations should include full blood count, U&Es, LFTs, thick and thin blood films, and blood cultures. Treatment involves correcting electrolyte imbalance, rehydration, and oral or intravenous administration of quinine (if not from drug resistant area). Malaria is a notifiable disease and it is a legal duty to inform the Consultant in Communicable Disease.

06.26 MICROBIOLOGY REQUEST FORM

INSTRUCTIONS Ms Simmons, 5/5/1992, a twenty-two-year-old office clerk, has presented with a two-day history of burning sensation when she passes urine. She has noticed that her urine is dark and smelly and is going to the toilet more frequently. She also mentions she has a dull suprapubic pain whenever she voids. She denies any nausea or vomiting and has not felt feverish. Past history includes previous UTI. She is currently on the COC pill and is allergic to penicillin.

STAGE	KEY POINTS AND ACTIONS	SCORE		
	Examiner asks candidate what their working diagnosis is	0	1	2
	The history is consistent with a presentation of urinary tract infection.			
	Examiner asks candidate what investigation they would like to perform			
Tests	Candidate mentions urine MC&S and chooses appropriate form.	0	1	–
Fills Out Form	Candidate chooses the correct request form (microbiology) and fills it out appropriately including:			
Name	Record patient's forename and surname.	0	1	–
DOB	Record patient's date of birth.	0	1	–
Date	Write down today's date.	0	1	–
Request	Request urine microscopy, culture, and sensitivity.	0	1	–
Details	Provide sufficient clinical details and mention penicillin allergy.	0	1	–
	Examiner asks candidate to explain to the patient how to collect a urine sample			
Requests MSU	Candidate instructs patient how to deliver a clean catch MSU.	0	1	2

EXAMINER'S EVALUATION							
Overall assessment of preparation of microbiology request	0	1	2	3	4	5
Total mark out of 15							

SAMPLE FORM

St. Somewhere or Another Hospital Trust
Clinical Laboratory Services – MICROBIOLOGY FORM

Surname	Simons
Forename	Fran
DOB	09.07.83 Gender: M / F........ Female
NHS No	808645x

Report Destination ....

Consultant / GP ....Dr. GP. Anybody.......................

Specialty ....General Practice..........................

Other ....

CLINICAL DETAILS

2 day history of dysuria and urinary frequency. Also has had lower abdominal pain. Allergic to Penicillin. ? UTI

TREATMENT

Nil antibiotics

EMERGENCY INVESTIGATIONS

1. MICROBIOLOGY FORM

2. SEND SAMPLE DIRECTLY TO x FLOOR

INVESTIGATIONS – PLEASE TICK

BLOOD CULTURE ☐

URINE ☐ ☒

CSF

SWAB (MC & S) ....

OTHERS .... SPECIFY

Urine Culture for Microscopy.
Culture and Sensitivity.

THIS REQUEST HAS A 'ROUTINE' PRIORITY

DOCTOR'S NAME (PRINT)........Dr Anybody.............

BLEEP No.............................DATE.........11.05.05........

Dr Anybody

SIGNATURE.....................................

06.27 DEATH CERTIFICATION

INSTRUCTIONS Philip Carter is an 85-year-old retiree. Two years ago he was diagnosed with multi-infarct dementia. He has had hypertension and diabetes for the past 15 years. One evening his wife found him collapsed on the floor unable to move his right side. He was brought into hospital and admitted under your team with a diagnosis of stroke. Despite the active efforts of your team, he died six days later. You last saw him the day before he died and there was no sign of pneumonia or heart failure. Complete the death certificate as accurately as possible.

NOTE: The doctor may only complete a death certificate if he or she has been in attendance on the deceased during the last illness and has seen the deceased within 14 days of death or after death. If no doctor meets these criteria the coroner must be informed.

STAGE	KEY POINTS AND ACTIONS	SCORE		
	FILL IN FORM			
Completion	Complete the patient's death certificate, writing in a legible manner. Use a black pen when filling in the form and complete as accurately as possible.	0	1	–
Detail	Fill in the patient's details on the death certificate, including the name of the deceased, the date of death, the age at death, and the place of death.	0	1	2
Last Seen	State the date when the patient was last seen alive by the attending doctor.	0	1	–
Statements	Ring one of the numbers adjacent to the correct statement.	0	1	2
	1. The certified cause of death takes account of information obtained from post mortem.			
	2. Information from post mortem may be available later.			
	3. Post mortem not being held.			
	4. I have reported this death to the coroner for further information.			
	Ring one of the letters adjacent to the correct statement.			
	a) Seen after death by me.			
	b) Seen after death by another medical practitioner but not by me.			
	c) Not seen after death by a medical practitioner.			

STAGE	KEY POINTS AND ACTIONS	SCORE
Cause of Death	Correctly identify and fill in, in the right order, the primary cause of death, secondary factors, and contributing causes. I (a) Disease or condition directly leading to death. This does not mean the mode of dying, such as heart failure, asphyxia, asthenia, etc. It means the disease, injury, or complication which caused the disease; e.g. myocardial infarction. (b) Other disease or condition if any, leading to 1(a). (c) Other disease or condition if any, leading to 1(b). II Other significant conditions that contributed to the death but are not related to the disease or condition causing it.	0 1 2
Employment	Tick the box if the death was related to the patient's employment.	0 1 –
Doctor's Details	Sign the death certificate printing your full name as well as your medical qualification as registered by the GMC. Fill in the date of issue of the death certificate.	0 1 2
Consultant	Provide the name of the consultant in charge of the patient's care.	0 1 –
Counterfoil	Complete the counterfoil section summarising the information stated above.	
Informant	Complete the notice to informant section.	
Coroner	Consider referring the case to the coroner if relevant.	0 1 2

Reasons to Refer a Patient's Death to the Coroner
- Unknown cause of death
- Patient was not seen by a doctor 14 days before death
- Death cause by medical treatment
- Suspicious death/Suicide
- Death within 24hrs of admission
- RTA, domestic/industrial accident

EXAMINER'S EVALUATION

	SCORE
Overall assessment of completing death certificate	0 1 2 3 4 5

Total mark out of 19

DATA
INTERPRETATION

07.1 CHEST RADIOGRAPH

INSTRUCTIONS Please review this radiograph and present your findings.

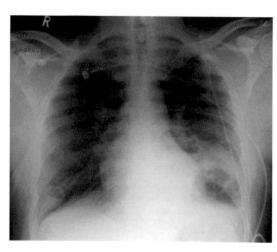

Source: Neel Sharma. *Data Interpretation Made Easy*.
London: Radcliffe Publishing; 2013.

Introduction (and buy time)

Name

Age/DOB

Date the radiograph was taken

STAGE	KEY POINTS AND ACTIONS	SCORE
	ASSESS THE QUALITY OF THE FILM	
	Penetration, Rotation, Inspiration, View, AP/PA/Lateral (PRIVA).	0 1
Penetration	The thoracic vertebrae should just be visible behind the heart shadow, as should the bronchovascular markings at the hilum.	0 1
Rotation	The medial heads of the clavicles should be an equal distance from the spinous process of the thoracic vertebrae.	0 1
Inspiration	The sixth (+/−1) anterior rib or the ninth (+/−) posterior rib should cross the level of the diaphragm of an inspiratory film (normal radiograph). More than 10 posterior ribs are indicative of a hyper-inflated chest while less than 8 indicate an expiratory film. (Expiratory films are useful when looking for a foreign body.)	0 1

STAGE	KEY POINTS AND ACTIONS	SCORE
View	The radiograph should encompass the entire lung field, from the apices to the costophrenic angles.	0 1 –
AP/PA/Lateral	Antero-posterior views are used in situations when the patient cannot sit up, but exaggerate the heart size. Postero-anterior views are the standard and give the most accurate view. Lateral films are rarely used; the one consistent indication is looking for an empyema. Look for erect or supine views.	0 1 –

THE INTERPRETATION

Gross Abnormality	State the most obvious thing if there is one; e.g. a large opacity, complete white-out, etc. 'The most obvious abnormality is….' Then assess the x-ray systematically using an ABCDE approach **A**irway **B**reathing **C**ardiac shadow **D**iaphragm **E**verything else 'I will now assess the radiograph systematically'.	
Airway	Identify the airway and its position. Determine if it is central (normal, consolidation), deviated away from (pleural effusion, tension pneumothorax), or deviated toward (lobe collapse, fibrosis) the abnormal side.	0 1 –

Deviated away	Central (normal)	Deviated toward
Pleural effusion	Normal	Lobe collapse
Tension pneumothorax	Consolidation	Fibrosis

BONUS: Look at the carina (where the trachea diverges into the left and right bronchus) – splaying here suggests mitral stenosis (due to enlargement of the left atrium).

Breathing	View the right and left lungs noting their volume (normal, reduced) and lucency.	0 1 2

Hypertranslucent (v.dark)	Radiolucent (normal)	Radio-opaque
Pneumothorax (with sharp line at edge of the lung – often seen best inverted view or rotated 90 degrees)	Normal	Consolidation, lung collapse, pleural effusion, pneumonectomy* *(fluid fills the space left behind)

Start from the apices and work down each side comparing the upper, middle, and lower zones of the lung, including behind the heart, for any abnormal shadowing or opacities. Describe any abnormal shadowing as nodular, reticular (crisscross lines – fibrosis), reticulo-nodular, or alveolar (fluffy appearance – pulmonary oedema). Note its size, shape, number, location, clarity of its margins, and its homogeneity.

< 5mm nodular shadowing	> 5mm nodular shadowing
Miliary TB	Lung cancer
Sarcoidosis	Metastases
Secondary carcinoma	Hydatid cyst
Varicella pneumonia	Wegener's granulomatosis (now known as granulomatosis with polyangiitis)

STAGE	KEY POINTS AND ACTIONS	SCORE

Observe for any ring shadows (abscess, or head on bronchi) or septal lines (Kerley B lines – short, thin horizontal lines found above the costophrenic angle, indicative of pulmonary oedema).

Silhouette Sign

The silhouette sign is a useful means of localising the pathology (collapse or consolidation) to a particular lobe. It states that if two densities are alike with margins adjacent to one another they will have their borders masked. If however they are separated by air, the boundaries of both will be seen.

0 1 2

Border	Lobe involved
Superior vena cava	Right upper lobe
Right heart border	Right middle lobe
Right hemidiaphragm	Right lower lobe
Aortic knuckle	Left upper lobe
Left heart border	Left lingular
Left hemidiaphragm	Left lower lobe

Look at the hilum; note the position of the hila, the left hilum is found higher than the right. The hila can be pulled upward or downward by lobe collapse or fibrosis. Enlarged, bulkier hila can be due to enlarged lymph nodes (TB, metastases, lymphoma, sarcoidosis), pulmonary artery hypertension, or bronchial carcinoma.

Look at the pulmonary vasculature (fanning out through the lung). Peripheral pruning of these vessels is a radiographic sign of pulmonary hypertension.

Cardiac Shadow

Comment on the size (cardiomegaly) and shape (pericardial effusion) of the heart. If the film is postero-anterior you can accurately assess the cardiodiaphragmatic ratio (CTR) which should be less than 50%; a CTR > 50% is suggestive of congestive cardiac failure. Note the presence of the left (left atrium and ventricle) and right (right atrium) heart borders. Obscuration of the left heart border is indicative of localised pathology in the lingular lobe (collapse, consolidation) and right heart border in the right middle lobe. Look for a double left heart border (left lower lobe collapse).

0 1 2

Diaphragm

Note the presence of the right and left hemidiaphragm margins and their level (9 posterior ribs). The right side is normally slightly higher than the left. A raised hemidiaphragm can be due to reduced lung volume, phrenic nerve paralysis, subphrenic abscess, or hepatomegaly. Ascertain that the surfaces of the hemidiaphragms curve downward. Extensive effusion or collapse can cause an upward curve. Check that the costophrenic and cardiophrenic angles are not blunted; blunting suggests an effusion of at least 200mL on an AP/PA view. Check for free air under the hemidiaphragms and air in the stomach.

0 1

Everything Else

Work up from the diaphragm and then out to the soft tissues.

Mediastinum

Note the presence of the aortic knuckle and the size, shape, and position of the mediastinum.

0 1

Causes of an enlarged mediastinum

Retrosternal thyroid	Neoplasm – four T's (Thyroid, thymoma, Teratoma, Thoracic tumour (lung cancer), Terrible lymphoma)
Aortic aneurysm	Oesophageal dilatation (achalasia – look for a fluid level behind the heart)

Soft Tissues

Look at the breast shadows (mastectomy), supraclavicular area, and axillae for any lesions. Note the presence of surgical emphysema.

0 1

Bone

Examine all the bones, including the vertebrae, humerus, scapulae, clavicle, and ribs for fractures, lesions (abscess, metastases), or rib notching (coarctation).

0 1

STAGE	KEY POINTS AND ACTIONS	SCORE
Artefacts	Look for any iatrogenic, incidental, or accidental objects including ECG lines, endotracheal tubes, NG tubes, CVP lines, chest drains, or a pacemaker.	0 1 –
Diagnosis	Summarise positive and important negative findings to the examiner including a possible differential diagnosis.	0 1 –

INVESTIGATION AND MANAGEMENT

State you would review previous films, take a full history and examination.
State you would manage any acute situation with an ABC approach.
For any tests start with bedside then simple and then complex investigations.
For any management start with conservative measures, then medical, and then surgical management.

EXAMINER'S EVALUATION

Overall assessment of presenting correct physical findings	0 1 2 3 4 5

Total mark out of 24

EXEMPLAR PRESENTATION

'Today I reviewed the chest radiograph of Mrs S, date of birth 30/7/45, taken on 21/12/13. The quality of the chest radiograph is good – it is not rotated, there is a good inspiration, the view is adequate, and a postero-anterior film has been taken with good penetration. The most obvious abnormality was a left upper zone opacity with well-defined margins, homogenous and approximately 9cm in width and a left lower zone opacity with a visible meniscus. Going through the radiograph systemically now the trachea is central, the right upper, middle, and lower zones are clear, the hilum is normal. The cardiac:thoracic ratio appears < 50% although I would like to formally measure it, and the shape is normal. The costophrenic angle is blunted on the left and clear on the right, there is no air under the diaphragm. The soft tissues appear normal, although there is only one breast shadow on the right side. There are no bony fractures. There is an area of lucency in the left humeral head. In summary this is a chest radiograph of a 68-year-old woman with an upper zone mass lesion, a left zone opacity in keeping with a pleural effusion and left humeral head changes suspicious of malignancy, with evidence of a previous mastectomy. These findings are most consistent with a diagnosis of metastatic breast cancer, with a differential diagnosis of a lung primary. I would like to take a full history and examination of the patient, review previous chest radiographs, and treat any acute medical need. Diagnostic investigations would include lung functions tests, a pleural tap for pH, glucose, protein, LDH, cytology, and microscopy, and a staging CT-Chest-Abdomen-Pelvis. Further management would be determined by the investigative findings, the patient's wishes, and the multi-disciplinary team'. ∎

NOTES ON THE CHEST X-RAY

Differential for a unilateral pleural effusion

Parapneumonic effusion

Malignancy (lung, mesothelioma)

Reactive (hepatitis)

Pulmonary infarction

Meigs syndrome (right sided)

Differential for a bilateral pleural effusion

Heart failure

Renal failure

Liver failure

Pacemakers

Can be many different devices implanted in the chest:

Pacemakers – single or dual chamber leads

+/– ICD – thick coil

CRT – cardiac resynchronization therapy – pacemaker + ICD + enlarged heart

Deep brain stimulator & vagal stimulator – leads lie cranially

Differential for cavitating lung lesions
[mnemonic—WEIRD HOLES]

Wegener's

Emboli

Infective – TB, E.Coli/Klebsiella abscess

Rheumatoid nodules

Degenerative cysts

Histiocytosis X

Oncological – SCC

Lymphangioleiomyomatosis – seen in tuberous sclerosis, F > M

Environmental/occupational – EAA, pleural plaques

Sarcoidosis

gns and symptoms

Pathology	CXR Appearance	Causes	Trachea	Other Signs
Lobar collapse	Source: Tristan Barrett, Nadeem Shaida, and Ashley Shaw. *Radiology for Undergraduate Finals and Foundation Years*. London: Radcliffe Publishing; 2010.	-Obstructive lesion (tumour, granuloma, abscess, foreign body) -Consolidation and secretions (mucous plugging)	Deviated toward side of volume loss	-Raised hemidiaphragm, deviated mediastinum Silhouette sign to localize lobe collapse
Pleural effusion	Source: Tristan Barrett, Nadeem Shaida, and Ashley Shaw. *Radiology for Undergraduate Finals and Foundation Years*. London: Radcliffe Publishing; 2010.	-Exudative (> 35g/dL protein) -Transudative (< 25g/dL protein) ALSO Chylothorax (lymph)Haemothorax (blood)	Deviated away in big effusions	-Meniscus -When it is flat suspect haemo-pneumothorax and an air-fluid level.
Consolidation	Source: Neel Sharma. *Data Interpretation Made Easy*. London: Radcliffe Publishing; 2013.	-Fluid filling the alveolar space -Usually inflammatory secondary to infection -May also be blood (pulmonary haemorrhage), tumour, aspirated food, and fluid	Central	-Silhouette sign -Lobar delineation -Air bronchogram (gas in bronchi against background of fluid in alveoli)
Pneumothorax	Source: Tristan Barrett, Nadeem Shaida, and Ashley Shaw. *Radiology for Undergraduate Finals and Foundation Years*. London: Radcliffe Publishing; 2010.	-Spontaneous – subpleural bulla (emphysema, COPD, PJP, Marfans), idiopathic (associated with tall, young men) -Trauma – penetrating, blunt (look for an air-fluid level and haemothorax in trauma)	-Central in open -Away in tension (medical emergency!)	-Hyper-translucent peripheries – absent lung markings and visible lung margin -Fractured ribs -Surgical emphysema in soft tissues
Pulmonary oedema		-Increased fluid in the extravascular space -Increased left ventricular pressure – left ventricular failure, mitral stenosis -Decompensated arrhythmias -Increased pulmonary vascular permeability – ARDS -Iatrogenic over fluid resuscitation	Central	**A**lveolar oedema (bat wings) Kerley **B** lines **C**ardiomegaly **D**ilated upper lobes (upper lobe diversion) **E**ffusions
Bronchial carcinoma	Source: Tristan Barrett, Nadeem Shaida, and Ashley Shaw. *Radiology for Undergraduate Finals and Foundation Years*. London: Radcliffe Publishing; 2010.	-Cigarette smoking (20% of all smoking related cancers) -Asbestos exposure (increases background risk by x 50 when smoking as well) -Silicosis	Central	Solitary spherical shaped opacity – anywhere in the lung Eccentric heterogenous centre and irregular edge. Cavitation seen particularly in squamous cell carcinoma. Mediastinal lymphadenopathy, collapse, pleural effusions (malignant spread), obstructive pneumonia. Bony destruction; e.g. humeral head, ribs, etc.
Hemithorax opacification (complete white-out)		-Consolidation -Massive pleural effusion -Total lung collapse -Pneumonectomy	Useful diagnostically – away in effusion, toward in collapse and pneumonectomy, neutral in consolidation	Look for associated signs of the above to differentiate between diagnoses – the trachea being the most useful.

07.2 ABDOMINAL RADIOGRAPH

INSTRUCTIONS Please review this radiograph and present your findings.

Introduction (and buy time)
Name
Age/DOB
Date the radiograph was taken

STAGE	KEY POINTS AND ACTIONS	SCORE
	ASSESS THE QUALITY OF THE FILM	
Type	Note the patient's position as being supine, erect, or decubitus. If unmarked assume the film is supine. Decubitus films are for detecting free air in the abdomen if there is some doubt with an erect chest x-ray.	0 1
View	The radiograph should visualize from the diaphragm to below the pelvis and the whole width of the abdomen. Sometimes in particularly obese patients two radiographs will be required.	0 1
Contrast	Note the absence or presence of contrast (barium/Gastrografin) and its type (barium swallow, barium meal, barium follow though, barium enema – single or double contrast). Also look for contrast in other areas; e.g. renal tract and bladder (urogram) or pancreas and biliary tree (ERCP, MRCP). Contrast is becoming increasingly rare on the plain film, but it is still useful anatomically and therefore appears disproportionately still in exams.	0 1
	THE INTERPRETATION	
Gross Abnormality	State the most obvious thing if there is one; e.g. obvious dilated bowel, IV pyelogram. 'The most obvious abnormality is….'	
Systematic Interpretation	Then go on to assess the radiograph systematically. One good way is by going through each density of tissue in the following order: A B B C D. **A**ir: Intraluminal – Gas pattern; Extraluminal – Free air in the abdomen **B**ody parts (soft tissues): Liver, spleen, kidney bladder **B**ones: Spine, lower ribs, and pelvis **C**alcifications **D**evices	

STAGE	KEY POINTS AND ACTIONS	SCORE

Air

Intraluminal   0 1 2

Assess the gas distribution in the abdomen and note the position of bowel loops. A ground glass or mottled appearance is often due to faecal shadowing (constipation).

Difference between large and small bowel

Large Bowel	Small Bowel
Found peripherally	Found centrally
Visible transverse folds called haustra that extend partially across the width of the bowel	Visible transverse valvulae conniventes that extend across the whole width of the bowel
Normally between < 5cm wide (except the caecum which is < 9cm)	< 3cm in diameter with wall thickness less than 3mm. The valvulae conniventes are also less than 3mm thick. There are approximately 3 air fluid levels per radiograph.

Note excessive amounts of air in the bowel and stomach. Measure the diameter of the small and large bowels, observing for dilatation. Small bowel obstruction is likely if bowel diameter is between 3 and 5cm whilst a width of more than 5cm (except caecum > 9cm) is highly suggestive of large bowel obstruction. Risk of perforation is greatly increased if the large bowel is greater than 9cm and the caecum more than 12cm.

Observe for a sentinel loop of bowel (collection of intraluminal gas) and note its position. Localised peritonitis can give rise to localized ileus; therefore the position of the sentinel loop can given an indication of the cause; i.e. right iliac fossa – appendicitis; left hypochondrium – pancreatitis.

Extraluminal

Inspect the x-ray for gas outside the stomach and bowel. Inspect for gas   0 1 2
within the peritoneal cavity (pneumoperitoneum – perforation, recent abdominal surgery), most likely found under the diaphragm, and for gas within the bowel wall (intramural gas – bowel infarct). Observe for air in the portal vein (bowel infarct), pancreas (acute necrotizing pancreatitis), biliary tree (biliary fistula, surgery), and urinary tract (enterovesical fistula).

Body Parts (soft tissues)   Look at the size and position of the liver, spleen, kidney, and bladder. (Remember   0 1 2
these aren't always visible on every film.) The kidney is found between T12 and L2 and is parallel to the psoas line. It measures around three vertebral bodies in length. Note the presence of psoas muscles shadows (absent – intraperitoneal disease). Also comment on the body habitus (this is relevant when thinking about the utility of abdominal ultrasound in the very obese).

Calcification   Look for calcification in the arteries (look for a large central calcification – this   0 1 2
may represent an abdominal aortic aneurysm, atherosclerosis), pancreas (chronic pancreatitis), gallbladder (chronic cholecystitis, biliary calculi – 20% radio-opaque), kidney, and ureters (nephrocalcinosis, renal calculi – 90% radio-opaque). When inspecting for renal calculi follow the urinary tract down from the transverse process of the lumbar vertebrae across the sacroiliac joint to the level of the ischial spine before it joins the bladder. Briefly inspect for calcification of the appendix (appendicitis – 15%), bladder (stone, tumour), and within the pelvis (calcified fibroids in the uterus and teratomas in the ovaries).

Devices   Identify any iatrogenic, incidental, or accidental objects such as surgical clips,   0 1 2
intrauterine contraceptive devices, stents, or filters (Greenfield filter – inferior vena cava filter).

STAGE	KEY POINTS AND ACTIONS	SCOR
Diagnosis	Summarise positive and important negative findings to the examiner including a possible differential diagnosis.	0 1

INVESTIGATION AND MANAGEMENT

State you would review previous films, take a full history and examination.
State you would manage any acute situation with an ABC approach.
For any tests, start with bedside, then simple, and then complex investigations.
For any management start with conservative measures, then medical, and then surgical management.

EXAMINER'S EVALUATION

Overall assessment of presenting correct physical findings	0 1 2 3 4

Total mark out of 20

NOTES ON THE ABDOMINAL X-RAY

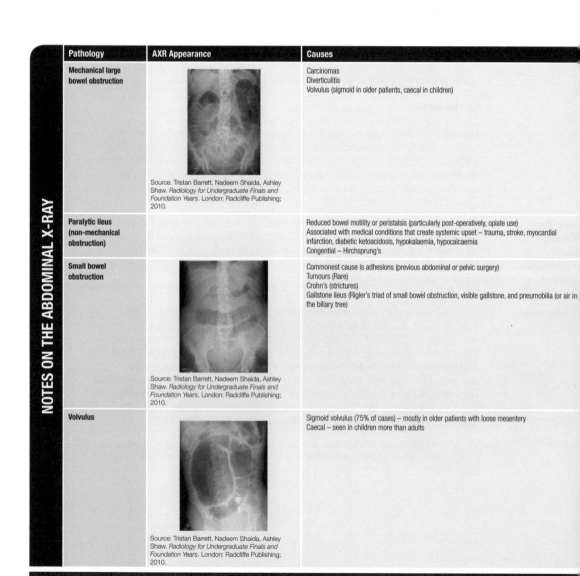

Pathology	AXR Appearance	Causes
Mechanical large bowel obstruction	Source: Tristan Barrett, Nadeem Shaida, Ashley Shaw. *Radiology for Undergraduate Finals and Foundation Years*. London: Radcliffe Publishing; 2010.	Carcinomas Diverticulitis Volvulus (sigmoid in older patients, caecal in children)
Paralytic ileus (non-mechanical obstruction)		Reduced bowel motility or peristalsis (particularly post-operatively, opiate use) Associated with medical conditions that create systemic upset – trauma, stroke, myocardial infarction, diabetic ketoacidosis, hypokalaemia, hypocalcaemia Congential – Hirchsprung's
Small bowel obstruction	Source: Tristan Barrett, Nadeem Shaida, Ashley Shaw. *Radiology for Undergraduate Finals and Foundation Years*. London: Radcliffe Publishing; 2010.	Commonest cause is adhesions (previous abdominal or pelvic surgery) Tumours (Rare) Crohn's (strictures) Gallstone ileus (Rigler's triad of small bowel obstruction, visible gallstone, and pneumobilia (or air in the biliary tree)
Volvulus	Source: Tristan Barrett, Nadeem Shaida, Ashley Shaw. *Radiology for Undergraduate Finals and Foundation Years*. London: Radcliffe Publishing; 2010.	Sigmoid volvulus (75% of cases) – mostly in older patients with loose mesentery Caecal – seen in children more than adults

EXEMPLAR PRESENTATION

'Today I reviewed the abdominal radiograph of Mr T, date of birth 22/8/67, taken on 21/1/15. The view is adequate. The most obvious abnormality is large dilated bowel loops, measuring > 8cm at its largest point, predominantly in the abdominal peripheries, with visible partially transverse haustra. There is no evidence of free air. Approaching the radiograph systemically now the intraluminal gas pattern in the small bowel is normal and there is no air in the rectum. There is no evidence of extraluminal air in the peritoneum or biliary tree. The liver is visible and appears mildly enlarged; the spleen and kidneys are visible and appear normally sized. The spine appears mildly scoliosed; there is a wedge-shaped change of the first lumbar vertebrae and several lucencies in the pelvis. The femoral heads appear in joint, aligned, and without obvious fracture. There is some calcification of both iliac arteries. There is no evidence of renal or biliary calculi. There is a urinary catheter in situ. In summary this is an abdominal radiograph of Mr T, taken on 21/1/15 with features of large bowel obstruction, and liver and bony changes suspicious of a metastatic process. These findings are most consistent with a diagnosis of metastatic left-sided bowel carcinoma. I would approach the patient with an ABC approach, fully resuscitating them. I would like to take a full history and examination of the patient including PR and spinal examination. If the patient was stable I would keep the patient nil-by-mouth, arrange an urgent CT-Abdomen and seek an immediate surgical review. Further management would be guided by initial biopsy and excision results, but would require an MDT approach'. ■

Other signs	Management
Widening of the diameter of the colon above 5cm (Caecum > 9cm). In 25% of patients the ileocaecal valve is incompetent and the small bowel will be dilated proximal to the obstruction also.	Depends on the cause – any loops of large bowel approaching 8-9cm are in danger of imminent perforation and require urgent surgical assessment. Sigmoid volvulus can often be reversed with sigmoidoscopy and air enema. Most other causes will require surgical correction.
Involves both large and small bowel. Also known as Ogilvie's syndrome.	Usually nothing – important to differentiate from mechanical obstruction by the absence of severe colicky pain and bowel sounds.
Dilated to 3-5cm; > 5cm danger of perforation. No large bowel dilatation, multiple air fluid levels (stepladder appearance) in central position. 'String of pearls' sign – where small amounts of trapped residual air occupy the fluid filled valvulae conniventes of the small bowel.	Again this depends on the cause. Typically a 'drip and suck' approach is taken with IVI and NG tube and monitoring. Any suggestion of worsening pain, increasing dilatation, or mesenteric ischaemia requires urgent surgery. Very dilated bowel will also require surgical intervention.
'Coffee' bean sign which represents the adjacent walls of dilated loop forming a dense white line. This line surrounds an extremely dilated sigmoid bowel and gives the beak sign – a sharp pointed end to the bowel caused by twisting of the mesenteric attachment.	Sigmoid volvulus requires sigmoidoscopy first and attempted correction, unless perforation has occurred. Caecal volvulus requires surgery.

07.3 INTERPRETING THE ECG

INSTRUCTIONS Please review this ECG of Mr Quam with a two-hour history of chest pain and present your findings.

NOTE: The ECG records the electrical activity of the heart through 10 leads attached to the surface of the skin. If the depolarization spreads in the direction of an electrode the ECG denotes this as a positive upward deflection, while if it moves away from it, the ECG records a downward negative deflection. The size of the deflection is relative to the degree of depolarization, which is proportional to the muscle mass.

(*SEE* PRACTICAL SKILLS SECTION FOR HOW TO SET UP AN ECG.)

STAGE	KEY POINTS AND ACTIONS	SCORE
	THE EVALUATION	

Interpreting

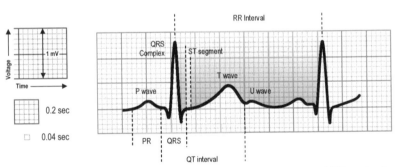

First check the calibration (1mV per 2 large squares) and print speed (25mm/sec) is the standard.

Rhythm

Check if the rate is regular or irregular first (this will help you determine the rate secondarily). Note any arrhythmias by looking at the presence of the P wave and the QRS complex as well as their relationship.

0 1 —

Rhythm	ECG findings
Sinus rhythm	Upright P waves (I,II) followed by QRS complex
Atrial fibrillation	No P wave with irregularly irregular timed QRS
Atrial tachycardia	Narrow QRS, > 100 bpm with abnormal P wave
Atrial flutter	Sawtooth pattern baseline with regular QRS
AV nodal rhythm	QRS complex present with P waves hidden
Ventricular rhythm	Broad complex QRS, > 150bpm

STAGE	KEY POINTS AND ACTIONS	SCORE
Rate	There is a 0.2 second period with a large square and 0.04 second period with each small square. For regular rhythms to calculate the heart rate roughly, divide the number of squares between two adjacent R waves into 300. Normal 60-100BPM Bradycardia < 60BPM Tachycardia > 100BPM For irregular rhythms you need to calculate the number of complexes in 10 seconds and multiply by 6 – this equates to 50 large squares, which is usually the length of a standard ECG or 25cm.	0 1 –
Cardiac Axis	Observe the direction of the cardiac axis to establish any deviation. If the QRS complexes are predominantly positive in I and II then the axis is normal.	0 1 –

Direction of deviation	ECG findings
L axis deviation (–30 degrees to –90 degrees)	QRS complex is positive in lead I but negative in lead II. Causes include left anterior hemi-block, inferior MI, WPW syndrome.
R axis deviation (+90 degrees to –150 degrees)	QRS complex is negative in lead I regardless of lead II.
Bizarre QRS axis arrangement (–150 to –90 degrees)	QRS complex is negative in both lead I and in lead II. Causes include limb lead error (R&L), dextrocardia.

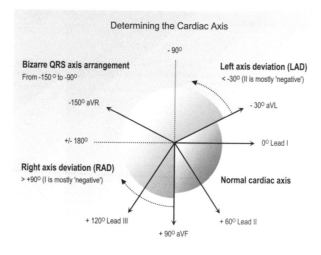

Determining the Cardiac Axis

Go through the QRS systematically wave by wave.

P Wave	P waves represent the depolarization of the right and left atriums. P waves should precede each QRS complex on the ECG. Their normal duration is less than 0.12 seconds (< 3 small squares) with amplitude of less than 2.5mm.	0 1 2

P wave abnormality	Cause
Absent	AF, SA block, AV nodal rhythm
Bifid P waves	Left atrial hypertrophy (P mitrale)
Peaked P waves	Right atrial hypertrophy (P pulmonale)

P-R Interval	Inspect for shortened or prolonged durations. P-R interval is the time taken from the onset of atrial depolarization (beginning of P waves) to the onset of ventricular depolarization (beginning of QRS).	0 1 2

P-R interval	Cause
0.12-0.20 seconds – (3-5 small squares)	Normal
< 0.12 – (< 3 small squares)	Shortened PR – faster conduction via accessory pathway (Wolff-Parkinson White)
> 0.2 seconds (> 5 small squares)	Delayed AV conduction (1st degree heart block)

STAGE	KEY POINTS AND ACTIONS	SCORE

Inspect successive PR intervals. Note the relationship between the P and QRS complex and observe for non-conducting P-waves (2nd degree block). A complete dissociation between the P and QRS complex is 3rd degree heart block.***

Different types of secondary heart block	Features
Mobitz type I	Lengthening of the PR interval with each successive QRS complex with eventual dropping of the P wave (Wenckebach phenomenon).
Mobitz type II*	Normal fixed PR intervals with occasional non-conducted P waves – this may be 2:1, 3:1, 4:1, or even 5:1 block and invariably reflects a disease of the His-Purkinje fibre system.

*/** /*** All of these rhythms require pacemaking because of the risk of progression to complete heart block, only Mobitz type I does not need pacing in the majority of cases.

QRS Complexes

The QRS complex represents the time required for the right and left ventricles to depolarize simultaneously. Note the width and height of the QRS complex and look for the presence of pathological Q waves.

0 1 2

Morphology		Features and cause
Duration < 0.12 seconds		Normal
Wide > 0.12 seconds		Ventricular origin (look for absent P waves and rate – if fast think ventricular tachycardia; if slow, think complete heart block and ventricular escape rhythm).
or i)		Or Supraventricular with aberrant conduction; e.g. bundle-branch block (M pattern seen above and W pattern seen below). (see below) Left and Right Bundle Branch Block (with wide QRS) Mnemonic—'WiLLiaM MaRRoW' WiLLiaM – A 'W' (i) pattern is seen in V1 and V2 with an 'M' pattern in leads V3 and V6. This is suggestive of a *left* bundle branch block. Causes: acute myocardial infarction, never normal
or ii)		MaRRoW- An 'M' (ii) or 'RSR' pattern is seen in V1 and V2 with a 'W' pattern in leads V3 and V6. This is suggestive of a *right* bundle branch block. This can be a normal variant, also seen in right heart strain (pulmonary hypertension, PE) and in old right-sided infarcts.
Paced QRS complexes (> 0.12 with pacing spikes)		No P waves Pacing spikes visible Usually ventricular origin therefore wide QRS
Deep Q waves ('pathological Q waves')		Suggest myocardial damage – in acute myocardial infarction these take hours to days to develop and will remain; in a stable patient without chest pain they more likely represent an old MI.

STAGE	KEY POINTS AND ACTIONS	SCORE

The ST Segment

In a normal ECG the ST segment is isoelectric, not above or below the baseline. Look for ST changes in more than one contiguous lead.

0 1 2

Elevation > 2mm in V1,V2,V3 or > 1mm or all other leads
ST-Elevated MI*, acute pericarditis (saddle shaped)
Depression > 0.5mm
Angina, digoxin therapy ('reverse tick' sign, NOT overdose), posterior infarct (V1-V2)

Position of myocardial infarct	Culpable vascular territory	ECG changes
Anterior	Left anterior descending artery	ST elevation in leads V2-V4
Antero-septal	Proximal left anterior descending artery	ST elevation in leads V1-V4
Inferior	Right coronary artery	ST elevation in leads II, III, and aVF
Lateral	Left circumflex artery	ST elevation in leads I, avL, V5, and V6
Posterior**	Right circumflex artery or right coronary artery	Tall R wave and ST depression in leads V1 and V2 with ST elevation in leads V7-9**

Ref: (http://circ.ahajournals.org/content/114/16/1755.full)

(*varies with male/female and age on definition-Further reading; http://www.escardio.org/guidelines-surveys/esc-guidelines/
GuidelinesDocuments/Guidelines_AMI_STEMI.pdf)
(** How to record a posterior ECG – V4,5,6 and moved into the following positions;
V4 left posterior axillary line to become V7
V5 to the tip of the scapulae to become V8
V6 to the paraspinal region in the same line to become V9
Record the ECG in the exact same manner but record V4-6 as V7-9 to avoid confusion.)

T Wave

The T wave represents ventricular repolarization and can be normally inverted in leads V1-V3 in Afro-Carribean ethnic groups and young people. Intermittent T-wave inversion in lead III is also normal if not isolated.

0 1 2

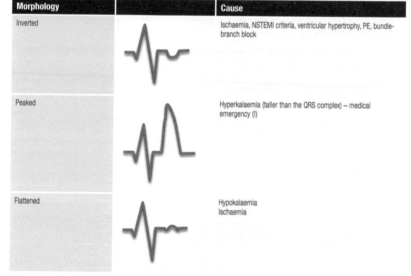

Morphology		Cause
Inverted		Ischaemia, NSTEMI criteria, ventricular hypertrophy, PE, bundle-branch block
Peaked		Hyperkalaemia (taller than the QRS complex) – medical emergency (!)
Flattened		Hypokalaemia Ischaemia

QT Interval

The QT interval is the duration of ventricular depolarization and repolarization. It is measured from the start of the QRS to the end of the T wave. It is more accurate to calculate the 'corrected' QT interval known as the QTc which takes into account the RR interval.

0 1 2

Normal   0.38-0.42 seconds
Prolonged > 0.42
Acute myocardial ischaemia, myocarditis, electrolyte abnormality (low K/Ca/Mg)

STAGE	KEY POINTS AND ACTIONS	SCORE

Additional Waves   Look carefully for the following waves:

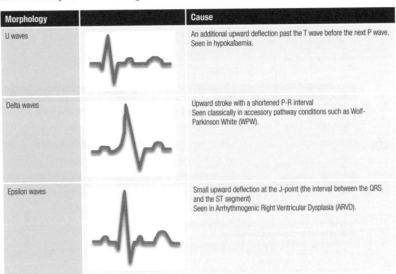

Morphology		Cause
U waves		An additional upward deflection past the T wave before the next P wave. Seen in hypokalaemia.
Delta waves		Upward stroke with a shortened P-R interval. Seen classically in accessory pathway conditions such as Wolf-Parkinson White (WPW).
Epsilon waves		Small upward deflection at the J-point (the interval between the QRS and the ST segment) Seen in Arrhythmogenic Right Ventricular Dysplasia (ARVD).

Summary   Summarise the ECG findings.   0   1   –

Diagnosis   'These findings are most consistent with a diagnosis of ....' And present a differential.   0   1   –

Management   State immediate and definitive management in this case. Don't forget to mention senior help.

EXAMINER'S EVALUATION

Overall assessment of interpretation of ECG   0   1   2   3   4   5

Total mark out of 22

SELECTED ECG RHYTHMS

VENTRICULAR FIBRILLATION

Ventricular fibrillation (VF) is a pulseless arrhythmia with irregular and chaotic electrical activity whereby the heart loses its ability to function as a pump. It is a medical emergency with immediate DC cardioversion indicated to avert impending death.

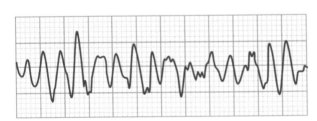

ATRIAL FIBRILLATION

Atrial fibrillation (AF) is a common arrhythmia with chaotic atrial activity. There are no clear P waves on the ECG tracing and the rhythm is irregularly irregular. Treatment strategy is divided into the stable patient and the unstable. Any patient who is unstable (fast rhythm, hypotension, shock, pulmonary oedema) requires urgent DC cardioversion under sedation. Stable patient treatment can be divided into rate control and rhythm control.

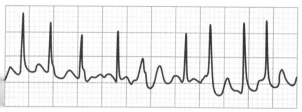

ATRIAL FLUTTER

Atrial flutter is common and invariably is due to organic disease of the heart. The atrial rate is commonly 300/min and there is usually a 2:1 block resulting in a ventricular response rate of 150/min. Atrial flutter can also occur with a 3:1 block and rate of 100/min. The ECG characteristically shows 'sawtooth' flutter waves on the baseline.

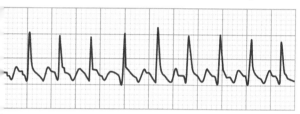

THIRD DEGREE HEART BLOCK

Third degree heart block (atrioventricular block) occurs when there is no association between atrial and ventricular activity. The ECG strip shows regular P waves and QRS complexes which have no association; watch for buried P waves in QRS complexes, this can be mistaken for second degree heart block occasionally. The ventricular escape rhythm occurs at a rate of around 40 beats per minute.

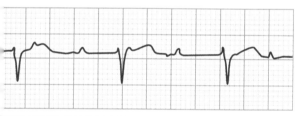

VENTRICULAR TACHYCARDIA

Ventricular tachycardia is defined by the presence of three or more consecutive ventricular beats. There may be a fusion beat present at the start of the trace. The ECG usually shows rapid ventricular rhythm (> 120BPM) with an abnormally broad QRS complex.

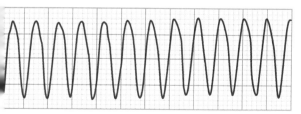

PREMATURE VENTRICULAR CONTRACTIONS

An isolated ventricular complex, without any obvious P wave, with a grossly different QRS morphology to the rest of the rhythm complex. Occasional ectopic beats are normal.

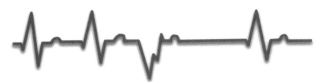

Other rhythms to look out for:

Rhythm	Features	Causes
Sinus bradycardia	Normal PQRST morphology with a rate < 60BPM.	-Normal: in sleeping individuals, athletes -Ischaemia to the sinus node -Hypothermia, hypothyroidism -Iatrogenic: beta blockade -Raised intracranial pressure (associated with hypertension – Cushing's reflex)
Sinus tachycardia	Normal PQRST morphology with rate > 100	-Physiological response to pain, distress or anxiety -Hyperthyroidism -PE -Dehydration or hemorrhage -Caffeine abuse -Alcohol or opiate withdrawal
Bifascicular block and Trifascicular block	Combination of RBBB and left axis deviation (bifascicular block) Combination of RBBB, left axis deviation, and 1st degree heart block	-Depends on the context -If symptomatic (hypotensive, syncopal) may require pacing -Reflects generalized damage to the myocardial conduction system
Ventricular bigeminy and trigeminy	One normal complex associated with either one premature complex (bigeminy) or in runs of three's (trigeminy – either two normal and one PVC or one normal and two PVCs)	-In a structurally normal heart – normal variant -In a damaged heart (post-MI for example), this rhythm is at risk of arrest and requires pacing/ICD insertion

07.4 INTERPRETING THE ABG

INSTRUCTIONS Please review this ABG of Mr Guillard, a 53-year-old gentleman, admitted with a COPD exacerbation with increasing shortness of breath on the ward.

NOTE – *SEE* PROCEDURES SECTION FOR HOW TO TAKE AN ABG

STAGE	KEY POINTS AND ACTIONS	SCORE
	EVALUATION	
Interpretation	Determine the status of the pH. Is there acidosis or alkalosis?	0 1 2

Acidosis	pH < 7.35
Neutral	pH 7.35–7.45
Alkalosis	pH > 7.45

STAGE	KEY POINTS AND ACTIONS	SCORE
PaO$_2$	Next assess the PaO$_2$ concentration. Is there respiratory failure?	0 1 2

PaO$_2$ < 10kPa in air indicates respiratory failure.
A rough rule to working out normal oxygenation on additional inspired oxygen can be thought of as

$$\text{Minimum normal PaO}_2 = \% \text{ inspired oxygen} - 10.$$
$$\text{E.g. in air a normal PaO}_2 = 20.95\% - 10$$
$$= 10.95 \text{ kPa}$$

Remember that any percentage of oxygen is difficult to calculate unless the patient is on controlled-oxygen delivery such as the Venturi system. Always write the % inspired oxygen on any blood gas result you take.

STAGE	KEY POINTS AND ACTIONS	SCORE
PaCO$_2$	If there is respiratory failure look next at the PaCO$_2$.	0 1 2

PaO$_2$	PaCO$_2$	Diagnosis
Low (< 10kPa in air)	Low (< 4.0kPa in air)	Type I respiratory failure: severe asthma, PE, pulmonary oedema
Low (< 10kPa in air)	High (> 6.0kPa in air)	Type II respiratory failure: life-threatening asthma, COPD (acute or chronic), obstructive sleep apneoa
High (> 15kPa in air)	Low (< 4.0kPa in air)	Hyperventilation
High (> 15kPa in air)	High (> 6.0kPa in air)	Over-oxygenation in patients with CO$_2$ retention; e.g. inappropriate oxygen therapy in a COPD patient with retention

STAGE	KEY POINTS AND ACTIONS	SCORE

Now look at the bicarbonate in association with the context of CO_2 and pH.

pH	CO₂	HCO₃	Diagnosis	Causes
Acidosis	High > 6.0kPa	> 26 mmol/L	Respiratory acidosis: Chronic CO_2 retention	Chronic COPD, chronic OSA
Acidosis	High > 6.0kPa	< 22mmol/L	Respiratory acidosis: Acute CO_2 retention with metabolic compensation	Severe asthma, COPD exacerbation
Acidosis	Low < 4.0kPa	< 22mmol/L	Metabolic acidosis: calculate the anion gap*	See below
Alkalosis	High > 6.0kPa	> 26mmol/L	Metabolic alkalosis	Dehydration Furosemide toxicity Vomiting Milk-alkali syndrome
Alkalosis	Low < 4.0kPa	Normal	Respiratory alkalosis	Type I respiratory failure: PE, severe asthma Hyperventilation

Metabolic Acidosis

The cause of a metabolic acidosis can be determined by the anion gap which is calculated (with potassium omitted) as

0 1 2

$$\text{Anion gap} = [Na] - [HCO_3 + Cl]$$
$$\text{Normal anion gap} = [140] - [25 + 100]$$
$$= 140 - 125$$
$$= 15$$

A normal anion gap should be between 11-16meq/L.

Normal anion gap metabolic acidosis (11-16meQ/L)	Raised anion gap acidosis (mnemonic—MUDPILERS) > 16meQ/L
Renal loss of bicarbonate – renal tubular acidosis	**M**ethanol poisoning
Gastrointestinal loss of bicarbonate – vomiting, diarrhea	**U**raemia
Addison's	**D**iabetic ketoacidosis
	Propylene glycol poisoning
	Isoniazid/Iron
	Lactic acidosis
	Ethylene glycol poisoning/Ethanol
	Rhabdomyolysis
	Salicylate poisoning

Summarise

Comment on any other electrolyte reported – if there is an obvious hypokalaemia or hyponatraemia point it out and request formal U&Es from the lab.

0 1 –

'The most obvious abnormality is a respiratory acidosis with a $PaCO_2$ of 10 and a pH of 7.2. This patient is very unwell. I would urgently review the patient in an ABC approach and get senior help. Immediate management would involve controlled oxygen and bronchodilators. This patient will need an urgent ITU review'.

EXAMINER'S EVALUATION

Overall assessment of arterial blood sampling

0 1 2 3 4 5

Total mark out of 14

section 08

EVIDENCE
APPRAISAL

EVIDENCE APPRAISAL

Introduction

This station may appear in different formats in either short or long station OSCEs, but it is an important skill as a doctor and one in which every graduate should have at least some grounding. The following structure will give you the basic approach and answer to the commonly asked questions; should you be interested there is a list of further references at the end of the chapter.

08.1 HOW TO APPROACH AN ABSTRACT

INSTRUCTIONS Please read the abstract and answer the examiner's questions.

STAGE	KEY POINTS AND ACTIONS		SCORE
	BACKGROUND		
Hypothesis	What was studied and is it important?	e.g. Oral corticosteroids in controlling severe asthma.	0 1 –
Population	What was the study population?	e.g. Adults ages 18-65 with severe asthma (as defined by…).	0 1 –
Intervention/Exposure	What was the effect being studied?	e.g. Oral corticosteroids versus placebo.	0 1 –
Outcome	How was the outcome of the study defined?	e.g. Improvement in self-reported symptom scores and peak flow.	0 1 –
	METHOD This will vary depending on the type of study (see below).		
Population	How was the population recruited? Were they randomized (if appropriate)? If not how were the study arms allocated? How many patients were in the study?	e.g. This was a multicentre study of all adult patients attending respiratory clinic with a primary diagnosis of asthma. e.g. 2792 patients were randomized to placebo or corticosteroid group.	0 1 –
Time	When was the study performed? How long was the follow-up time? How were participants followed up?	e.g. Patients were followed up for a median 4.5 years at 3-monthly appointments with questionnaires.	0 1 –

STAGE	KEY POINTS AND ACTIONS		SCORE
Intervention/Exposure	Were the patients blinded to the intervention? (single blinding) Were the study doctors (or equivalent) blinded to the intervention? (double-blinding)	e.g. Double-blind study design.	0 1 –
Outcome	Was the primary outcome defined in the protocol? How were the outcomes measured?	e.g. Peak flow and self-reported symptom scores.	0 1 –
RESULTS			
Statistics	What did the study show? Was the statistical analysis appropriate for the data? (see below) Was the result significant? (see below)	e.g. Mean peak-flow improvement in the treatment group was 120.6 versus 35.3 in the placebo group (odds ratio 3.416 95% confidence interval 2.53-4.59, p = 0.0002).	0 1 –
Conclusions	Were the conclusions appropriate? Were they relevant?	e.g. Treatment with oral corticosteroids significantly improved peak flow in patients with asthma compared with placebo.	0 1 –
CRITICAL ANALYSIS			
General	Any conflict of interest from the authors?	e.g. All authors are on retention for Steroids Incorporated.	0 1 –
Method	Was the study size large enough to reflect the population? (power of the study) Were there any potential confounders? (see below) Was the study type appropriate to the exposure/intervention? Were the arms as comparable as possible?	e.g. A power calculation showed a requisite study size of at least 1562 patients; final recruitment was 2801. e.g. All patients previously not on steroids; follow-up time too short. e.g. This study was a randomized controlled trial to test drug versus placebo. e.g. The arms were randomized.	0 1 –
Results	Were the outcomes defined before the study, or added after the data had been collected? (posthoc analysis) Were the statistical tests appropriate?	e.g. Paired parametric data analysed with Student's Paired T-test.	0 1 –
SUMMING UP			
Overall	Was the study well-designed large enough and relevant to my practice?		
EXAMINER'S EVALUATION			
Overall assessment of interpreting an abstract			0 1 2 3 4 5
Total mark out of 18			

NOTES ON EVIDENCE APPRAISAL

Types of study

The hierarchy of evidence is a commonly asked about concept in epidemiology and one worth studying for both the written and the practical examination.

Type of study	Methodology	Pros	Cons	Good for...	Bad for...
Meta-analysis	Quantitative and reproducible statistical method of combining and analysing multiple trials on a single subject	1. Very large numbers 2. Can statistically account for heterogeneity between studies 3. Can generate new knowledge without the risk to patients involved in further trials 4. Cheap	1. Prone to publication bias (this can be looked at using a funnel plot) 2. Combining studies is not always possible, or helpful 3. Time-consuming	Analysing similar smaller trials on a single intervention to give a more robust answer	Combining very different tr types or studying different outcomes
Systematic review	Qualitative and reproducible method of subjectively appraising multiple trials on a single subject	1. Very large numbers 2. Can appraise diverse study types 3. Cheap 4. Identifies need for further research 5. Reproducible search strategy	1. Qualitative not quantitative 2. Prone to bias analysis (especially by experts in the field) 3. Time-consuming 4. Cannot combine study to give a uniform answer	Analysing diverse trial types or different outcomes on a single subject	Combining similar trials to generate new knowledge (better to perform a meta-analysis)
Randomized controlled trial	1. Participants are appropriately randomized to study arms 2. Each study arm is as similar to the others as possible except for the intervention 3. Participants and study organisers are blinded as far as possible	1. Strict methodology 2. 'Gold-standard' for testing an intervention in a population 3. Reproducible 4. Can show 'cause and effect'	1. Easily confounded 2. Very expensive 3. Long follow-up required 4. Time-consuming +++	1. Comparing the effect of a treatment against placebo 2. Comparing the effect of a treatment against the current gold standard	1. Situations where it woul not be ethical to randomize patients 2. Very small populations; e.g. rare diseases 3. Rare outcomes (very larg numbers required)
Cohort study	A specific cohort of patients is identified and then followed up for a specific outcome (prospective) or identified from records and followed up from then (retrospective)	1. Can show causation	1. Expensive 2. Non-randomized	Good for studying rare diseases or exposures; e.g. radiation exposure	Bad for studying a rare outcome
Case-control	A specific group of patients is identified and termed 'cases' and compared with a group of matched 'controls' that is ideally as similar as possible to the case group and associations are made retrospectively	1. Can show association 2. Cheap	1. Difficult to identify true 'controls' 2. Difficult to determine what constitutes a 'case' 3. Cannot demonstrate causality	Good for studying rare outcomes	Bad for studying a rare disease
Cross-sectional survey	A survey is conducted of a population at a single point in time to look at present or past interventions/exposures and outcomes.	1. Can show association 2. Quick 3. Can study many variables simultaneously with one survey	1. Prone to 'response bias' 2. Cannot demonstrate causality	Good for identifying associations in specific populations; e.g. low-income families	Demonstrating causation

Confounders

Commonly asked about, confounders are defined as factors associated with both the exposure and the outcome, tha are not controlled or accounted for, outside of the intervention being studied. Factors that are usually controlled are age and sex, but additional confounders will depend on the study. This is not the same as Bias (see below).

Bias

Biases are systematic flaws in the design of the study which lead to an unfair result. These could be in any part of the study design and need to be carefully looked for in the methodology in order to trust the result. There are many different forms of bias but learning the most common ones will give you the biggest yield in the OSCE.

Type of bias	Description	Example
Selection bias	How the participants are recruited to the study	Those with more severe disease are more likely to be excluded from the trial, exaggerating the interventions effect.
Measurement bias	How the outcome is measured	Unblinded studies may overestimate a drop in blood pressure by repeating office readings in the treatment group and not in the control.
Analysis bias	How the results are analysed and statistically accounted for	Patients lost to follow-up are excluded, despite those being more likely to experience side effects or find no benefit from the intervention, therefore overestimating the treatment benefit and underestimating the dangers. Performing a 'posthoc' analysis of the data to find a significant association or subgroup and publishing that, outside of what the study design and primary outcome was.
Publication bias	In meta-analysis how available data is for collation and comparison	A treatment effect is overestimated because all trials showing negative results are unpublished and not included in the analysis.

Statistics

This is an extremely complex subject; for the OSCE you only need the very basics.

Term	Definition	How to phrase it to a patient	Example
Risk	Number of events in the group/number of patients in that group	The proportion of patients experiencing a particular event	There were 4 deaths in the control group of 100 patients, this is a risk of 0.04 or 4% or 1 in 25.
Relative risk	Risk in the treatment group/risk in the control group	The probability of an event occurring in the treatment group compared with the control group	The risk of death in the treatment group was 0.02 compared with a risk of death of 0.04 in the control group. This is a relative risk of 0.02/0.04 = 0.5 or 50% or 1 in 2.
Absolute risk reduction	Risk in the control group/risk in the treatment group *(X wrong!)*	The difference in probability of an event happening between the control group and the treatment group	The risk of death in the treatment group was 0.02 and in the control group it was 0.04. The absolute risk reduction was 0.02 or 2% or 2 in 100.
Number needed to treat	1/ARR	For every x number of patients exposed to the intervention, one less event will be avoided	The absolute risk reduction is 2%; therefore the number needed to treat to avoid 1 death is 1/0.02 = 50.
p value	The probability the observations were due to chance alone and no true association exists	The result is considered likely to be true if there is less than a 5% (<0.05) probability it is due to random chance	The p-value was reported as 0.03 which is considered statistically significant.
Confidence intervals	The range of values between which with 95% probability the true value in the **population** lies	The result is considered likely to be non-significant if the confidence intervals cross 1 for relative risk or odds ratio or 0 for the RRR or ARR.	The 95% confidence intervals for the ARR were 0.002-0.1 which indicates a likely significant observation.

ARR = risk in treatment group - risk in control group

08.2 EXPLAINING AN ARTICLE TO A PATIENT

INSTRUCTIONS You are a foundation year House Officer in GP. Mr D is a 65-year-old man with heart disease who has brought an article to discuss with you. Please answer his questions.

ABSTRACT

Statin therapy in adults under 50: A randomized controlled trial

Background

Statins have been shown to reduce cardiovascular risk in certain cohorts of patients. A high number of adults is increasingly experiencing early myocardial infarcts. The role of statins in this subgroup is unknown.

Method

A total of 460 adults were recruited into the trial from three general medical clinics in Norway, of which 400 were suitable. Of these, 200 patients were randomized to receive a once daily dose of simvastatin 20mg, and 200 patients were randomized to a placebo. The study was double-blinded. Median follow-up was 5.2 years. The primary outcome was proven myocardial infarction.

Results

The event rate was 1/200 in the treatment group, and 2/200 in the placebo group. Relative risk reduction of 50% (p = 0.25).

Conclusions

Statin therapy reduced the risk of myocardial infarct in patients under 50.

STAGE	KEY POINTS AND ACTIONS	SCORE
	INTRODUCTION	
Introduction	Introduce yourself. Elicit name, age, and occupation. Establish rapport.	0 1 –
Understanding	Elicit patient's understanding and reason for coming today. 'I understand that you are here today to discuss an article about heart disease. What can you tell me about the article'?	0 1 –
Concerns	Elicit patient's concerns about the article and conclusions; i.e. heart disease and new medication. 'Do you have any particular concerns about the article that you would like me to clarify'?	0 1 –
	EXPLAINING	
Study Outline	Explain the population, exposure, and outcome being studied. 'This is a study in adults under 50 from Norway looking at the use of statin-based drugs on the risk of heart attack'.	0 1 –
Type of Study	'This is a randomized controlled trial. Two groups of adults under 50, similarly matched for age and sex, were randomly selected to either take a statin or a placebo – a sugar-pill with no effect. Both groups were then followed up for five years to see if any had a heart attack'.	0 1 –
Size of the Study	'The study was quite small: 200 adults in each group'.	0 1 –
Study Results and the Risk	'The study found one person had a heart attack in the treatment group and two people had heart attacks in the placebo group. It has given a figure here of 50% decreased risk reduction or a 1 in 200 chance of heart attack with the treatment, and a 1 in 100 chance without. The p-value is 0.25'.	0 1 –
Limitations of the Study	'This was quite a small study, although it appears well constructed. Only three people had heart attacks out of 400; it is difficult to say if this was due to the treatment or due to chance because of the small numbers. This number here, the p-value, shows that there is a 25% probability these results were due to chance. In medical terms we wouldn't say this study is useful in making treatment decisions'.	0 1 –
What This Means for the Patient	'This study was specifically in people under 50; this means the results are difficult to apply to you as a 65-year-old man. The results, because the study is so small, are not very useful'.	0 1 –
Explore the Patient Questions and Concerns	'Is that useful? Is there anything you wanted to ask me about that'?	0 1 –
Make a Plan	'I understand you are interested in doing the maximum to look after your heart. Let's make an appointment to talk about this, and I will give you some leaflets to read in the meantime'.	0 1 –
Finishing Off	Thank the patient.	

EXAMINER'S EVALUATION	
Overall assessment of explanation of article	0 1 2 3 4 5
Total mark out of 16	

INDEX

A

AAAA PPPP mnemonic, 14
AABCD mnemonic, 318
ABCDEFGH mnemonic, 79
ABCDEF mnemonic, 48
ABCDE mnemonic, 60, 313
abdomen
  in abdomen examination, 54–56
  contour, 53
  in lymphatic system examination, 118
abdomen examination, 52–60
  additional notes, 57–60
  auscultation, 56
  exemplar presentation, 57
  face signs, 54
  hands signs, 53
  inspection, 52–54
  notes for OSCE, 57–60
  palpation, 54–56
  percussion, 56
abdominal aortic aneurysm, 104
abdominal distension, 55
abdominal masses, 116
abdominal pain history taking, 31–34
  associated history, 32–33
  communication skills, 33
  differential diagnosis, 34
  exemplar presentation, 34
abdominal radiograph, 318–21
  assessing quality of the film, 318
  exemplar presentation, 321
  interpretation of, 318–32
  investigation and management, 320
  mnemonics, 320
  notes, 320–1
abducens nerve, 63
ABG, 329–30
ABO incompatibility, 152
ABPI, 186–8
abscess, 48
  breast, 37
  perinephric, 59
  psoas, 32
absolute risk reduction, 335
abstract, reading and understanding, 332–5
  critical analysis of, 333
  determining study method, 332–3
  study results, 333
accessory nerve, 65
accident & emergency history taking, 2–4
accommodation, visual, 63, 89
ACE inhibitors, 277
acoustic neuroma, 97
acronyms, prescribing, 226
acute asthma attack
  prescribing for, 232–3
    acute medical management, 233
    continuing medical management, 233
    infusion therapy, 233
    as required medicines, 233
acute cholecystitis, 34
acute coronary syndrome
  prescribing for, 236–7
    acute medical management, 237
    continuing medical management, 237
    general prescribing, 237
    infusion therapy, 237
    as required medicines, 237
acute ischaemia, 103
acute left ventricular failure
  prescribing for, 238–9
    acute medical management, 239
    continuing medical management, 239
    general prescribing, 239
    infusion therapy, 239
    as required medicines, 239
acute liver failure, 60
acute lymphadenitis, 116
acutely unwell patient, managing, 193–222
acute medical management
  for acute asthma attack, 233
  for acute coronary syndrome, 237
  for acute left ventricular failure, 239
  for COPD exacerbation, 235
  for GI bleed, 227–8
  for hyperkalaemia, 240
acute pancreatitis, 34
adenosine, 200
AED, 177–8
AFRO-C mnemonic, 61
AIDS, 247
air conduction, 64, 95

air in abdominal radiograph, 319
airway
  in basic life support, 177
  in chest radiograph, 313
airway patency in the acutely unwell patient, 194
  with DKA, 214
  with hypoglycaemia, 210
  with palpitations, 198
  with pulmonary embolism, 202
  with sepsis, 206
  with upper GI bleed, 218
alcohol. *See also* ethanol
  and diabetes, 280
  in lower limb neurological examination, 79
  and warfarin therapy, 283
alcohol antiseptic for hand washing, 143
allergies, 153, 155
  in the acutely unwell patient, 196, 200, 204
    with sepsis, 208
    with upper GI bleed, 220
  document on prescriptions, 224
AMPLE mnemonic, 196, 200, 204, 208, 220
anaemia, 49, 306
  in cardiovascular examination, 41
anaesthetic
  for arterial blood sampling, 185
  for male catheterisation, 159
anal sphincter, 130
analysis bias, 334
anaphylaxis, 152
aneurysmal arteries, 104
angina, 3, 6, 9, 13, 17, 21, 25, 28, 32, 35
anhydrosis, 67
ankle brachial pressure index, 186–8
  equipment, 186
  evaluation, 187
  procedure, 186–7
ankle brachial pulse index (ABPI), 102
ankle dorsiflexion, 75
ankle plantarflexion, 75
ankle pulse, 187
ankle reflexes, 76
ankle swelling, 105
antalgic gait, 138
antibiotics, 208
anticongulation valves, 45
anti-emetic, 227, 228
anus in rectal examination, 129
aorta in abdomen examination, 56
aortic area in auscultation, 43
aortic dissection, 10
aortic regurg, 46

aortic sclerosis, 46
aortic stenosis, 45, 46
apex beat, 43
A Place to Meet mnemonic, 43
appendicitis, 32, 34
APPENDICITIS mnemonic, 32
apthous ulcers, 54
arms
  movements in GALS examination, 138
  muscle weakness in thyroid examination, 121
arrythmia in the acutely unwell patient, 200
arterial blood gas, 329–30
  in oxygen therapy, 180
arterial blood sampling, 184–5
  equipment, 184
  procedure, 184–5
arterial circulation examination, 101–4
  auscultation, 102
  inspection, 101
  notes on, 103–4
  palpation, 101–2
  special tests, 102
arteries
  aneurysmal, 104
  identification in arterial blood sampling, 185
  measuring blood flow through peripheral, 188
asbestosis/abscess, 48
ascites, 56, 60
ascultation
  in cardiovascular examination, 43–44
  in confirmation of death, 189
  in respiratory examination, 49–51
associated history
  in abdominal pain, 32–33
  in blood pressure management, 275–6
  in breast lump, 35–36
  in breathlessness, 13
  in chest pain, 9
  in diabetic management, 279–80
  in general history taking, 2
  in general surgery, 25
  in headaches, 21
  in loss of consciousness, 17
  in rheumatology, 6
  in steroid therapy, 285
  in urology, 28
  in warfarin therapy, 282
asterixis, 48, 53
asthma, 3, 6, 9, 13, 17, 21, 25, 28, 32, 45, 182
asthma inhaler, 267–8
ataxia, 81
athetosis, 68

atrial fibrillation, 327
atrial flutter, 327
atrophic glossitis, 54
attic in the ear, 96
automated external defibrillator, 177–8
AVPU mnemonic, 195, 204, 207, 211, 216
axilla, 118, 126

B

back passage in rectal examination,
      129–30
barium enema, explaining, 257–8
basal cell carcinoma, 98
basement membrane puncture marks, 69
basic life support, 176–8
BBCC mnemonic, 60
bedside inspection, 52
beer bottle shaped legs, 105
Bell's palsy, 66
BELL'S Palsy mnemonic, 66
benign prostatic hypertrophy, 29, 131
beta blockers, 277
bias in a study, 334
bicarbonate in arterial blood gas, 330
biceps, 70
big toe extension, 75
bilateral cerebellar lesions, 83
bilateral inguinal swelling, 136
bilateral pleural effusion, 316
bilateral sensory loss of the legs, 80
biliary colic, 34
biological therapies for breast cancer, 127
bisferien pulse, 42
bitemporal hemianopia, 62
bladder cancer, 29
bladder in abdomen examination, 56
blind spot, 62, 89
blink reflex, 66
blood
administrating, 151
compatibility for blood transfusion, 150
drawing, 144–5, 169–70
in urine, 27, 174
blood culture bottles, 145, 167
blood cultures, taking, 166–8
equipment, 166
notes, 168
procedure, 166–7
blood glucose monitoring, 171–2
equipment, 171
procedure, 171–2
blood group for blood transfusion, 151

blood pressure
management
associated history, 275–6
medical advice, 276–8
and steroids, 286
blood pressure, taking, 169–70
blood request, 304–6
blood supply for ulcers, 110
blood tests for warfarin, 283
blood transfusion, 150–2
equipment, 150
procedure, 151
reactions, 152
bloody diarrhoea, 7
BONDS mnemonic, 27
bone conduction, 64, 95
bounding pulse, 49
brachial pulse, 187
brachioradialis, 70
branchial cyst, 114, 115
breaking bad news to a patient, 291–2
breast abscess, 37
breast cancer, 37, 127
breast cyst, 37
breast examination, 124–8
exemplar presentation, 127
inspection, 124–5
notes for OSCE, 127–8
palpation, 125–6
breast lump, 126, 127
history taking, 35–37
associated history, 35–36
communication skills, 36
differential diagnosis, 37
exemplar presentation, 37
breathing
in the acutely unwell patient, 194–5
with DKA, 214–15
with hypoglycaemia, 210–11
with palpitations, 198
with pulmonary embolism, 202–3
with sepsis, 206
with upper GI bleed, 218
in basic life support, 177
in chest radiograph, 313
breathlessness, 179
history taking, 12–15
associated history, 13–14
communication skills, 14
differential diagnosis, 14
exemplar presentation, 15
British Hypertensive Society guidelines, 276

Broca's aphasia, 86
Broca's dysphasia, 85
bronchial carcinoma, 48, 317
bronchiectasis, 48, 50
bruits, 102, 106
Buerger's angle, 102
Buerger's test, 102
bulbar palsy, 67
B vitamin deficiency, 79

C

cachexia, 116
café au lait spots, 68, 74
calcification, 319
calcium antagonists, 278
cancer. *See also* specific types of cancer
  in lower limb neurological examination, 79
  nose, 100
  thyroid, 123
cannulation, 146–7
  equipment, 146
capillary refill, 40, 101, 110
carbon dioxide retention, 48
cardiac axis, 323
cardiac murmurs, 44, 46
cardiac shadow in chest radiograph, 314
cardiac syncope, 18
cardiovascular examination, 40–47
  additional points, 44–45
  anticoagulation and prosthetic valves, 45
  aortic stenosis, 45
  auscultation, 43–44
  chest examination, 43
  exemplar presentation, 46
  face inspection, 41
  hand signs, 40–41
  hepatojugular reflex, 42
  inspection, 40–42
  jugular venous pressure, 42
  murmurs, 44, 46
  notes for OSCE, 45
  oedema, 44–45
  palpation, 43
  pulse assessment, 41–42, 46
carotid body tumor, 114, 115
carotid impulse, 42
carotid pulse, 41
case-control study, 334
catheter, 208
  in male catheterisation, 159–60
cause of death, 310
cavitating lung lesions, 316

ceftriazone as an intramuscular medication, 157
central cyanosis, 54
central retinal vein occlusion, 93
cerebellar examination, 81–83
  differential diagnosis, 83
  exemplar presentation, 83
  inspection, 81–82
cerebellar lesions, 83
cerebral manifestations, 306
cervical lymph nodes, 117–18
cervix in rectal examination, 130
CHAPLIN mnemonic, 306
chemotherapy for breast cancer, 127
chest
  in abdomen examination, 54
  cardiovascular examination, 43
  sounds on auscultation, 49–50
  in thyroid examination, 122
chest leads in an ECG, 191
chest pain, 202, 236
  history taking, 8–11
    associated history, 9
    communication skills, 10
    differential diagnosis, 10
    exemplar presentation, 11
    risk factors, 9, 10
chest radiograph, 312–17
  assessing quality of film, 312–13
  exemplar presentation, 315
  interpretation of, 313–15
  investigation and management, 315
  notes, 316
  signs and symptoms, 317
Childs-Pugh classification, 60
cholangitis, 34
cholecystitis, 34
cholesterol. *See* high cholesterol
chorea, 68, 74
chronic leg ischaemia, 103
chronic myeloid leukaemia, 58
chronic obstructive pulmonary disease. *See* COPD
ciliospinal reflex, loss of, 67
circulation in the acutely unwell patient, 195
  with DKA, 215
  with hypoglycaemia, 211
  with palpitations, 199
  with pulmonary embolism, 203
  with sepsis, 207
  with upper GI bleed, 219
circumduction gait, 138
claudication, 186
clinical skills, 141–92

ankle brachial pressure index, 186–8
arterial blood sampling, 184–5
basic life support, 176–8
blood glucose monitoring, 171–2
blood transfusion, 150–2
cannulation, 146–7
confirmation of death, 189–90
hand washing, 142–4
intramuscular injection, 155–7
intravenous injection, 153–4
iv infusion, 148–9
male catheterisation, 158–60
nasogastric intubation, 161–3
oxygen therapy, 179–81
recording an ECG, 191
setting up a nebuliser, 182–3
surgical gown and scrub, 164–5
taking a blood pressure, 169–70
taking blood cultures, 166–8
urine dipstick, 173–5
venepuncture, 144–5
clonus, 75
clubbing of hands, 40–41, 48, 53
cluster headache, 22
cog-wheeling, 69
cohort study, 334
colic, 34
  ureteric, 32
collapsing pulse, 42
colorectal carcinoma, 32
colour vision, 61, 63, 88
communication skills, 245–310
  for barium enema, 257–8
  for blood pressure management, 275–8
  for blood request, 304–6
  for breaking bad news, 291–2
  for breathlessness history taking, 14
  for chest pain history, 10
  for cross cultural, 299–301
  for CT head scan, 251–2
  for dealing with an angry patient, 293–4
  for death certification, 309–10
  for diabetic management, 279–81
  for epileptic starting a family, 288–90
  for general medical history, 3
  for general surgery, 26
  for GTN spray, 271–2
  for headaches, 22
  for hernia repair, 262–3
  for HIV test counselling, 246–8
  for inhaler technique, 267–8
  for instilling eye drops, 273–4
  for interprofessional, 297–8
  for laparoscopic cholecystectomy, 264–6
  for loss of consciousness history taking, 18
  for microbiology request form, 307–8
  for MRI scan, 253–4
  for negotiation, 295–6
  for OGD endoscopy, 255–6
  for peak flow, 249–50
  for radiology request, 302–3
  for rheumatological history, 7
  for spacer device, 269–70
  for steroid therapy, 285–7
  for transurethral resection of the prostate,
    259–61
  for warfarin therapy, 282–4
computerised tomography (CT), 251–2
conductive aphasia, 85
conductive dysphasia, 86
conductive hearing, 95
confidence intervals, 335
confirmation of death, 189–90
confounders in a study, 334
confrontation in testing visual fields, 88
connective tissue disorders, 79, 104
consolidation in chest radiograph, 317
continuing medical management
  for acute asthma attack, 233
  for acute coronary syndrome, 237
  for acute left ventricular failure, 239
  for COPD exacerbation, 235
  for hyperkalaemia, prescribing for, 240
contraception, 246
co-ordination
  in lower limb neurological examination, 76
  in upper limb neurological examination, 70–71
COPD, 50, 179, 184
  exacerbation, prescribing for, 234–5
    acute medical management, 235
    continuing medical management, 235
    infusion therapy, 235
    as required medicines, 235
corneal reflex, 63
coroner, 310
cotton wool spots, 92
cough impulse, 134
CPR in basic life support, 177, 178
cranial nerve, 66
cranial nerve syndromes, 67
critical ischaemia, 103
Crohn's disease, 32
cross cultural communication, 299–301
  medical advice, 300

cross-sectional survey, 334
CRVO, 93
c-spine, 139
CT head scan, explaining, 251–2
culture and communication skills, 299–301
cyclizine as an intramuscular medication, 157
cyst
   branchial, 114, 115
   breast, 37
   degenerative, 316
   epididymal, 132, 135
   ovarian, 32
   pre-auricular dermoid, 94
   thyroglossal, 114, 115
cystic fibrosis, 48
cystic hygroma, 114, 115

D

data interpretation, 311–30
   of abdominal radiograph, 318–21
   of the ABG, 329–30
   of chest radiograph, 312–17
   of the ECG, 322–8
D-Dimer, 205
deafness, 95
dealing with an angry patient, 293–4
death
   certification, 309–10
   confirmation of, 189–90
decreased oxygen, 48
deep palpitation, 55
deep Q waves, 324
deep vein thrombosis, 108
defibrillator, 177–8
degenerative cysts, 316
Delta waves, 326
De Quervains' thyroiditis, 123
diabetes, 3, 6, 9, 13, 17, 21, 25, 28, 32, 35
   complications of, 279
   impacting the eye, 91
   measuring blood glucose, 172
   risk factors, 280
   and steroids, 286
diabetes mellitus, 79, 216
diabetic foot, 103–4, 111
diabetic ketoacidosis, 214–17
diabetic management
   associated history, 279–80
   medical advice, 280–1
diabetic meter, 171–2
diabetic retinopathy, 91
diability in the acutely unwell patient, 195

with DKA, 215–16
with hypoglycaemia, 211–12
with palpitations, 199
with pulmonary embolism, 203–4
with sepsis, 207
with upper GI bleed, 219
diaphragm in chest radiograph, 314
diet
   and diabetes, 280
   and hypertension, 276
   and warfarin therapy, 283
dietary history in headaches, 22
dilated subcutaneous veins, 116
direct and consensual pupil response, 62, 89
dissociated sensory loss of the legs, 80
diuretics, 278
diverticulitis, 32, 34
DKA in the acutely unwell patient, 214–17
   airway patency, 214
   breathing, 214–15
   circulation, 215
   diability, 215–16
   exemplar presentation, 217
   exposure, 216
   management, 216–17
double vision, 63
drawing blood, 144–5, 166–7
drip
   calculation, 149
   in iv infusion, 149
   rate of blood, 151
drug administration
   in intramuscular injection, 156
   in intravenous injection, 154
drug allergies. See allergies
drug charts, 224–6
   label for GI bleed, 227
   sample, 229–31, 242–4
drug history
   in abdominal pain history taking, 32
   in breast lump history taking, 36
   in breathlessness, 13
   in diabetes, 280
   in general surgery, 25
   in headaches, 21
   in loss of consciousness, 17
   in steroid therapy, 285
   in urological history taking, 28
drug-induced hyperthyroidism, 123
drugs. See recreational drugs
dry macular degeneration, 92
dullness shifting, 56

Dupuytren's syndrome, 53
dysarthria, 85
dysdiachokinesia, 70, 81
dyspepsia, 286
dysphasia, 84
dysphonia, 85
dystrophies, 80

E

earache, 66
ear examination, 94–97
  assessing hearing, 94–95
  inspection, 94
  notes for OSCE, 97
  otoscopy, 95–96
  palpation, 94
  structures in ear, 96
ECG, 191
  evaluating, 322–6
  interpretation, 322–8
  selected rhythms, 326–8
ectopic pregnancy, 32
eczema, 105
elbow extension, 69
elbow flexion, 69
electrocardiogram. See ECG
elicit reflexes, 70, 75
emboli, 316
embolic phenomena, 47
emergency history taking, 2–4
empyema, 48
endocarditis, 40
endometriosis, 32
endoscopy test, 255–6
endrocine, 79
enlarged spleen, 56
enopthalmos, 67
epididymal cyst, 132, 135
epididymis, 132, 136
epididymo-orchitis, 136
epilepsy, 3, 6, 9, 13, 17, 21, 25, 28, 32, 35
epileptic starting a family
  communicating about, 288–90
  complications, 289
  impact of taking epileptic medications, 289
episcleritis, 7
epistaxis, 100
epitrochlear lymph nodes, 118
epsilon waves, 326
equipment
  for ankle brachial pressure index, 186
  for arterial blood sampling, 184
    for blood glucose, 171
    for blood transfusion, 150
    for cannulation, 146
    for intramuscular injection, 156
    for intravenous injection, 154
    for iv infusion, 148
    for male catheterisation, 158
    for nasogastric intubation, 161
    for oxygen therapy, 179
    surgical gown and scrub, 164
    for taking blood cultures, 166
    for venepuncture, 144
ethanol, 3, 6, 9, 13, 17, 21, 25, 28. See also alcohol
events in the acutely unwell patient, 196
  with palpitations, 200
  with pulmonary embolism, 204
  with sepsis, 208
  with upper GI bleed, 220
evidence appraisal, 331–7
  explaining an article to a patient, 336–7
  how to approach an abstract, 332–5
examinations, 39–140
  abdomen, 52–60
  arterial circulation, 101–4
  breast, 124–8
  cardiovascular, 40–47
  cerebellar, 81–83
  ear, 94–97
  eye, 87–93
  inguinal scrotal, 132–6
  lower limb neurological, 74–80
  lymphatic system, 116–20
  musculoskeletal system, 137–40
  neck lump, 113–15
  nerve, 61–67
  nose, 98–100
  rectal, 129–31
  respiratory, 48–51
  speech, 84–86
  thyroid, 121–3
  ulcers, 109–12
  upper limb neurological, 68–73
  venous circulation, 105–8
exemplar presentation, 91
  in abdomen examination, 57
  abdominal radiograph, 321
  breast examination, 127
  breathlessness, 15
  in cerebellar examination, 83
  for chest pain, 11
  chest radiograph, 315

DKA in acutely unwell patients, 217
general schemata for management of the acutely unwell patient, 197
headaches, 23
loss of consciousness, 19
lower limb neurological examination, 78
lymphatic system examination, 119
nerve examination, 66
palpitations in the acutely unwell patient, 201
pulmonary embolism in the acutely unwell patient, 205
sepsis of the acutely unwell patient, 209
in speech examination, 86
upper GI bleed in the acutely unwell patient, 221
in upper limb neurological examination, 73
urological history taking, 30
venous circulation examination, 107
exercise, 12
and hypertension, 276
expeditions/excursions, 3, 6, 9, 13, 17, 21, 25, 28, 33
expiry date of blood unit, 151
explaining an article to a patient, 336–7
exposure in the acutely unwell patient, 195–6, 219–20
with DKA, 216
with hypoglycaemia, 212
with palpitations, 199
with pulmonary embolism, 204
with sepsis, 207
expressive dysphasia, 86
external canal of the ear, 97
external genitalia in inguinal scrotal examination, 132–3
extraluminal air, 319
extravasation, 149
eye drops, instilling
procedure, 273–4
eye examination, 87–93
additional points, 90
exemplar presentation, 91
eye movements, 89
fundoscopy, 89–90
inspection, 87
notes for OSCE, 91–93
pupillary reflexes, 89
visual acuity, 87–88
visual fields, 88–89
eye movements, 89

F

face
in abdomen examination, 54
in lymphatic system examination, 117
signs in thyroid examination, 121–2
face mask for oxygen therapy, 179–81
facial muscles, 64
facial nerve, 63–64
factitious hyperthyroidism, 123
faeces in abdomen examination, 55
false pregnancy in abdomen examination, 55
family history, 28
in abdominal pain history taking, 32
in breast lump history taking, 36
in breathlessness history taking, 13
in diabetes history taking, 280
in general surgery history taking, 25
in headaches history taking, 21
in loss of consciousness history taking, 17
in urology history taking, 28
fasciculation, 68, 74
fat in abdomen examination, 55
femoral artery, 134
femoral hernias, 136
festinant gait, 138
fetus in abdomen examination, 55
fibroadenoma, 37, 128
fibroadenosis, 128
fibroids in abdomen examination, 55
fibrosing alveolitis, 48
finger
abduction, 70
extension, 69
flexion, 70
finger-nose test, 70, 82
flatus in abdomen examination, 55
fluid, 208
in abdomen examination, 55
overload, 152
fluid bag, 148–9
fluid thrill, 56
Fontaine classification of chronic leg ischaemia, 103
foot ulcers, 103
Fred's Tabby Cat Seeks Mice mnemonic, 80
Friedreich's ataxia, 79
9 Fs mnemonic, 55
full bladder in abdomen examination, 55
full-sized tumours in abdomen examination, 55
fundoscopy, 89–90

G
gag reflex, 65
gait, 76
in GALS examination, 137–8

gait ataxia, 81
GALS examination, 137–40
   gait, 137–8
   inspection, 137
   movement in, 139
   notes, 140
gastrointestinal. See GI
Gaucher's disease, 58
GCS, 195, 204, 207, 211, 216
general medical history
   communication skills, 4
   drug history, 3
   family history, 3
   history, 2
   mnemonics, 3
   social history, 3
   system review, 3
general schemata for management of the acutely
      unwell patient, 194–7
   airway patency, 194
   breathing, 194–5
   circulation, 195
   diability, 195
   exemplar presentation, 197
   exposing for examination, 195–6
   gathering patient's history, 196
general surgery for breast cancer, 127
general surgery history taking, 24–26
   associated history, 25
   communications skills, 26
   history, 24–25
genitalia in inguinal scrotal examination, 132–3
GI bleed, prescribing for, 227–31
   acute medical management, 227–8
   drug chart label, 227, 229–31
   general prescribing, 228
   as required medicines, 228
glandular fever, 119
Glasgow Coma Scale (GCS), 195, 204, 207, 211,
      216
glossopharyngeal nerve, 65
gloves, surgical, 165
glyceryl trinitrate spray (GTN), 271–2
goitre, 122, 123
gout, 6
gown, surgical, 165
grand mal seizure, 18
Graves' disease, 122
groin, lumps in, 136
gross abnormality, 313, 318
GROSS mnemonic, 6
GTN spray procedure, 271–2

Guillain-Barré syndrome, 79
guttering, venous, 102

H
haematocele, 132
haematological dysfunction, 16
haematological malignancies, 58
haematuria, 29
hand inspection
   in abdomen examination, 53
   in cardiovascular examination, 40–41
   in lymphatic system examination, 117
   in respiratory examination, 48
   in thyroid examination, 121
   in upper limb neurological examination, 69
hand washing, 164–5
   procedure, 142–3
   questions, 143
headaches
   differential diagnosis, 22
   exemplar presentation, 23
   history taking, 20–23
      associated history, 21–22
      communication skills, 22
head injury, 21
hearing, 64, 95
   assessment in ear examination, 94–95
   loss of, 97
heart, auscultation of, 43–44
heart failure, 42
heart rate in an ECG, 323
heaves & thrills, 43
heel/shin test, 76, 82
heel to toe walking, 138
hemiplegia, 80
hemisensory loss, 79
hemithorax opacification, 317
hepatojugular reflex, 42
hepatomegaly, 57
hepatosplenomegaly, 59
hereditary motor sensory neuropathy, 79
hernia repair
   explaining, 262–3
   post-op advice, 263
hernias, 56
   examination, 133–4
   femoral, 136
Hernias Very Much Like To Swell mnemonic, 134
high cholesterol, 3, 6, 9, 13, 17, 21, 25, 28, 32, 35
high-stepping gait, 138
hip extension, 75
hip flexion, 75

histiocytosis X, 316
history taking, 1–38
    in abdominal pain, 31–34
    in accident & emergency, 1–4
    in the acutely unwell patient, 196, 200
    in breast lump, 35–37
    in breathlessness, 12–15
    in chest pain, 8–11
    in general surgery, 24–26
    in headaches, 20–23
    in loss of consciousness, 16–19
    in rhematology, 5–7
    in urology, 27–30
HIV test counselling
    communication skills for, 246–8
HIV testing, 247
Hodgkin's disease, 119
Hoffmann's reflex, 70
home environment, 3, 6, 9, 21, 25, 28, 33
hormonal therapies for breast cancer, 127
Horner's syndrome, 66–67
HOSE PIPERS mnemonic, 3, 6, 9, 13, 17, 21,
        25–26, 28–29, 33
Hudson mask, 181
hydrocele, 132, 135
hydronephrosis, 59
hyperglycaemia, 216
hyperkalaemia, prescribing for, 240–4
    acute medical management, 240
    continuing medical management, 240
    general prescribing, 241
    infusion therapy, 240
    as required medicines, 240
hypertension, 3, 6, 9, 13, 17, 21, 25, 28, 32, 35
    medications for, 277
    risk factors, 275
    stages of, 276
    treatment of, 276–7
hypertensive retinopathy, 92
hyperthyroidism, 122–3
hypoglossal nerve, 65
hypoglycaemia, 306
    in the acutely unwell patient, 210–3
        airway patency, 210
        breathing, 210–11
        circulation, 211
        diability, 211–12
        exposure, 212
        management of, 212–13
hypokalaemia, 216
hypopigmented patches, 69, 74
hypothyroidism, 123

hypotonia, 69, 82
hypoxia, 48

I

iatrogenic fluid, 42
iliac fossa pain, 32
immunological phenomena, 47
impotence, 260
inattention, 88
    visual, 62
indirect hernias, 136
indirect inguinal hernia, 132
infection, 28, 260
infectious mononucleosis, 58, 119
infertility, 260
inflammatory bowel disease, 32
infusion therapy
    for acute asthma attack, 233
    for acute coronary syndrome, 237
    for acute left ventricular failure, 239
    for COPD exacerbation, 235
    for hyperkalaemia, 240
inguinal lymph nodes, 118
inguinal scrotal examination, 132–6
    external genitalia, 132–3
    hernias, 133–4
    inspection, 132–3
    notes for OSCE, 135
inhaler technique
    explaining, 268
    procedure, 267–8
inspection
    in abdomen examination, 52–54
    in arterial circulation examination, 101
    in breast examination, 124–5
    in cardiovascular examination, 40–42
    in cerebellar examination, 81–82
    in ear examination, 94
    in eye examination, 87
    in GALS examination, 137
    in inguinal scrotal examination, 132–3
    in lower limb neurological examination, 74–76
    in lymphatic system, 116–9
    in neck lump examination, 113
    in nerve examination, 61–65
    in nose examination, 98–99
    in rectal examination, 129
    in respiratory examination, 48–49
    in speech examination, 84–85
    in thyroid examination, 121–2
    in ulcers examination, 109–11
    in upper limb neurological examination, 68–69

in venous circulation examination, 105–6
instilling eye drops, 273–4
intention tremor, 82
intermittent claudication, 103
internuclear opthalmoplegia, 63
interprofessional communication skills, 297–8
intraluminal air, 319
intramuscular injection, 155–7
   administering the drug, 156
   equipment, 156
   procedure, 155
ntravenous infusion, 148–9
ntravenous injection, 153–4
   administering the drug, 154
   equipment, 154
   procedure, 153–4
ntussusception, 32
rritable bowel disease (IBD), 7, 32
schaemic heart disease, 10, 103
schaemic ulcers, 111
v infusion, 148–9
   equipment, 148
   procedure, 148–9

aundice, 3, 6, 9, 13, 17, 21, 25, 28, 35
aw jerk, 63
oint distribution, 5
ugular impulse, 42
ugular venous pressure, 42, 49
unctions in venous circulation examination, 106
VP, 42, 49

eratoconjunctiva sicca, 7
etosis breath, 54
idneys
   in abdomen examination, 55–56
   enlarged, 59
ings College criteria for liver transplant, 60
nee extensors, 75
nee flexion, 75
nee reflexes, 75
oilonychia, 53
orotkoff sounds, 170

boratory services
   request form, 305
   for urine analysis, 174
crimation, 66
ctate, 208

lactic acidosis, 306
laparoscopic cholecystectomy
   complications, 265
   explaining, 264–5
   post-op advice, 265
last meal in the acutely unwell patient, 196, 200
   with pulmonary embolism, 204
   with sepsis, 208
   with upper GI bleed, 220
leadpipe tone, 69
left homonymous hemianopia, 62
left iliac fossa pain, 32
left lower lobe pneumonia, 32
legs
   in GALS examination, 138
   in lymphatic system examination, 118
   sensory loss of, 80
   in thyroid examination, 122
leg varicosities, 56
leishmaniasis, 58
leukonychia, 53
lifestyle and diabetes, 280
light palpation, 55
light touch
   in lower limb neurological examination, 76
   in ulcers examination, 110
   in upper limb neurological examination, 71
limb ataxia, 81
lipodermatosclerosis, 105
liver
   in abdomen examination, 55, 56
   enlargement, 57
   transplant, 60
liver failure, 60
lobar collapse, 317
long saphenous vein, 106
long wrist extensors, 69
long wrist flexors, 69
loss of consciousness
   exemplar presentation, 19
   history taking, 16–19
      differential diagnosis, 18
      history, 16–17
low blood sugar. See hypoglycaemia
lower limb neurological examination, 74–80
   additional points, 77–78
   co-ordination, 76
   exemplar presentation, 78
   inspection, 74–76
   motor power, 75
   motor skills, 75
   notes, 79–80

reflexes, 75–76
sensation, 76–77
sensory deficits, 79–80
tone, 75
lower motor neurone lesion, 64
lower motor neurone signs, 71, 76, 80
lower right homonymous quadrantanopia, 62
lumbar spine flexion, 139
lump
    detection, 24
    in the groin, 136
    in neck, 113–15
lung bases, 44
lung lesions, 316
lymphadenopathy, 115, 116, 118
lymphangioleiomyomatosis, 316
lymphangitis, 116
lymphatic system examination, 116–20
    differential diagnosis, 119–20
    exemplar presentation, 119
    inspection, 116–9
    palpation, 117
lymph nodes, 54, 56, 110, 114
    axillary, 118
    in breast examination, 126
    carcinoma of, 120
    cervical, 117–18
    diseases of, 119–20
    enlarged, 118
    epitrochlear, 118
    features of, 117
    and hernia examination, 134
    inguinal, 118
    in inguinal scrotal examination, 133
    popliteal, 118
lymphoma, 58

M
macroglossia, 54
macula, 90
macular degeneration, 92
magnetic resonance imaging (MRI), 253–4
malar flush, 40
malaria, 58, 306
male catheterisation, 158–60
    equipment, 158
    procedure, 159–60
malleus, 96
management of the acutely unwell patient,
        193–222
    with DKA, 214–17
    general schemata, 194–7

with hypoglycaemia, 210–3
with palpitations, 198–201
with pulmonary embolism, 202–5
with sepsis, 206–9
with upper GI bleed, 218–22
mask in a nebuliser, 182–3
massive respiratory collapse, 50
MCA stroke, 73
measurement bias, 334
mechanical large bowel obstruction, 320
median nerve, 71
mediastinum, 314
medical history
    for abdominal pain, 32
    for chest pain, 9
    for diabetes, 280
    general medical history, 2–3
    for general surgery, 25
    for headaches, 21
    for rheumatology, 6
    for steroid therapy, 285
Medical Research Council (MRC) scale for muscle
        power, 70
medications
    for the acutely unwell patient, 196, 200
        with pulmonary embolism, 204
        with sepsis, 208
        with upper GI bleed, 220
    for intramuscular injections, 157
menstrual history, 35
Mercedes Benz' scar, 53
Merkel's, 32
meta-analysis study, 334
metabolic acidosis, 330
microbiology request form, 307–8
middle cerebral artery stroke, 73
middle ear, 97
migraine, 22
miosis, 67
mitral area in ascultation, 44
mitral regurg, 46
mitral stenosis, 46
MJTHREADS mnemonic, 3, 6, 9, 13, 17, 21, 25,
        28, 32, 35
1234567 mnemonic, 76
mnemonics
    1234567, 76
    AAAA PPPP, 14
    ABBCD, 318
    ABCDE, 60, 313
    ABCDEF, 48
    ABCDEFGH, 79

abdominal radiograph, 320
AFRO-C, 61
AMPLE, 196, 200, 204, 208, 220
APPENDICITIS, 32
AVPU, 195, 204, 207, 211, 216
BBCC, 60
BELL'S Palsy, 66
BONDS, 27
CHAPLIN, 306
Fred's Tabby Cat Seeks Mice, 80
9 Fs, 55
GROSS mnemonic, 6
Hernias Very Much Like To Swell, 134
HOSE PIPERS, 3, 6, 9, 13, 17, 21, 25–26,
        28–29, 33
MJTHREADS, 3, 6, 9, 13, 17, 21, 25, 28, 32, 35
NOSE, 100
ONE RESPS, 12
PIPER, 47
PIS, 27–28
A Place To Meet, 43
PQRST, 42
Ride Your Green Bike, 191
RILE, 44
SAMPLE, 67
SHOVE IT, 132
Six Ps, 103
SOCRATES, 8, 20–21, 31
SSSS, 176
SUPERCLOTS, 32
ToP RaCk, 69, 75–76
WEIRD HOLES, 316
Model for End Stage Liver Disease (MELD) score,
        60
modified Duke criteria for endocarditis, 47
monoarticular joints, 5
mononeuropathy, 79
mononuclear field loss, 62
mononucleosis, 119
monoplegia, 80
mood change, 286
mortality in sepsis, 209
motor deficits in lower limb neurological
        examination, 80
movement in GALS examination, 139
MRI scan, explaining, 253–4
multi-nodular goitre, 123
multiple sclerosis, 73
murmurs, cardiac, 44, 46
Murphy's sign in abdomen examination, 55
muscle power, 69–70, 75
    grading, 70

muscles of mastication, 63
muscle wasting, 68, 74
musculoskeletal pain, 10
musculoskeletal system, 137–40
myelofibrosis, 58
myocardial infarction, 3, 6, 9, 13, 17, 21, 25, 28,
        32, 35
myopathies, 80

N
nasal cannulae, 180
nasal deviation acquired, 99
nasal polyps, 100
nasogastric intubation, 161–3
    equipment, 161
    procedure, 162–3
nasopharyngeal carcinoma, 100
National Institute for Health and Care Excellence
        (NICE) hypertension guidelines, 276
near vision, 62, 88
nebuliser, setting up, 182–3
neck
    in thyroid examination, 122
    triangles of, 114
neck lump examination, 113–15
    auscultation, 114
    differential diagnosis, 114–15
    inspection, 113
    notes for OSCE, 114–15
    palpation, 113–14
    percussion, 114
neck mass, 100
necrosis of renal tubules, 306
neglect in sensation, 72, 78
negotiation skills, 295–6
neoplasia, 32, 99
neoplastic ulcers, 112
nerve examination, 61–67
    additional points, 65
    exemplar presentation, 66
    inspection, 61–65
    notes for OSCE, 66–67
nerve palsies, 66, 89
nerve root supply, 76
nerves. See also specific nerves
    thickened, 69, 74
nerve supply for ulcers, 110
nervous system, 74–80
    examination, 68–69
    lower limb, 74–80
    upper limb, 68–73
neurofibromas, 68, 74

neuropathic ulcers, 111
NICE hypertension guidelines, 276
nicotine stains, 40, 48
nipple discharge, 126
nitrites in urine, 174
nominal aphasia, 85, 86
non-ABO compatibility, 152
non-proliferative retinopathy, 91
non-variceal upper GI bleeding, 220
nose examination, 98–100
 inspection, 98–99
 notes for OSCE, 99–100
 palpation, 99
 special tests, 99
NOSE mnemonic, 100
nystagmus, 82

O
Objective Structured Clinical Examinations. *See* OSCE
obstructed nasal passage, 100
occupation, 3, 6, 9, 13, 17, 21, 25, 28, 33
oculomotor nerve, 63
oedema, 116
 in cardiovascular examination, 44–45
 in respiratory examination, 50
OGD endoscopy, 255–6
olfactory nerve, 61
oligoarticular joints, 5
ONE RESPS mnemonic, 12
opthalmoscopy, 61, 63
optic atrophy, 93
optic disc, 90, 93
optic nerve, 61
orchitis, 132
OSCE notes
 in abdomen examination, 57–60
 in breast examination, 127–8
 in cardiovascular examination, 45
 in ear examination, 97
 in eye examination, 91–93
 in inguinal scrotal examination, 135
 in neck lump examination, 114–15
 in nerve examination, 66–67
 in nose examination, 99–100
 in respiratory examination, 50
 in speech examination, 86
 in upper limb neurological examination, 73
 in venous circulation examination, 108
osteoarthritis, 6
osteoporosis and steroids, 286
otosclerosis, 97

otoscopy, 95–96
ovarian cyst, 32
oxygen therapy, 179–81
 equipment for, 179
 procedure for, 179–80

P
paced QRS complexes, 324
pacemakers, 316
$PaCo_2$ concentration, 329
Paget's disease of the breast, 124, 125
pain, 2, 20, 24
 abdominal, 31–34
 breast lump, 35
 chest, 8
 headache, 20–21
 LIF, 32
 in lower limb neurological examination, 77
 rheumatological, 5
 RIF, 32
 stomach, 27
 in ulcers examination, 110
 in upper limb neurological examination, 72
Palmar erythema, 53
palpation
 in abdomen examination, 54
 in arterial circulation examination, 101–2
 in breast examination, 125–6
 in cardiovascular examination, 43
 in ear examination, 94
 in inguinal scrotal examination, 132–3
 in lymphatic system examination, 117
 in neck lump examination, 113–14
 in nose examination, 99
 in rectal examination, 130
 in respiratory examination, 49
 in venous circulation examination, 106
palpitations in the acutely unwell patient, 198–201
 airway patency, 198
 AMPLE history, 200
 breathing, 198
 circulation, 199
 diability, 199
 exemplar presentation, 201
 exposure, 199
 managing arrthymia, 200
pancreatitis, 34
PaO_2 concentration, 329
papilloedema, 93
paralytic ileus, 320
paraplegia, 80
Parkinson's, 73

pars flaccida, 96
pars tensa, 96
past medical history
    in the acutely unwell patient
        with pulmonary embolism, 204
        with sepsis, 208
        with upper GI bleed, 220
    in history taking, 196, 200
past pointing test, 82
patent ductus arteriosus murmur, 46
patient
    dealing with an angry one, 293–4
    explaining an article to, 336–7
    managing acutely unwell, 193–222
    preparing for male catheterisation, 159
PDA murmur, 46
peak flow
    communication skills for, 249–50
    procedure, 249–50
pelvic inflammatory disease, 32
percuss, 114
    in hernia examination, 134
percussion
    in abdomen examination, 56
    in respiratory examination, 49, 51
percussion note, 49
pericardial constriction, 42
pericardial effusion, 42
pericarditis, 10
perinephric abscess, 59
period pain, 32
peripheral artery disease, 188
peripheral cyanosis, 40, 48
peripheral nerves, 71
peripheral neuropathy, 73
peripheral pulses, 101–2, 107, 110, 199, 207, 219
peri-ungual fibromas, 69
Perthes' test, 107
pets, 3, 6, 9, 13, 17, 21, 25, 28, 33
pigmentation in skin, 105
pillows, 12
PIPER mnemonic, 47
PIS mnemonic, 27–28
pitting oedema, 106
plantar response, 76
pleural effusion, 50, 317
pneumonectomy, 50
pneumonia, 32, 50
pneumothorax, 50, 317
polyarticular joints, 5
polycystic kidney disease, 59
polyneuropathy, 79

popliteal lymph nodes, 118
positive culture for endocarditis, 47
postural hypotension, 18
power grading of muscles, 70, 75
PQRST mnemonic, 42
pre-auricular dermoid cyst, 94
pregnancy
    by an epileptic, 288–90
    and warfarin therapy, 283
premature ventricular contractions, 328
presbyacusis, 97
prescribing acronyms, 226
prescribing medications, 223–44
    for acute asthma attack, 232–3
    for acute coronary syndrome, 236–7
    for acute left ventricular failure, 238–9
    for COPD exacerbation, 234–5
    general tips, 224–6
    for GI bleed, 227–31
    for hyperkalaemia, 240–4
P-R interval, 323
procedure
    for ankle brachial pressure index, 186–7
    for arterial blood sampling, 184–5
    for basic life support, 176
    for blood glucose, 171–2
    for blood transfusion, 151
    for hand washing, 142–3
    for intramuscular injection, 155
    for intravenous injection, 153–4
    for iv infusion, 148–9
    for male catheterisation, 159–60
    for nasogastric intubation, 162–3
    for oxygen therapy, 179–80
    for peak flow, 249–50
    for recording an ECG, 191
    for setting up a nebuliser, 182–3
    for surgical gown and scrub, 164–5
    for taking a blood pressure, 169–70
    for taking blood cultures, 166–7
    for urine dipstick, 173–4
    for venepuncture, 144–5
proliferative retinopathy, 91
proprioception, 72, 77, 110
prostate, 131
    in rectal examination, 130
    transurethral resection of, 259–61
prostate carcinoma, 131
prosthetic valves, 45
prostrate cancer, 29
protein in urine, 174
pseudobulbar palsy, 67

psoas abscess, 32
psych, 3, 6, 9, 13, 17, 21, 25, 28, 33
ptosis, 67
publication bias, 334
pulmonary area in ascultation, 43
pulmonary embolism, 42, 50
　in the acutely unwell patient, 202–5
　　airway patency, 202
　　AMPLE history, 204
　　breathing, 202–3
　　circulation, 203
　　diability, 203–4
　　exemplar presentation, 205
　　exposure of, 204
　　management of, 204
pulmonary embolus, 10
pulmonary fibrosis, 50
pulmonary hypertension, 42
pulmonary oedema, 306, 317
pulse, 41, 46
　ankle, 187
　in arterial circulation examination, 101–2
　brachial, 187
　peripheral, 107, 110, 199, 207, 219
　in respiratory examination, 49
pupil dilation, 195
pupillary reflexes, 61, 62, 89
p value, 335
P wave, 323
pyrexia, 47

Q
QRS complexes, 324
QT interval, 325
quadriplegia, 80

R
radial nerve, 71
radiology request, 302–3
　form, 303
radiotherapy for breast cancer, 127
raised intracranial pressure, 22
randomized controlled trial, 334
Raynaud's phenomenon, 7
3rd nerve palsy, 89
reactive hyperaemia, 102
receptive dysphasia, 86
recording an ECG, 191
　procedure, 191
recreational drugs, 3, 6, 9, 13, 17, 21, 25, 28, 33
rectal examination, 129–31
　inspection, 129

palpation, 130
rectum in rectal examination, 130
rectus sheath haematoma, 32
red reflex, 90
reflexes
　in cerebellar examination, 82
　pupillary, 89
　in upper limbs, 70
　visual, 61, 62
relative risk, 335
renal artery in abdomen examination, 56
renal malignancy, 59
renal stones, 32
respiratory examination, 48–51
　additional points, 50
　auscultation in, 49–51
　common conditions, 50
　exemplar presentation, 51
　hand signs, 48
　inspection, 48–49
　notes for OSCE, 50
　palpation, 49
　percussion in, 49, 51
　pulse assessment, 49
respiratory rate, 203, 215
retina's quadrants, 90
retinopathy, 91–92
rheumatic fever, 3, 6, 9, 13, 17, 21, 25, 29, 32, 35
rheumatoid arthritis, 6, 291–2
rheumatoid nodules, 316
rheumatological history
　associated history, 6–7
　drug history, 7
　extra-articular, 7
　family history, 7
　history, 5–7
　medical history, 6
　social history, 6
　system review, 7
rhinitis, 99
rhythms in an ECG, 322, 326–8
Ride Your Green Bike mnemonic, 191
RIF pain, 32
right iliac fossa mass, 55
right iliac fossa pain, 32
RILE mnemonic, 44
Rinne's test, 64, 95
rising in GALS examination, 138
risk as a statistic, 335
Rockall scoring system, 222
Romberg's test, 76, 82, 138
Rovsing's sign in abdomen examination, 55

S

salbutamol inhaler, 182–3, 267–8
saline drop, 148–9
salpingitis, 32
SAMPLE mnemonic, 67
saphenofemoral junction, 106
saphenopopliteal junction, 106
saphenous veins, 106
sarcoidosis, 6, 316
scars
  at fistula sites, 53
  in lower limb neurological examination, 74
  presence of in cardiovascular examination, 40
  in upper limb neurological examination, 68
  in venous circulation examination, 105
scissoring gait, 138
scleritis, 7
scrotal lump, 133
scrotal swellings, 132
secondary carcinoma, 120
selection bias, 334
seminoma, 135
senile macular degeneration, 92
sensation
  in face, 63
  in lower limb neurological examination, 76–77
  in upper limb neurological examination, 71–72
sensorineural hearing, 95
sensory deficits in lower limb neurological
    examination, 79–80
sepsis, 152, 209
  in the acutely unwell patient, 206–9
    airway patency, 206
    AMPLE history, 208
    breathing, 206
    circulation, 207
    diability, 207
    exemplar presentation, 209
    exposure, 207
    management, 208
  severe, 209
septic shock, 209
serous otitis media externa, 100
serum albumin ascites gradient (SAAG), 60
setting up a nebuliser, 182–3
severe sepsis, 209
sexual history, 3, 6, 9, 13, 17, 21–22, 25–26,
    28–29, 33
  for HIV test counselling, 246
sexual intercourse, 260
  types of, 246
shake in basic life support, 176

shortness of breath, 2, 14, 202, 232, 234, 238
short sapphenous vein, 106
shoulder abduction, 69
shoulder adduction, 69
shout for help in basic life support, 176
SHOVE IT mnemonic, 132
sigmoid diverticulitis, 32
silhouette sign in chest radiograph, 314
sinusitis, 22
SIRS, 209
sitting in GALS examination, 137
Six **P**s, 103
Sjögren's syndrome, 7
skin
  in lower limb neurological examination, 74
  thinning, 286
  in upper limb neurological examination, 68
  venous circulation examination, 105
SLE, 6, 7
sleep, 12
slow pursuit in nerve examination, 63, 89
slow rising pulse, 42
slurred speech, 83
smell
  changes in, 61
  loss of, 99
smoking, 3, 6, 9, 13, 17, 21, 25
  and diabetes, 280
  and hypertension, 276
Snellen chart, 87
social history, 28–29
  in abdominal pain history taking, 32, 33
  in breast lump history taking, 36
  in breathlessness, 13
  in chest pain, 9
  in general history taking, 3
  in general surgery, 25
  in headaches, 21–22
  in loss of consciousness history taking, 17
  in rheumatological history, 6
  in steroid therapy, 285
  in urological history taking, 28–29
SOCRATES mnemonic, 8, 20–21, 31
soft tissues in abdominal radiograph, 319
spacer device
  explaining, 270
  procedure, 269–70
spastic rigidity, 69
speech, slurred, 82
speech examination, 84–86
  additional points, 85
  exemplar presentation, 86

inspection, 84–85
notes for OSCE, 86
spermatic cord, 132, 134
spermatocele, 132
spinal root lesions, 79
spironolactone, 278
spleen
    in abdomen examination, 55–56
    enlargement, 58
splenomegaly, 56, 58
sputum, 51
SSSS mnemonic, 176
stamping gait, 138
stapes in the ear, 97
STAT fluids, 227
statistics used in studies, 335
sternomastoid tumor, 114, 115
steroid card, 286
steroid therapy
    associated history, 285
    medical advice, 286
stiffness, 5
stones, renal, 32
stools, 24–25
stress and hypertension, 276
stroke, 3, 6, 9, 13, 17, 21, 25, 28, 32, 35
struma ovarii, 123
ST segment, 325
studies
    bias in, 334
    confounders, 334
    critical analysis of, 333
    results of, 333
    statistics used in, 335
    types of, 334
study method determination, 332–3
subarachnoid haemorrhage, 22
SUPERCLOTS mnemonic, 32
superior vena caval (SVA) obstruction, 42, 49
support group, 248
supraventricular tachycardia, 200
surgery. See general surgery
surgical gown and scrub, 164–5
    equipment, 164
    hand washing, 164–5
    procedure, 164–5
surgical history
    in abdominal pain history taking, 32
    in breast lump history taking, 36
    in general surgery, 25
    in urological history taking, 28
SVT, 200

swelling
    in face and neck, 116
    of joints, 5
swinging light test, 62, 89
sympathetic nerve fibres, 66–67
systematic review study, 334
systemic inflammatory response syndrome (SIRS),
    209
systemic lupus erythematosus. See SLE

T
tactile fremitus, 51
tamponade, 42
tap test, 107
taste, loss of, 66
TB. See tuberculosis
temperature
    in lower limb neurological examination, 77
    in upper limb neurological examination, 72
temporal arteritis, 22
tenderness in the nose, 99
tendon reflexes, 76
tension headache, 22
teratoma, 135
testicle, 134
testicular cancer, 135
testicular torsion, 32
testicular tumour, 132
testis, 132
thickened nerves, 69, 74
third degree heart block, 327
4th nerve palsy, 89
6th nerve palsy, 89
thrombophlebitis, 105
thumb abduction, 70
thyroglossal cyst, 114, 115
thyroid cancer, 123
thyroid examination, 121–3
    face signs, 121–2
    hand signs, 121
    inspection, 121–2
    muscle weakness in arms, 121
    notes, 122–3
tongue in abdomen examination, 54
ToP RaCk mnemonic, 69, 75–76
torsion, 32
    of testis, 132
tourniquet, 166–7
tourniquet test, 107, 108
toxic adenoma, 123
transfusion. See blood transfusion
transfusion related acute lung injury (TRALI), 152

transthroacic echo, 47
transurethral resection of the prostate, 259–61
    complications of, 260
    explaining, 259–60
    post-op advice, 260–1
tremors, 68, 74
    intention, 82
Trendelenburg gait, 138
Trendelenburg's test, 107
triangles of the neck, 114
triceps, 70
tricuspid area in ascultation, 44
tricuspid regurgitation, 42, 46
tricuspid stenosis, 42
trigeminal nerve, 63
trochlear nerve, 63
truncal ataxia, 81
tuberculosis, 3, 6, 9, 13, 17, 21, 25, 28, 32, 35, 58
tuberculosis lymphadenitis, 120
T wave, 325
two-point discrimination, 72, 77
tympanic membrane, 96

U

ulcers, 105
    characteristics of, 109–10
    edge of, 110
    examination, 109–12
    ischaemic, 111
    neoplastic, 112
    neuropathic, 111
    venous, 111
ulnar nerve, 71
ultrasound scans in pregnant epileptic, 290
unilateral cerebellar lesions, 83
unilateral pleural effusion, 316
upper GI bleed in the acutely unwell patient,
        218–22
    airway patency, 218
    AMBLE history, 220
    breathing, 218
    circulation, 219
    diability, 219
    exemplar presentation, 221
    exposure, 219–20
    management, 220–1
upper left homonymous quadrantanopia, 62
upper limb neurological examination, 68–73
    additional points, 72
    co-ordination, 70–71
    exemplar presentation, 73
    inspection, 68–69

    motor skills, 69
    notes for OSCE, 73
    power, 69–70
    reflexes, 70
    sensation, 71–72
    tone, 69
upper motor neurone lesion, 64
upper motor neurone signs, 71, 76, 80
ureteric colic, 32
urinary tract infection, 29
urine
    characteristics, 27–28
    infection, 174
    testing, 173–4
urine dipstick, 173–5
    evaluation of, 174, 175
urolithiasis, 29
urological history taking, 27–30
    associated history, 28
    communication skills, 29
    exemplar presentation, 30
uvula deviation, 65
U waves, 326

V

vaccines as an intramuscular medication, 157
vagus nerve, 65
Valsalva manoeuvre, 44
variceal upper GI bleeding, 221
varicocele, 132, 136
varicose veins, 105, 108
vasovagal episode, 18
veins, 106
venepuncture, 144–5, 166–7
    equipment for, 144
    procedure, 144–5
venous circulation examination, 105–8
    auscultation, 106–7
    exemplar presentation, 107
    inspection, 105–6
    notes for OSCE, 108
    palpation, 106
    special tests, 107
venous guttering, 102
venous stars, 105
venous ulcers, 111
ventilate in basic life support, 177
ventricular fibrillation, 326
ventricular septral defect murmur, 46
ventricular tachycardia, 327
Venturi face mask, 179, 181
Venturi valves, 180

vestibular cochlear nerve, 64
vibration sense, 10, 72, 77
Virchow's node, 133
vision notation and interpretation, 88
visual acuity
   in eye examination, 87–88
   in nerve examination, 61–62
visual defects, 62
visual fields, 61, 62
   in eye examination, 88–89
visual periphery, 90
vocal fremitus, 49
volvulus, 320
vomiting, 24, 218, 220
VSD murmur, 46

W
walking in GALS examination, 138
warfarin therapy

   associated history, 282
   examiner's evaluation, 284
   medical advice, 283–4
Weber's test, 64, 95
Wegener's, 316
weight
   and diabetes, 280
   and hypertension, 276
WEIRD HOLES mnemonic, 316
Well's score, 205
Wernicke's aphasia, 86
Wernicke's receptive dysphasia, 84
wet macular degeneration, 92
wide based gait, 138

X
xanthelasma, 41
x-ray. *See* chest radiograph; specific types of
   radiographs